Fucoidans

Fucoidans

Editor

You-Jin Jeon

MDPI • Basel • Beijing • Wuhan • Barcelona • Belgrade • Manchester • Tokyo • Cluj • Tianjin

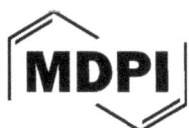

Editor
You-Jin Jeon
Department of Marine Life Sciences, Jeju National University
Korea

Editorial Office
MDPI
St. Alban-Anlage 66
4052 Basel, Switzerland

This is a reprint of articles from the Special Issue published online in the open access journal *Marine Drugs* (ISSN 1660-3397) (available at: https://www.mdpi.com/journal/marinedrugs/special_issues/fucoidans).

For citation purposes, cite each article independently as indicated on the article page online and as indicated below:

LastName, A.A.; LastName, B.B.; LastName, C.C. Article Title. *Journal Name* **Year**, *Volume Number*, Page Range.

ISBN 978-3-0365-2410-8 (Hbk)
ISBN 978-3-0365-2411-5 (PDF)

© 2021 by the authors. Articles in this book are Open Access and distributed under the Creative Commons Attribution (CC BY) license, which allows users to download, copy and build upon published articles, as long as the author and publisher are properly credited, which ensures maximum dissemination and a wider impact of our publications.

The book as a whole is distributed by MDPI under the terms and conditions of the Creative Commons license CC BY-NC-ND.

Contents

About the Editor vii

Preface to "Fucoidans" ix

K. K. Asanka Sanjeewa and You-Jin Jeon
Fucoidans as Scientifically and Commercially Important Algal Polysaccharides
Reprinted from: *Mar. Drugs* 2021, 19, 284, doi:10.3390/md19060284 1

Jiaojiao Tan, Jing Wang, Lihua Geng, Yang Yue, Ning Wu and Quanbin Zhang
Comparative Study of Fucoidan from *Saccharina japonica* and Its Depolymerized Fragment on Adriamycin-Induced Nephrotic Syndrome in Rats
Reprinted from: *Mar. Drugs* 2020, 18, 137, doi:10.3390/md18030137 5

Masanobu Takahashi, Kento Takahashi, Sunao Abe, Kosuke Yamada, Manami Suzuki, Mai Masahisa, Mari Endo, Keiko Abe, Ryo Inoue and Hiroko Hoshi
Improvement of Psoriasis by Alteration of the Gut Environment by Oral Administration of Fucoidan from *Cladosiphon Okamuranus*
Reprinted from: *Mar. Drugs* 2020, 18, 154, doi:10.3390/md18030154 15

Ahmed Zayed and Roland Ulber
Fucoidans: Downstream Processes and Recent Applications
Reprinted from: *Mar. Drugs* 2020, 18, 170, doi:10.3390/md18030170 29

Ilekuttige Priyan Shanura Fernando, Kalu Kapuge Asanka Sanjeewa, Hyo Geun Lee, Hyun-Soo Kim, Andaravaas Patabadige Jude Prasanna Vaas, Hondamuni Ireshika Chathurani De Silva, Chandrika Malkanthi Nanayakkara, Dampegamage Thusitha Udayangani Abeytunga, Dae-Sung Lee, Jung-Suck Lee and You-Jin Jeon
Fucoidan Purified from *Sargassum polycystum* Induces Apoptosis through Mitochondria-Mediated Pathway in HL-60 and MCF-7 Cells
Reprinted from: *Mar. Drugs* 2020, 18, 196, doi:10.3390/md18040196 51

Thilina U. Jayawardena, Lei Wang, K. K. Asanka Sanjeewa, Sang In Kang, Jung-Suck Lee and You-Jin Jeon
Antioxidant Potential of Sulfated Polysaccharides from *Padina boryana*; Protective Effect against Oxidative Stress in In Vitro and In Vivo Zebrafish Model
Reprinted from: *Mar. Drugs* 2020, 18, 212, doi:10.3390/md18040212 65

Xu Bai, Yu Wang, Bo Hu, Qi Cao, Maochen Xing, Shuliang Song and Aiguo Ji
Fucoidan Induces Apoptosis of HT-29 Cells via the Activation of DR4 and Mitochondrial Pathway
Reprinted from: *Mar. Drugs* 2020, 18, 220, doi:10.3390/md18040220 79

María Elena Reyes, Ismael Riquelme, Tomás Salvo, Louise Zanella, Pablo Letelier and Priscilla Brebi
Brown Seaweed Fucoidan in Cancer: Implications in Metastasis and Drug Resistance
Reprinted from: *Mar. Drugs* 2020, 18, 232, doi:10.3390/md18050232 93

Makoto Tomori, Takeaki Nagamine and Masahiko Iha
Are *Helicobacter pylori* Infection and Fucoidan Consumption Associated with Fucoidan Absorption?
Reprinted from: *Mar. Drugs* 2020, 18, 235, doi:10.3390/md18050235 111

Philipp Dörschmann, Maria Dalgaard Mikkelsen, Thuan Nguyen Thi, Johann Roider, Anne S. Meyer and Alexa Klettner
Effects of a Newly Developed Enzyme-Assisted Extraction Method on the Biological Activities of Fucoidans in Ocular Cells
Reprinted from: *Mar. Drugs* **2020**, *18*, 282, doi:10.3390/md18060282 . . . . **123**

Wanchun Su, Lei Wang, Xiaoting Fu, Liying Ni, Delin Duan, Jiachao Xu and Xin Gao
Protective Effect of a Fucose-Rich Fucoidan Isolated from *Saccharina japonica* against Ultraviolet B-Induced Photodamage In Vitro in Human Keratinocytes and In Vivo in Zebrafish
Reprinted from: *Mar. Drugs* **2020**, *18*, 316, doi:10.3390/md18060316 . . . . **139**

Huaide Liu, Jing Wang, Quanbin Zhang, Lihua Geng, Yue Yang and Ning Wu
Protective Effect of Fucoidan against MPP$^+$-Induced SH-SY5Y Cells Apoptosis by Affecting the PI3K/Akt Pathway
Reprinted from: *Mar. Drugs* **2020**, *18*, 333, doi:10.3390/md18060333 . . . . **151**

Tien-Chiu Wu, Yong-Han Hong, Yung-Hsiang Tsai, Shu-Ling Hsieh, Ren-Han Huang, Chia-Hung Kuo and Chun-Yung Huang
Degradation of *Sargassum crassifolium* Fucoidan by Ascorbic Acid and Hydrogen Peroxide, and Compositional, Structural, and In Vitro Anti-Lung Cancer Analyses of the Degradation Products
Reprinted from: *Mar. Drugs* **2020**, *18*, 334, doi:10.3390/md18060334 . . . . **169**

Xindi Shan, Xueliang Wang, Hao Jiang, Chao Cai, Jiejie Hao and Guangli Yu
Fucoidan from *Ascophyllum nodosum* Suppresses Postprandial Hyperglycemia by Inhibiting Na$^+$/Glucose Cotransporter 1 Activity
Reprinted from: *Mar. Drugs* **2020**, *18*, 485, doi:10.3390/md18090485 . . . . **191**

Natalie L. Benbow, Samuel Karpiniec, Marta Krasowska and David A. Beattie
Incorporation of FGF-2 into Pharmaceutical Grade Fucoidan/Chitosan Polyelectrolyte Multilayers
Reprinted from: *Mar. Drugs* **2020**, *18*, 531, doi:10.3390/md18110531 . . . . **209**

Soukaina Bouissil, Zainab El Alaoui-Talibi, Guillaume Pierre, Halima Rchid, Philippe Michaud, Cédric Delattre and Cherkaoui El Modafar
Fucoidans of Moroccan Brown Seaweed as Elicitors of Natural Defenses in Date Palm Roots
Reprinted from: *Mar. Drugs* **2020**, *18*, 596, doi:10.3390/md18120596 . . . . **229**

About the Editor

You-Jin Jeon is a Professor at the School of Marine Biomedical Science at Jeju National University in South Korea. He received his BS, MS, and PhD from Pukyong National University, and conducted his postdoctoral research studies at Department of Biochemistry, Memorial University of Newfoundland in Canada, and at Agricultural, Food and Nutritional Science, University of Alberta in Canada. Prof. Jeon has been serving in the Korea Society of Marine Biotechnology as President, and currently holds an industrial position as Technical Director of Aqua Green Tech Co. Ltd. He is working with marine biomass to develop functional food materials and cosmeceuticals for human use. He has published more than 500 international and 120 Korean domestic articles, as well as more than 100 patents. He has a total citation number of 21,604, as well as an 84 h-index and a 400 i10-index. Since 2016, these have been 16,291, 62, and 351. Now, he is a member of the Korean Academy of Science and Technology.

Preface to "Fucoidans"

Fucoidans are a group of fucose-containing sulfated polysaccharides found in many species of brown seaweed, with numerous bioactive properties. These days, fucoidans in the market are highly attractive, because fucoidans isolated from different brown seaweeds have been scientifically and industrially studied for their potential biological activities, such as anti-inflammatory, immunomodulatory, antioxidant, anticoagulant, antivirus, and anticancer. Besides, the chemical structures of fucoidans are unique, due to fucose-rich polysaccharides, containing sulfate groups. These sulfated polysaccharides are not found in land plants. Therefore, this book entitled "Fucoidans" will help with the understanding and application of fucoidans, not only in research, but also in industrial applications.

You-Jin Jeon
Editor

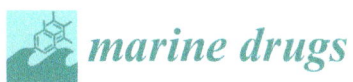

Editorial

Fucoidans as Scientifically and Commercially Important Algal Polysaccharides

K. K. Asanka Sanjeewa and You-Jin Jeon *

Department of Marine Life Science, Jeju National University, Jeju 690-756, Korea; asanka.sanjeewa001@gmail.com
* Correspondence: youjinj@jejunu.ac.kr

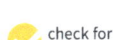

Citation: Sanjeewa, K.K.A.; Jeon, Y.-J. Fucoidans as Scientifically and Commercially Important Algal Polysaccharides. *Mar. Drugs* 2021, 19, 284. https://doi.org/10.3390/md19060284

Received: 14 May 2021
Accepted: 18 May 2021
Published: 21 May 2021

Publisher's Note: MDPI stays neutral with regard to jurisdictional claims in published maps and institutional affiliations.

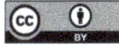

Copyright: © 2021 by the authors. Licensee MDPI, Basel, Switzerland. This article is an open access article distributed under the terms and conditions of the Creative Commons Attribution (CC BY) license (https://creativecommons.org/licenses/by/4.0/).

1. Introduction

As a highly bioactive seaweed substance with many promising physiological activities, fucoidan has attracted attention from many industries all over the world. Even though fucoidans are a rich source of bioactive properties, the structural properties and bioactive mechanisms of fucoidans are poorly understood. Therefore, novel studies that either characterize the physical properties or biological activities of fucoidans will fill the knowledge gap between industrial applications and the scientific background of those applications.

Both purified and partially purified fucoidans isolated from brown seaweeds present high potential as preventative and therapeutic agents against a number of chronic diseases due to their anti-inflammatory, antioxidant, anticancer, neuroprotective, antiviral, antimicrobial, and anticoagulative properties.

This Special Issue is aimed at presenting updated information on well-documented studies of the structural characterization and major biological actions relevant for medical, cosmeceutical, and pharmaceutical applications that fucoidans isolated from brown seaweed can offer.

2. What Is Fucoidan

Fucoidan is a type of sulfated polysaccharide which contains a significant portion of L-fucose. Fucoidans are mainly extracted from brown seaweeds and one of the well-known bio-active polysaccharides collected from seaweeds [1]. Earlier Fucoidan was named as "fucoidin" when it was first separated from seaweeds by Kylin in 1913. According to the IUPAC rules correct term is fucoidan. However, some people still use fucosan, fucan, and sulfated fucan instead of fucoidan [2]. In recent years, fucoidan has been extensively studied due to its beneficial and interesting biological activities [3]. Specifically, fucoidan possess numerous bioactive properties such as, anti-inflammatory, immunomodulatory, antioxidant, anticoagulant, antivirus, anticancer, and gastric protective properties.

3. The Structure Characterization

With the effort of the scientific community, several fucoidans' structures have been elucidated, and their biological activities have been identified [3]. The structure of fucoidans is complex in nature and it is very difficult to elucidate the general structure due to their heterogenous nature [4]. However, the majority of algal fucoidans consist of a linear backbone of random 1 → 3 or 1 → 4 linked α-L-fucopyranose residues periodically interrupted by other monosaccharides. Sulfate ester groups are arbitrarily substituted at 2, 3 and/or 4 positions of fucopyranose units, making it a highly heterogenous polymer [1,5].

4. How to Prepare

Fucoidan contents of brown seaweeds depend on a lot of factors such as variety, harvesting season, and maturity stage of seaweeds. In general, polysaccharides available in seaweeds can be extracted using water with or without some special enzymes, and separated by adding organic solvents [6]. However, extractions of cell wall polysaccharides are little bit difficult with the solvent extraction process. To extract cell wall polysaccharides such as fucoidan requires lyases in order to increase the extraction efficiency. Therefore, an enzyme-assisted extraction technique can be employed as an alternative method to enhance the extraction efficiency of fucoidan for industrial use [7].

In the article by Dörschmann, P. et al. [8], the authors enzymatically extracted *Saccharina latissima* fucoidan and isolated its low-molecular weight fraction. The results showed that the enzyme-treated fucoidans and the fractionated low-molecular-weight fucoidans are very promising for beneficial age-related macular degeneration-relevant biological activities. In order to modify fucoidans in molecular weights, fucoidans can be hydrolyzed by enzymes or phyco-chemical treatments and the resultant smaller fucoidans or fucoidan oligomers might improve bioactivities. In this Special Issue, a native fucoidan extracted from *Sargassum crassifolium* pretreated by single-screw extrusion was degraded by ascorbic acid or hydrogen peroxide. The lower-molecular-weight fucoidan prepared by ascorbic acid exhibits the highest cytotoxicity to A-549 cells and a strong ability to suppress Bcl-2 expression [9]. Tan, J. et al. [10] isolated fucoidan from *Saccharina japonica* and prepared its depolymerized fragment by oxidant degradation. The molecular weights of Fucoidan and its depolymerized fragment were 136 and 9.5 kDa, respectively. The low-molecular-weight fucoidan had higher renoprotective activity on adriamycin-induced nephrotic syndrome. On the other hand, Zayed, A. and Ulber, R. [11] mentioned in their review article that since a universal protocol for fucoidans production has not been established yet, all the currently used processes were presented and justified. The review article in the fucoidans field provided an updated overview regarding the different downstream processes, including pre-treatment, extraction, purification and enzymatic modification processes, and shows the recent non-traditional applications of fucoidans in relation to their characters.

5. Important Bioactivities

With the growing interest towards functional materials from natural sources, fucoidans isolated from different seaweeds have been scientifically and industrially studied aiming at assessing their potential biological activities such as anti-inflammatory, immunomodulatory, antioxidant, anticoagulant, antivirus, and anticancer properties [5,12]. Besides the cellular level activities, studies also focused on non-classical studies from fucoidans such as angiogenesis, treatment of intestinal diseases (inflammatory bowel disease and gastric ulcers), treatment of metabolic syndrome, and bone health supplements [13,14]. In this Special Issue, many articles provided bioactivities and physiological functionalities of fucoidans; for example, fucoidans of Moroccan brown seaweed act as an elicitor of natural defenses in date palm roots [15] and fucoidan from *Ascophyllum nodosum* suppresses postprandial hyperglycemia by inhibiting Na+/glucose cotransporter 1 activity [16]. It is well known that fucoidans show a protective effect against apoptosis [17] and ultraviolet B-induced photodamage [18]. On the other hand, one of the important bioactivities of fucoidans is an anticancer effect. Two articles in the Special Issue published anticancer activities of fucoidan via inducing apoptosis of cancer cells [19,20]. M. E. Reyes et al. reviewed brown seaweed fucoidan in cancer, in particular introduced implications in metastasis and drug resistance [21]. Typical bioactivities of fucoidans are antibacterial and antioxidant. Fucoidans in this Special Issue exhibited antibacterial effect against *Helicobacter pylori* infection [22] and antioxidant effect against oxidative stress [23]. Fucoidans can be effective on skin. Takahashi, M. et al. [24] have studied the improvement of psoriasis by alteration of the gut environment by oral administration of fucoidan. Furthermore, fucoidans were recently utilized to create a multilayer film with chitosan to bind fibroblast growth factor-2 for pharmaceutical-grade use [25].

6. Conclusions

Functional food is considered to be any food or food component that provides health benefits beyond basic nutrition. Recently, considerable attention has been directed by consumers towards functional ingredients from food, because of the lack of side effects.

Compared with other polysaccharides, fucoidans are sulfated polysaccharides and are very active in their functions. In order to be commercially and widely available as functional food additives, a large number of fucoidans have been investigated in recent years.

Funding: This work was supported by the 2021 education, research and student guidance grant funded by Jeju National University.

Conflicts of Interest: The author declares no conflict of interest.

References

1. Fernando, I.P.S.; Dias, M.; Madusanka, D.M.D.; Han, E.J.; Kim, M.J.; Jeon, Y.J.; Ahn, G. Fucoidan refined by *Sargassum confusum* indicate protective effects suppressing photo-oxidative stress and skin barrier perturbation in UVB-induced human keratinocytes. *Int. J. Biol. Macromol.* **2020**, *164*, 149–161. [CrossRef] [PubMed]
2. Li, B.; Lu, F.; Wei, X.; Zhao, R. Fucoidan: Structure and bioactivity. *Molecules* **2008**, *13*, 1671–1695. [CrossRef] [PubMed]
3. Sanjeewa, K.K.A.; Jayawardena, T.U.; Kim, S.-Y.; Kim, H.-S.; Ahn, G.; Kim, J.; Jeon, Y.-J. Fucoidan isolated from invasive *Sargassum horneri* inhibit LPS-induced inflammation via blocking NF-κB and MAPK pathways. *Algal Res.* **2019**, *41*, 101561. [CrossRef]
4. Asanka Sanjeewa, K.K.; Jayawardena, T.U.; Kim, H.S.; Kim, S.Y.; Shanura Fernando, I.P.; Wang, L.; Abetunga, D.T.U.; Kim, W.S.; Lee, D.S.; Jeon, Y.J. Fucoidan isolated from *Padina commersonii* inhibit LPS-induced inflammation in macrophages blocking TLR/NF-kappaB signal pathway. *Carbohydr. Polym.* **2019**, *224*, 115195. [CrossRef]
5. Ale, M.T.; Mikkelsen, J.D.; Meyer, A.S. Important determinants for fucoidan bioactivity: A critical review of structure-function relations and extraction methods for fucose-containing sulfated polysaccharides from brown seaweeds. *Mar. Drugs* **2011**, *9*, 2106–2130. [CrossRef]
6. Wijesinghe, W.A.J.P.; Jeon, Y.-J. Biological activities and potential industrial applications of fucose rich sulfated polysaccharides and fucoidans isolated from brown seaweeds: A review. *Carbohydr. Polym.* **2012**, *88*, 13–20. [CrossRef]
7. Sanjeewa, K.K.; Fernando, I.P.; Kim, E.A.; Ahn, G.; Jee, Y.; Jeon, Y.J. Anti-inflammatory activity of a sulfated polysaccharide isolated from an enzymatic digest of brown seaweed Sargassum horneri in RAW 264.7 cells. *Nutr. Res. Pr.* **2017**, *11*, 3–10. [CrossRef]
8. Dörschmann, P.; Mikkelsen, M.D.; Thi, T.N.; Roider, J.; Meyer, A.S.; Klettner, A. Effect of a newly developed enzyme-assisted extraction method on the biological activities of fucoidans in ocular cells. *Mar. Durgs* **2020**, *18*, 282. [CrossRef]
9. Wu, T.-C.; Hong, Y.-H.; Tsai, Y.-H.; Hsieh, S.-L.; Huang, R.-H.; Kuo, C.-H.; Huang, C.-Y. Degradation of Sargassum crassifolium fucoidan by ascorbic acid and hydrogen peroxide and compositional, structural, and in vitro anti-lung cancer analyses of the degradation products. *Mar. Durgs* **2020**, *18*, 334. [CrossRef]
10. Tan, J.; Wang, J.; Geng, L.; Yue, Y.; Wu, N.; Zhang, Q. Comparative study of fucoidan from Saccharina japonica and its depolymerized fragment on Adriamycin-induced nephrotic syndrome in rats. *Mar. Durgs* **2020**, *18*, 137. [CrossRef]
11. Zayer, A.; Ulber, R. Fucoidans: Downstream processes and recent applications. *Mar. Durgs* **2020**, *18*, 170.
12. Phull, A.R.; Kim, S.J. Fucoidan as bio-functional molecule: Insights into the anti-inflammatory potential and associated molecular mechanisms. *J. Funct. Foods* **2017**, *38*, 415–426. [CrossRef]
13. Wang, Y.; Xing, M.; Cao, Q.; Ji, A.; Liang, H.; Song, S. Biological Activities of Fucoidan and the Factors Mediating Its Therapeutic Effects: A Review of Recent Studies. *Mar. Durgs* **2019**, *17*, 183. [CrossRef]
14. Vo, T.-S.; Kim, S.-K. Fucoidans as a natural bioactive ingredient for functional foods. *J. Funct. Foods* **2013**, *5*, 16–27. [CrossRef]
15. Bouissil, S.; Alaoui-Talibi, Z.E.; Pierre, G.; Rchid, H.; Michaud, P.; Delattre, C.; Modafar, C.E. Fucoidans of Moroccan brown seaweed as elicitors of natural defenses in data palm roots. *Mar. Drugs* **2020**, *18*, 596. [CrossRef]
16. Shan, X.; Wang, X.; Jiang, H.; Cai, C.; Hao, J.; Yu, G. Fucoidan from *Ascophyllum nodosum* suppresses postprandial hyperglycemia by inhibiting Na+/glucose cotransporter 1 activity. *Mar. Drugs* **2020**, *18*, 485. [CrossRef]
17. Liu, H.; Wang, J.; Zhang, Q.; Geng, L.; Yang, Y.; Wu, N. Protective effect of fucoidan against MPP+-induced Sh-Sy5Y cells apoptosis by affecting the PI3K/Akt pathway. *Mar. Drugs* **2020**, *18*, 333. [CrossRef]
18. Su, W.; Wang, L.; Fu, X.; Ni, L.; Duan, D.; Xu, J.; Gao, X. Protective effect of a fucose-rich fucoidan isolated from Saccharina japonica against ultraviolet B-induced photodamage in vitro in human keratinocytes and in vivo in zebrafish. *Mar. Drugs* **2020**, *18*, 316. [CrossRef]
19. Bai, X.; Wang, Y.; Bu, B.; Cao, Q.; Xing, M.; Song, S.; Ji, A. Fucoidan induces apoptosis of HT-29 cells via the activation of DR4 and mitochondrial pathway. *Mar. Drugs* **2020**, *18*, 220. [CrossRef] [PubMed]
20. Fernando, I.P.S.; Sanjeewa, K.K.A.; Lee, H.G.; Kim, H.-S.; Vaas, A.P.J.P.; Silva, H.I.C.D.; Nanayakkara, C.M.; Abeytonga, D.T.U.; Lee, D.-S.; Lee, J.-S.; et al. Fucoidan purified from *Sargassum polycystum* induces apoptosis through mitochondria-mediated pathway in HL-60 and MCF-7 cells. *Mar. Drugs* **2020**, *18*, 196. [CrossRef]
21. Reyes, M.E.; Riquelme, I.; Salvo, T.; Zanella, L.; Letelier, P.; Brebi, P. Brown seaweed fucoidan in cancer: Implication in metastasis and drug resistance. *Mar. Drugs* **2020**, *18*, 232. [CrossRef] [PubMed]
22. Tomori, M.; Nagamine, T.; Iha, M. Are Helicobacter pylori infection and fucoidan consumption associated with fucoidan absorption? *Mar. Drugs* **2020**, *18*, 235.

23. Jayawardena, T.U.; Wang, L.; Sanjeewa, K.K.A.; Kang, S.I.; Lee, J.-S.; Jeon, Y.-J. Antioxidant potential of sulfated polysaccharides from *Padina boryana*; Protective effect against oxidative stress in in vitro and in vivo zebrafish model. *Mar. Drugs* **2020**, *18*, 212. [CrossRef]
24. Takahashi, M.; Takahashi, K.; Abe, S.; Yamada, K.; Suzuki, M.; Masahisa, M.; Endo, M.; Abe, K.; Inoue, R.; Hoshi, H. Improvement of psoriasis by alteration of the gut environment by oral administration of fucoidan from *Cladosiphon okamuranus*. *Mar. Drugs* **2020**, *18*, 154. [CrossRef]
25. Benbow, N.; Karpiniec, S.; Krasowska, M.; Beattie, D.A. Incorporation of FGF-2 into pharmaceutical grade fucoidan/chitosan polyelectrolyte multilayers. *Mar. Drugs* **2020**, *18*, 531. [CrossRef]

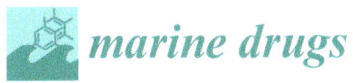

Article

Comparative Study of Fucoidan from *Saccharina japonica* and Its Depolymerized Fragment on Adriamycin-Induced Nephrotic Syndrome in Rats

Jiaojiao Tan [1,2,3], Jing Wang [1], Lihua Geng [1], Yang Yue [1], Ning Wu [1] and Quanbin Zhang [1,2,3,*]

1. Key Laboratory of Experimental Marine Biology, Center for Ocean Mega-Science, Institute of Oceanology, Chinese Academy of Sciences, Qingdao 266071, China; qdrdtanjiaojiao@163.com (J.T.); jingwang@qdio.ac.cn (J.W.); lhgeng@qdio.ac.cn (L.G.); yueyang@qdio.ac.cn (Y.Y.); wuning@qdio.ac.cn (N.W.)
2. Laboratory for Marine Biology and Biotechnology, Qingdao National Laboratory for Marine Science and Technology, Qingdao 266237, China
3. University of the Chinese Academy of Sciences, Beijing 100049, China
* Correspondence: qbzhang@qdio.ac.cn; Tel.: +86-532-82898708

Received: 27 January 2020; Accepted: 25 February 2020; Published: 27 February 2020

Abstract: Nephrotic syndrome (NS) is a clinical syndrome with a variety of causes, mainly characterized by heavy proteinuria, hypoalbuminemia, and edema. At present, identification of effective and less toxic therapeutic interventions for nephrotic syndrome remains to be an important issue. In this study, we isolated fucoidan from *Saccharina japonica* and prepared its depolymerized fragment by oxidant degradation. Fucoidan and its depolymerized fragment had similar chemical constituents. Their average molecular weights were 136 and 9.5 kDa respectively. The effect of fucoidan and its depolymerized fragment on adriamycin-induced nephrotic syndrome were investigated in a rat model. The results showed that adriamycin-treated rats had heavy proteinuria and increased blood urea nitrogen (BUN), serum creatinine (SCr), total cholesterol (TC), and total triglyceride (TG) levels. Oral administration of fucoidan or low-molecular-weight fucoidan for 30 days could significantly inhibit proteinuria and decrease the elevated BUN, SCr, TG, and TC level in a dose-dependent manner. At the same dose (100 mg/kg), low-molecular-weight fucoidan had higher renoprotective activity than fucoidan. Their protective effect on nephrotic syndrome was partly related to their antioxidant activity. The results suggested that both fucoidan and its depolymerized fragment had excellent protective effect on adriamycin-induced nephrotic syndrome, and might have potential for the treatment of nephrotic syndrome.

Keywords: fucoidan; low-molecular-weight fucoidan; adriamycin; nephrotic syndrome

1. Introduction

Chronic kidney disease has become a significant public health concern. Nephrotic syndrome (NS) is a special type of chronic kidney disease, which could be caused by a variety of factors. It is characterized by heavy proteinuria (more than 3.5 g/d), hypoalbuminemia, and edema [1]. Affected patients without effective treatment will in time develop end-stage renal disease. The adriamycin-induced nephrotic syndrome, which was first reported by Bertani et al. in 1982, is a classical nephrotic syndrome model [2]. Adriamycin is a quinone-containing anthracycline antibiotic and can be reduced to a semiquinone radical by metabolism in the kidney. The latter reacts with oxygen to produce reactive oxygen, inducing lipid peroxidation in the glomerular epithelial cells and destruction of the structure and function of the filtration membrane, and leading to progressive and irreversible proteinuria, hypoalbuminemia and hyperlipidemia [3]. An acute adriamycin-induced nephropathy model is induced by a single tail vein injection of 5–7.5 mg/kg adriamycin. This model, similar to human minimal change nephrotic syndrome, has been well characterized as an experimental model for nephrotic syndrome [4].

Treatment of nephrotic syndrome can slow its progression to end-stage renal disease. However, the therapies of nephrotic syndrome remain limited [5]. Many clinical and experimental studies have shown that the pathogenesis of nephrotic syndrome is associated with immune dysfunction. Immunosuppressive treatment, including corticosteroids, is the first-line treatment for nephrotic syndrome [6]. However, steroid resistance or steroid dependence is very common and frequently causes immune dysfunction and complicated infection, leading to end-stage renal failure [7]. Therefore identification of effective and less toxic therapeutic interventions for nephrotic syndrome remains to be an important issue.

The brown seaweed, *Saccharina japonica*, is a common seafood in China and Japan. It was documented as a traditional herb in traditional Chinese medicine for over a thousand years. The hot-water decoction of *S. japonica* is orally administered solely or combined with other herb extracts, and used for treatment of edema, a symptom of renal disease. Based on its therapeutic effect, our previous studies revealed that fucoidan, the water-soluble sulfated fucose-containing polysaccharide from *S. japonica*, was the main active component to treat edema. Fucoidan from *S. japonica* had renoprotective effect on chronic renal failure, diabetic nephropathy and acute kidney disease [8–11]. Nephrotic syndrome is a special type of chronic kidney disease, whether fucoidan have protective effect on nephrotic syndrome is still unclear.

As reviewed by Berteau and Mulloy [12], algal fucoidan represents a rather heterogeneous group of sulfated polysaccharides with complex and heterogeneous structures devoid of regularity. The structure of fucoidan extracted from *S. japonica* was much more complicated [13]. Its backbone was primarily consisted of (1→3)-linked-α-L-fucopyranose residues and a few (1→4)-α-L-fucopyranose linkages. The branch points were at C-4 of 3-linked -α-L-fucopyranose residues by β-D-galactopyranose unites or at C-2 of 3-linked -α-L-fucopyranose residues by non-reducing terminal fucose units. Sulfate groups occupied at position C-4 or C-2, sometimes C-2, 4 to fucose residues, and C-3 and/or C-4 to galactose residues. Besides fucose, fucoidan from *S. japonica* also contains minor galactose, mannose, glucose, rhamnose, and xylose. Fucoidans have been reported to have diverse bioactivities, such as antioxidant [14], anti-inflammatory [15], reno-protective [8], antitumor [16], and anticoagulant [17] activities. The molecular weight has been demonstrated to play an important role in the biological activities of polysaccharides. Comparing with unfractioned heparin, low-molecular-weight heparin has improved bio-availability, a longer half-life, and more predictable dose response, which make their use increasing common in the treatment and prophylaxis [18]. The relationship between molecular weight and bioactivities of fucoidan was reported in recent years. A low-molecular-weight fucan fraction extracted from the brown seaweed *Ascophyllum nodosum* exhibited dose-related venous antithrombotic activity [19]. A high level of inhibitory activity on complement can be achieved with low-molecular-weight fucoidan molecules [20]. If fucoidans with different molecular weight have a different effect on nephrotic syndrome still needs investigation.

In this study, we isolated a fucoidan from *S. japonica* and prepared its depolymerized fragment by oxidant degradation. The effect of fucoidan and its depolymerized fragment on adriamycin-induced nephrotic syndrome were investigated in a rat model.

2. Results and Discussion

2.1. Chemical Properties

Fucoidan was extracted from *S. japonica* by hot-water extraction. The yield of fucoidan was 1.2%. Fucoidan was further degraded into low-molecular-weight fucoidan (LMWF) by oxidant degradation by the combination of hydrogen peroxide and ascorbic acid at room temperature. The average molecular weights of fucoidan and its depolymerized fragment LMWF were 136 and 9.5 kDa, respectively.

It is reported that ascorbate and hydrogen peroxide could induce scission of plant cell wall polysaccharides [21]. In this study, this method was used for the degradation of native fucoidan, and the changes of molecular mass indicated that fucoidan was successfully degraded into depolymerized fragment.

The chemical properties of fucoidan and its depolymerized fragment are shown in Table 1. The results indicated that both fucoidan and its depolymerized fragment had similar chemical constituents. The fucose content of fucoidan and LMWF were 31.6% and 29.6%, respectively. Their sulfate contents were 33.58% and 32.66%, respectively. Besides fucose, other monosaccharides including galactose, mannose, glucose, rhamnose, and xylose were present in fucoidan and LMWF, and they also had similar neutral monosaccharide ratios.

Table 1. Chemical constituents of fucoidan and low-molecular-weight fucoidan (LMWF) prepared from *S. japonica*.

Samples	Fucose %	Uronic Acid %	Sulfate %	Neutral Monosaccharide (Molar Ratio)					
				Fuc	Gal	Man	Glc	Rha	Xyl
LMWF	31.60	5.69	33.58	1.000	0.303	0.088	0.072	0.035	0.053
Fucoidan	29.12	6.07	32.66	1.000	0.296	0.068	0.087	0.039	0.046

The IR spectra of fucoidan and LMWF are shown in Figure 1. Both samples had same infrared absorption properties, suggesting that both fucoidan and its depolymerized fragment contained the same functional groups. As shown in Figure 1, the band at 3600-3000 cm^{-1} was assigned to the deformation of O-H. The strong band around 1251 cm^{-1} was attributed to the asymmetric stretching of S=O, the absorption band around 835 cm^{-1} indicated the presence of sulfate groups. The strong absorption at approximately 1020–1050 cm^{-1} corresponded to the C-O-C/C-OH stretching frequency. Meanwhile, from the spectra, it was found that the band around 1251 cm^{-1} of fucoidan and LMWF had similar intensity, which means their sulfate contents were similar, which was consistent to the results of chemical analysis. The results indicated that oxidation degradation had no damage to the backbone structure of fucoidan.

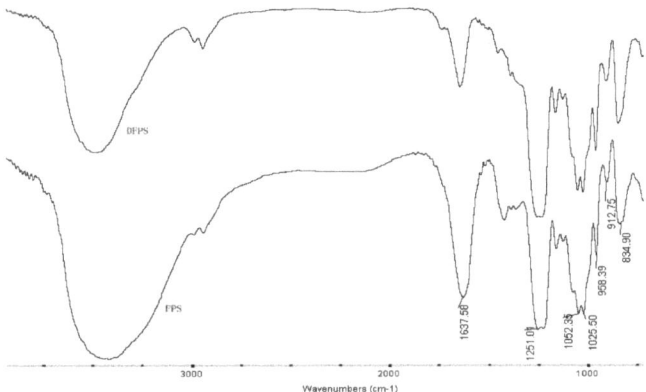

Figure 1. Infrared spectra of fucoidan and low molecular weight fucoidan (LMWF). FPS—fucoidan; DFPS:—low-molecular-weight fucoidan.

Based on the above analysis, it can be concluded that after degradation, the chemical constituents of fucoidan and its depolymerized fragment had no significant changes, only the molecular weight was greatly decreased.

2.2. *Evaluation of Rats Weight Alteration*

The adriamycin-induced nephrotic syndrome is a classical nephrotic syndrome model. In this study, the general condition of the animals was observed during the experiments. Compared with the normal rats, rats treated with adriamycin showed abnormal behavioral activities, including reduced feed intake, easy tiredness, emaciation, tarnish, and depilation. Some animals had obvious diarrhea.

Body weight changes of all rats were examined once a week during the experiment; the weight changes before and after drug administration are shown in Table 2. Significant changes in body weight were observed among the normal and other groups during the treatment period. The body weight of the model group was significantly lower ($p < 0.01$) than that of the normal group. Compared with the model group, the body weight of rats in positive control group administrated with dexamethasone was much lower, while rats treated with fucoidan and LMWF at the dose of 100 mg/kg gained weight significantly. Rats treated with LMWF at the dose of 100 mg/kg gained a higher weight than fucoidan-treated rats at two weeks after drug administration ($p < 0.05$). LMWF treatment at the dose of 50 and 25 mg/kg also increased the body weight of rats, but had no statistical difference.

Table 2. Effect of fucoidan and low molecular weight fucoidan (LMWF) treatment on body weight of rats ($\overline{X} \pm S$, g).

Groups	Dosage (mg/kg)	Weeks after Drug Administration				
		0	1	2	3	4
Normal	-	344.4 ± 12.2	366.3 ± 21.9	387.5 ± 23.5	401.2 ± 24.8	408.8 ± 26.9
Model	-	296.2 ± 26.9 $^{\Delta\Delta}$	293.0 ± 16.7 $^{\Delta\Delta}$	294.4 ± 19.8 $^{\Delta\Delta}$	303.9 ± 19.6 $^{\Delta\Delta}$	309.5 ± 21.8 $^{\Delta\Delta}$
dexamethasone	0.1	293.2 ± 30.8	250.0 ± 18.6 **	223.3 ± 14.1 **	225.9 ± 16.3 **	225.4 ± 14.2 **
Fucoidan	100	292.8 ± 15.3	315.5 ± 24.4 *	307.7 ± 14.1	323.3 ± 11.3 *	332.9 ± 17.1 *
LMWF	100	279.8 ± 13.0	318.6 ± 29.4 *	329.3 ± 31.5 *	332.9 ± 34.1 *	339.5 ± 35.9 *
LMWF	50	286.7 ± 21.3	309.6 ± 29.7	321.5 ± 30.5 *	315.1 ± 33.2	317.3 ± 37.9
LMWF	25	285.2 ± 19.3	309.5 ± 20.2	320.6 ± 24.8 *	319.9 ± 27.8	314.5 ± 28.1

$^{\Delta}$: $p < 0.05$, $^{\Delta\Delta}$: $p < 0.01$ (vs normal group); *: $p < 0.05$, **: $p < 0.01$ (vs model group).

The daily feed intake of rats was significantly reduced after adriamycin treatment (Table 3). Compared with the model group, rats treated with fucoidan and LMWF at the dose of 100 mg/kg had much higher feed intake. It partly explains why these rats had higher body weight.

Table 3. Effect of fucoidan and low molecular weight fucoidan (LMWF) treatment on feed intake of rats ($\overline{X} \pm S$, g).

Groups	Dosage (mg/kg)	Weeks after Drug Administration				
		0	1	2	3	4
Normal	-	26.8 ± 1.3	36.1 ± 1.0	34.0 ± 0.9	37.2 ± 0.3	38.1 ± 1.3
Model	-	16.8 ± 0.3 $^{\Delta}$	23.1 ± 0.1 $^{\Delta}$	23.9 ± 1.4 $^{\Delta}$	24.0 ± 0.9 $^{\Delta}$	23.7 ± 0.4 $^{\Delta}$
dexamethasone	0.1	16.9 ± 1.6 $^{\Delta}$	17.4 ± 0.0 *	19.4 ± 3.4	16.6 ± 1.9	19.1 ± 2.9
Fucoidan	100	17.4 ± 1.4 $^{\Delta}$	28.2 ± 2.0 *	29.5 ± 2.1 *	32.0 ± 2.0 *	32.7 ± 3.8 *
LMWF	100	18.3 ± 1.6 $^{\Delta}$	32.9 ± 2.7 *	30.5 ± 1.0 *	31.9 ± 5.0 *	34.9 ± 2.4 *
LMWF	50	18.5 ± 0.7 $^{\Delta}$	23.5 ± 1.6	29.3 ± 1.3	28.0 ± 5.4	28.4 ± 0.9
LMWF	25	18.1 ± 1.8 $^{\Delta}$	22.9 ± 2.4	28.2 ± 0.9	26.7 ± 4.9	24.7 ± 1.8

$^{\Delta}$: $p < 0.05$ (vs normal group); *: $p < 0.05$ (vs model group).

2.3. Urinary Protein Excretion

Proteinuria is the most important feature of nephrotic syndrome. To measure the urinary protein levels, the rats were placed in individual metabolic cages for 24 h urine collection once a week. We detected the 24 h urinary protein excretion of all rats. As shown in Table 4, two weeks after adriamycin administration (0 week in Table 4, the beginning time of drug administration), the 24 h urinary protein of the model group was significantly higher than that of the normal group and became higher over time. This phenomenon proved that adriamycin treatment can be used to form a rat model of nephropathy with continuous aggravation, which is similar to nephrotic syndrome. The urinary protein excretion of rats treated with fucoidan or LMWF (50 or 100 mg/kg) was significantly reduced after administration, which was significantly different from that of the model rats. The results suggested that both fucoidan and LMWF could ameliorate the symptoms of hyperalbuminuria and gradually recover the damage of glomerular filtration membrane caused by adriamycin. Compared with fucoidan, LMWF at dose of 100 mg/kg had a much lower urinary protein excretion ($p < 0.05$, three weeks after drug administration), suggesting that low-molecular-weight fucoidan could inhibit the production of proteinuria with a higher activity.

Table 4. Effect of fucoidan and LMWF treatment on 24 h urinary protein of rats ($\overline{X} \pm S$, mg/mL).

Groups	Dosage (mg/kg)	Weeks after Drug Administration (mg/mL)				
		0	1	2	3	4
Normal	-	0.58 ± 0.40	0.73 ± 0.51	0.73 ± 0.47	0.65 ± 0.35	0.59 ± 0.36
Model	-	22.42 ± 22.55 ΔΔ	36.60 ± 14.54 ΔΔ	43.98 ± 26.64 ΔΔ	48.41 ± 22.18 ΔΔ	54.60 ± 31.27 ΔΔ
dexamethasone	0.1	19.98 ± 14.87 ΔΔ	23.56 ± 10.47 *	25.25 ± 9.85 *	26.63 ± 16.98 *	28.62 ± 19.15 *
Fucoidan	100	20.45 ± 10.00 ΔΔ	20.19 ± 12.37 *	23.21 ± 13.54 *	26.13 ± 9.63 *	27.82 ± 12.28 *
LMWF	100	20.11 ± 10.86 ΔΔ	19.26 ± 12.12 *	21.88 ± 13.28 *	21.71 ± 12.76 **	25.31 ± 9.58 *
LMWF	50	23.28 ± 19.18 ΔΔ	22.90 ± 12.39 *	24.40 ± 7.89 *	29.34 ± 9.67 *	29.15 ± 8.79 *
LMWF	25	25.16 ± 20.65 ΔΔ	33.19 ± 15.96	30.42 ± 21.03	31.00 ± 14.17	36.91 ± 20.51

Δ: $p < 0.05$, ΔΔ: $p < 0.01$ (vs normal group); *: $p < 0.05$, **: $p < 0.01$ (vs model group).

2.4. Blood Biochemical Indexes

At the end of the experiment, the blood biochemical indexes of rats were detected. The blood levels of total protein (TP), albumin, blood urea nitrogen (BUN), serum creatinine (SCr), total cholesterol (TC), and total triglyceride (TG) of the model rats were significantly changed (Table 5). It is worth noting that the blood lipid level of the model rats was remarkably elevated. Compared with the normal rats, the blood level of total cholesterol and total triglyceride of the model rats induced by adriamycin were increased by 9.4-fold and 6.4-fold, respectively. These results indicated that adriamycin treatment could induce significant hyperlipidemia.

Table 5. Effect of fucoidan and low molecular weight fucoidan (LMWF) on blood biochemical indexes of NS rats ($\overline{X} \pm S$).

Groups	Dosage (mg/kg)	T-P (g/L)	ALB (g/L)	SCr (μmol/L)	BUN (mmol/L)	TG (mmol/L)	T-CHO (mmol/L)
Normal	-	68.63 ± 5.77	32.71 ± 8.78	77.23 ± 5.26	7.21 ± 0.92	0.48 ± 0.13	1.50 ± 0.38
Model	-	50.85 ± 18.50 Δ	16.14 ± 3.68 ΔΔ	101.33 ± 20.96 ΔΔ	16.14 ± 7.60 ΔΔ	4.99 ± 1.38 ΔΔ	11.12 ± 3.07 ΔΔ
dexamethasone	0.1	59.34 ± 16.39	18.87 ± 4.95	86.37 ± 3.18	10.41 ± 2.42 *	3.80 ± 2.02	9.48 ± 3.20
Fucoidan	100	64.46 ± 6.94	21.40 ± 6.61 *	85.60 ± 11.42	10.52 ± 1.59 *	2.86 ± 1.29 **	8.10 ± 4.01
LMWF	100	66.49 ± 11.28 *	26.26 ± 10.11 *	79.53 ± 15.50 *	8.64 ± 2.93 *	2.39 ± 1.54 **	7.23 ± 2.99 **
LMWF	50	61.86 ± 4.16	22.50 ± 8.27 *	86.77 ± 10.29	10.64 ± 2.28	2.90 ± 1.38 **	8.01 ± 1.71 **
LMWF	25	61.35 ± 4.53	19.93 ± 2.85 *	79.85 ± 4.88	9.40 ± 1.55 *	2.94 ± 1.73 **	8.63 ± 2.84 *

Δ: $p < 0.05$, ΔΔ: $p < 0.01$ (vs normal group); *: $p < 0.05$, **: $p < 0.01$ (vs model group). T-P: total protein; ALB: albumin; SCr: serum creatinine; BUN: blood urea nitrogen; TG: triglyceride; T-CHO: total cholesterol.

Blood urea nitrogen and serum creatinine are two major indexes of renal function. As expected, adriamycin-induced rats had higher BUN and SCr levels, indicating that the kidney of the model rats was damaged by adriamycin administration. Blood total protein and albumin level of model rats were decreased by adriamycin, suggesting that hypoalbuminemia occurred in the model rats. However, the alteration of these biochemical indexes could be significantly reversed by fucoidan and LMWF treatment in a dose-dependent manner. Fucoidan, dexamethasone and LMWF (50 mg/kg) decreased the levels of BUN and SCr at the similar magnitude, while LMWF at the dose of 100 mg/kg had the highest decrease in SCr level ($p < 0.05$, vs fucoidan group). Both fucoidan and LMWF could significantly increase the blood albumin level and decrease TG and TC levels, and LMWF at the dose of 100 mg/kg had a more potent activities ($p < 0.05$). But the positive control dexamethasone could not alter the level of blood albumin, TG, and TC.

These results showed that both fucoidan and its depolymerized fragment could improve the renal function, elevate blood albumin level, and inhibit hyperlipidemia. Low-molecular-weight fucoidan had a more potent activity.

Adriamycin is a kind of amino nucleoside substance. After adriamycin transformed to semiquinone free radicals in organism, the radicals can react with oxygen to produce reactive oxygen species (ROS). The ROS further induces lipid peroxidation of glomerular epithelial cells and destroys the structure and function of the filtration membrane, leading to proteinuria and subsequent nephrotic syndrome [4]. It has been observed that a high cholesterol diet can aggravate the lipid metabolism disorder of adriamycin-induced renal injury [22]. On the contrary, serious proteinuria could lead to the incidence of hypoproteinemia, which further causes malnutrition, especially protein malnutrition. Hypoproteinemia can also reduce the plasma osmotic pressure, especially the colloidal osmotic pressure around the hepatocytes, stimulate the hepatocytes to synthesize lipoproteins, and finally results in the disorder of lipid metabolism and hyperlipidemia.

The renoprotective effect of fucoidan or LMWF may be due to its antioxidant activity. Fucoidan and low-molecular-weight fucoidan were proved to have in vitro free radical scavenging activities [23]. The antioxidant activity of fucoidan may be helpful in eliminating the reactive oxygen species initiated by adriamycin and maintaining the structure and function of glomerular basement membrane, thus inhibiting the occurrence and development of proteinuria. In order to verify the correlation between the renoprotection and anti-oxidation of fucoidan and its depolymerized fragment, we further detected the lipid peroxidation in kidney of rats.

2.5. Lipid Peroxidation

The levels of malondialdehyde (MDA) and superoxide dismutase (SOD) of the kidney tissue were measured in all groups. The MDA production was increased in kidney tissue of adriamycin-treated model rats (Table 6). While adriamycin treatment decreased the SOD level of the kidney tissue of rats. Treating adriamycin-induced rats with LMWF significantly and dose-dependently increased the SOD level and decreased the MDA level in kidney tissue. Fucoidan treatment also increased the SOD level and decreased the MDA level. LMWF at the dose of 100 mg/kg was more potent in decreasing the MDA level ($p < 0.05$), while both fucoidan and LMWF had similar activities on SOD at the same dose (100 mg/kg).

Table 6. Effect of fucoidan and low molecular weight fucoidan (LMWF) on malondialdehyde (MDA) and superoxide dismutase (SOD) levels in kidney ($\overline{X} \pm S$).

Groups	Dosage (mg/kg)	MDA (nmol/mg prot)	SOD (u/mg prot)
Normal	-	1.03 ± 0.35	86.31 ± 5.50
Model	-	1.65 ± 0.66 $^\Delta$	72.92 ± 12.66 $^\Delta$
dexamethasone	0.1	1.07 ± 0.35 *	77.48 ± 11.22
Fucoidan	100	1.12 ± 0.44 *	84.45 ± 10.44 *
LMWF	100	0.94 ± 0.33 **	83.72 ± 8.15 *
LMWF	50	1.16 ± 0.27 *	82.89 ± 7.27 *
LMWF	25	1.37 ± 0.22	79.68 ± 9.91

$^\Delta$: $p < 0.05$ (vs normal group); *: $p < 0.05$, **: $p < 0.01$ (vs model group).

MDA is a main marker of endogenous lipid peroxidation [24]. The increase of MDA production indicates that peroxidative damage increases after adriamycin induction. Antioxidant enzymes are considered to be a primary defense that prevents biological macromolecules from oxidative damage. SOD is an important enzymatic antioxidant defense mechanisms that protects against oxidative processes initiated by the superoxide anion.

The results demonstrated that both fucoidan and its depolymerized fragment were successful in inhibiting lipid peroxidation in the kidney of adriamycin-induced rats, as observed in the reduction of MDA production and increase of SOD level. The results were in accordance with previous studies on the antioxidant activities of fucoidan and low-molecular-weight fucoidans [24]. The renoprotective effect of fucoidans was at least partly due to its antioxidant activities.

2.6. Effect of Molecular Weight on Adriamycin-Induced Nephrotic Syndrome

The molecular weight has been demonstrated to play an important role in the biological activities of polysaccharides [25]. Low-molecular-weight heparin is a classic example. Comparing with unfractioned heparin, low-molecular-weight heparin has improved bio-availability, a longer half-life, and more predictable dose response, which make its use increasingly common in the treatment and prophylaxis of thromboembolism [18]. High and low-molecular-weight fucoidans were also reported to have differential effect on the severity of collagen-induced arthritis in mice [26]. A daily oral administration of high-molecular-weight fucoidan (HMWF, 100 ± 4 kDa) enhanced the severity of arthritis, inflammatory responses in the joint cartilage, and the levels of collagen-specific antibodies, while low-molecular-weight fucoidan (LMWF, 1 ± 0.2 kDa) reduced the severity of arthritis and the levels of Th1-dependent collagen-specific IgG2a.

Our group previously reported that fucoidan from *S. japonica* has a protective effect on chronic renal failure, diabetic nephropathy, and acute kidney injury [8–11]. This study revealed that fucoidan and low-molecular-weight fucoidan also have a protective effect on adriamycin-induced nephrotic syndrome. LMWF at the same dose had a better protective effect than fucoidan. Since fucoidan and LMWF had similar sugar constituents but different molecular weight, the difference in renoprotection between fucoidan and LMWF was mainly attributed to their discrepancy in molecular weight. The exact mechanism of the renoprotective effect of fucoidan and LMWF needs further investigation in the following study.

3. Materials and Methods

3.1. Materials

Adriamycin was purchased from Meilun Biological Technology Co., Ltd. (Dalian, China). Dexamethasone Acetate tablet (Lot No.170545) was purchased from Tianjin Tianyao Pharmaceutical Co. Ltd. (Tianjin, China). All other chemicals and reagents were obtained from general commercial sources.

3.2. Preparation of Fucoidan and Its Depolymerized Fragment

Saccharina japonica Aresch (Formerly name: *Laminaria japonica*, Laminariaceae), cultured in the coast of Rongcheng, Shandong Province, China, was collected in July 2017. The fresh seaweed was washed with clean seawater and sun dried. Fucoidan was extracted from *S. japonica* in hot water at 100 °C for 2 h. The extraction liquid was filtered and 1% $CaCl_2$ was added to precipitate soluble alginate. After centrifugation, the supernatant was dialyzed using a dialysis membrane (molecular weight cutoff (MWCO) 3500 Da) against pure water, concentrated under reduced pressure and finally precipitated with ethanol. The precipitate was washed twice with ethanol and dried to get fucoidan.

Low-molecular-weight fucoidan (LMWF) was prepared using free radical degradation with the combination of hydrogen peroxide and ascorbic acid. Briefly, fucoidan was dissolved in distilled water to a final concentration of 0.5%, ascorbic acid and hydrogen peroxide was added to the solution to a final concentration of 30 mM, and stirred at room temperature for 2 h. The solution was filtered, dialyzed against pure water (MWCO 3500 Da), concentrated under reduced pressure and subsequently precipitated with ethanol (75%, final concentration).

3.3. Chemical Analysis

Fucose content was determined using cysteine hydrochloride–sulfuric acid method with L-fucose as the standard [27]. Sulfate content was analyzed using ion chromatography with potassium sulfate as the standard. Total sugar content was measured by phenol-sulfuric acid method. Uronic acid was tested using modified carbazole method with D-glucuronic acid as the standard [28]. Monosaccharide composition was estimated with high-performance liquid chromatography (HPLC) according to the method of Zhang et al. [29]. The proportion of monosaccharide was evaluated by calculating the molar ratio of other monosaccharide to fucose. Infrared spectra were recorded with a Nicolet-750

FT-IR spectrometer. Average molecular weight was determined by high performance gel filtration chromatography (HPGPC) on TSK G4000 PW_{xl} or G3000 PWxl column eluted with 0.7% Na_2SO_4 using a series of dextrans with different molecule weight as standard.

3.4. Animals and Experimental Design

Adult male Sprague-Dawley rats (220–240 g) were provided by Experimental Animal Center of Shandong University. The animals were maintained on a 12 h dark/light cycle at about 22 °C and relative humidity (60–70%), allowed free access to standard rat chows and water during the experiments. The experiments were performed in complete compliance with the National Guide for the Care and Use of Laboratory Animals, and were approved by the Experimental Animal Ethics Committee of Institute of Oceanology, Chinese Academy of Sciences, China (approval code SCXK(Lu)20190002).

The adriamycin-induced nephrotic syndrome model in rats was performed according to Bertani et al. protocol [2]. A single dose of adriamycin (6.0 mg/kg body weight) was injected via the femoral vein to induce nephrotic syndrome (NS) model. After injection of adriamycin, 24 h urinary protein content was measured once a week. Two weeks following the adriamycin injection, proteinuria was detected, then the rats were randomly divided into six groups (n = 10): Group 1 was the model group which consisted of NS rats; Group 2 consisted of 10 NS rats and the rats were treated with daily oral gavage of fucoidan at dosage of 100 mg/kg body weight; Group 3, 4, and 5 consisted of NS rats and were treated daily oral gavage of LMWF at dosage of 100, 50, and 25 mg/kg body weight, respectively. Group 6 was the positive control group, and NS rats in this group were administrated with dexamethasone acetate at dose of 0.1 mg/kg body weight. Group 7 was the normal group (n = 10) and rats were orally administrated with 10 mL/kg/d of saline. All rats were raised in the same environment and were allowed unlimited access to water and conventional rat chow during the experiments. During the experiments, the animals were weighed twice a week, the general state of animals was recorded every day, including body hair, stool, and mental state.

To measure urinary protein levels, the rats were placed in individual metabolic cages for 24 h urine collection once a week.

On the thirtieth experimental day the animals were anaesthetized by ether and blood samples were taken from the eye-pit of rats. After the blood sample was taken, the rats were killed and the kidneys were weighted and taken for routine histological examination.

3.5. Blood Biochemical Indexes

Serum was separated and the levels of serum creatinine, blood urea nitrogen (BUN), total protein, albumin, total cholesterol, and total triglyceride were analyzed with Beckman biochemical analyzer. The protein of the kidney was determined using Coomassie Brilliant Blue (G-250) by the method of Bradford using a bovine serum albumin (BSA) standard.

3.6. Assessment of MDA and SOD Levels

The kidney levels of SOD and MDA were analyzed using kits from NanJing JianCheng (NanJing JianCheng Bio Inst, China), and the protocols were all followed the introduction of the kit.

3.7. Statistical Analysis

Data were presented as means ± SD. ANOVA was used to analyze the data and the Student's t-test was used to determine the level of significance of differences in population means. A significant difference was accepted with $p < 0.05$.

4. Conclusions

Fucoidan was extracted from *S. japonica*, and further degraded into low-molecular-weight fucoidan by oxidant degradation. The average molecular weights of fucoidan and low-molecular-weight fucoidan were 136 and 9.5 kDa, respectively. The in vivo animal experiment revealed that fucoidan and low-molecular-weight fucoidan had protective effect on adriamycin-induced nephrotic syndrome. Fucoidan and LMWF treatment could significantly inhibit adriamycin-induced proteinuria and decrease the elevated BUN, SCr, TG, and TC level of rats in a dose-dependent manner. LMWF at the same dose had a better protective effect than fucoidan. Since fucoidan and LMWF had similar sugar constituents but different molecular weight, the difference in renoprotection between fucoidan and LMWF was mainly attributed to their discrepancy in molecular weight. Their renoprotective effect maybe partly related to their antioxidant effect.

Author Contributions: Conceptualization, Q.Z. and J.T.; methodology, J.T.; validation, J.W and N.W.; formal analysis, J.T. and L.G.; investigation, J.T. and Y.Y.; resources, Q.Z. ; data curation, Q.Z. and J.W.; writing—original draft preparation, J.T.; writing—review and editing, Q.Z.; project administration, Q.Z.; funding acquisition, Q.Z. All authors have read and agreed to the published version of the manuscript.

Funding: This work was supported by the National Key R&D Plan of China (Grant No. 2018YFD0901104), Major Scientific and Engineering Projects of Innovation in Shandong Province (Grant No.2019JZZY010818), STS Program of Chinese Academy of Sciences (KFJ-STS-QYZD-195) and K.C. Wong Education Foundation, CAS.

Conflicts of Interest: The authors declare no conflicts of interest.

References

1. Kaneko, Y.; Narita, I. Nephritis and nephrotic syndrome. *Nihon Jinzo Gakkai Shi.* **2013**, *55*, 35–41.
2. Bertani, T.; Poggi, A.; Pozzoni, R.; Delaini, F.; Sacchi, G.; Thoua, Y.; Mecca, G.; Remuzzi, G.; Donati, M.B. Adriamycin-induced nephrotic syndrome inrats: sequenceof pathological events. *Lab. Investig.* **1982**, *46*, 16–23.
3. Faleiros, C.M.; Francescato, H.D.C.; Papoti, M.; Chaves, L.; Silva, C.G.A.; Costa, R.S.; Coimbra, T.M. Effects of previous physical training on adriamycin nephropathy and its relationship with endothelial lesions and angiogenesis in the renal cortex. *Life Sci.* **2017**, *169*, 43–51. [CrossRef] [PubMed]
4. Lee, V.W.; Harris, D.C. Adriamycin nephropathy: A model of focal segmental glomerulosclerosis. *Nephrology* **2011**, *16*, 30–38. [CrossRef] [PubMed]
5. Pena-Polanco, J.E.; Fried, L.F. Established and emerging strategies in thetreatment of chronic kidney disease. *Semin. Nephrol.* **2016**, *36*, 331. [CrossRef] [PubMed]
6. Cohen, G.; Hörl, W.H. Immune dysfunction in uremia—An update. *Toxins* **2012**, *4*, 962–990. [CrossRef] [PubMed]
7. Beaudreuil, S.; Lorenzo, H.K.; Elias, M.; Nnang, O.E.; Charpentier, B.; Durrbach, A. Optimal management of primary focal segmental glomerulosclerosis inadults. *Int. J. Nephrol. Renovasc. Dis.* **2017**, *10*, 97–107. [CrossRef] [PubMed]
8. Zhang, Q.; Li, Z.; Xu, Z.; Niu, X.Z.; Zhang, H. Effects of fucoidan on chronic renal failure in rats. *Planta Med.* **2003**, *69*, 537–541. [PubMed]
9. Zhang, Q.; Li, N.; Zhao, T.; Qi, H.; Xu, Z.; Li, Z. Fucoidan inhibits the development of proteinuria in active Heymann nephritis. *Phytother. Res.* **2005**, *19*, 50–53. [CrossRef]
10. Wang, J.; Liu, H.; Li, N.; Zhang, Q.; Zhang, H. The protective effect of fucoidan in rats with streptozotocin-induced diabetic nephropathy. *Mar. Drugs* **2014**, *12*, 3292–3306. [CrossRef]
11. Li, X.; Wang, J.; Zhang, H.; Zhang, Q. Renoprotective effect of low-molecular-weight sulfated polysaccharide from the seaweed *Laminaria japonica* onglycerol-induced acute kidney injury in rats. *Int. J. Biol. Macromol.* **2017**, *95*, 132–137. [CrossRef] [PubMed]
12. Berteau, M.; Mulloy, B. Sulfated fucans, fresh perspectives: Structures, functions, and biological properties of sulfated fucans and an overview of enzymes active toward this class of polysaccharide. *Glycobiology* **2003**, *13*, 29–40. [CrossRef] [PubMed]
13. Wang, J.; Zhang, Q.; Zhang, Z.; Zhang, H.; Niu, X. Studies on a novel fucogalacan sulfate extracted from the brown seaweed *Laminaria japonica*. *Int. J. Biol. Macromol.* **2010**, *47*, 126–131. [CrossRef] [PubMed]
14. Jin, W.; Zhang, W.; Wang, J.; Yao, J.; Xie, E.; Liu, D.; Duan, D.; Zhang, Q. A study of neuroprotective and antioxidant activities of heteropolysaccharides from six *Sargassum* species. *Int. J. Biol. Macromol.* **2014**, *67*, 336–342. [CrossRef]

15. Takahashi, H.; Kawaguchi, M.; Kitamura, K.; Narumiya, S.; Kawamura, M.; Tengan, I.; Nishimoto, S.; Hanamure, Y.; Majima, Y.; Tsubura, S.; et al. An exploratory study on the anti-inflammatory effects of fucoidan in relation to quality of life in advanced cancer patients. *Integr. Cancer Ther.* **2018**, *17*, 282–291. [CrossRef]
16. Jin, W.; Zhang, W.; Wang, J.; Zhang, Q. The neuroprotective activities and antioxidant activities of the polysaccharides from *Saccharina japonica*. *Int. J. Biol. Macromol.* **2013**, *58*, 240–244. [CrossRef]
17. Tran, P.H.L.; Tran, T.T.D. Current designs and developments of fucoidan-based formulations for cancer therapy. *Cur. Drug Metab.* **2019**, *20*, 933–941. [CrossRef]
18. Gouin-Thibault, I.; Pautas, E.; Siguret, V. Safety profile of different low-molecular weight heparins used at therapeutic dose. *Drug Saf.* **2005**, *28*, 333–349. [CrossRef]
19. Boisson-Vidal, C.; Chaubet, F.; Chevolot, L.; Sinquin, C.; Theveniaux, J.; Millet, J.; Sternberg, C.; Mulloy, B.; Fischer, A.M. Relationship between antithrombotic activities of fucans and their structure. *Drug Dev. Res.* **2000**, *51*, 216–224. [CrossRef]
20. Tissot, B.; Montdargent, B.; Chevolot, L.; Varenen, A.; Descroix, S.; Gareil, P.; Daniel, R. Interaction of fucoidan with the proteins of the complement classical pathway. *Biochim. Biophys. Acta* **2003**, *1651*, 5–16. [CrossRef]
21. Fry, S.C. Oxidative scission of plant cell wall polysaccharides by ascorbate-induced hydroxyl radicals. *Biochem. J.* **1998**, *332*, 504–515. [CrossRef] [PubMed]
22. Song, H.; Li, X.; Zhu, C.; Wei, M. Glomerulosclerosis in adriamycin-induced nephrosis is accelerated by a lipid-rich diet. *Pediatr. Nephrol.* **2000**, *15*, 196–200. [CrossRef] [PubMed]
23. Wang, J.; Zhang, Q.; Zhang, Z.; Li, Z. Antioxidant activity of sulfated polysaccharide fractions extracted from *Laminaria japonica*. *Int. J. Biol. Macromol.* **2008**, *42*, 127–132. [CrossRef] [PubMed]
24. Inal, M.E.; Kanbak, G.; Sunal, E. Antioxidant enzyme activities and malindialdehyde levels related to aging. *Clin. Chim. Acta* **2001**, *305*, 75–80. [CrossRef]
25. Nishino, T.; Aizu, Y.; Nagumo, T. The influence of sulfate content and molecular weight of a fucan sulfate from the brown seaweed *Ecklonia kurome* on its antithrombin activity. *Thromb. Res.* **1991**, *64*, 723–731. [CrossRef]
26. Park, S.; Chun, K.; Kim, J.; Suk, K.; Jung, Y.; Lee, W. The differential effect of high and low-molecular-weight fucoidans on the severity of collagen-induced arthritis in mice. *Phytother. Res.* **2010**, *24*, 1384–1391. [CrossRef]
27. Dische, Z.; Shettles, L.B. A specific color reaction of methylpentose and a spectrophotometric micromethod for their determination. *J. Biol. Chem.* **1948**, *175*, 595–603.
28. Bitter, T.; Muir, H.M. A modified uronic acid carbazole reaction. *Anal. Biochem.* **1962**, *4*, 330–334. [CrossRef]
29. Zhang, J.; Zhang, Q.; Wang, J.; Shi, X.; Zhang, Z. Analysis of monosaccharide compositions in fucoidan by pre-column derivation HPLC. *Chin. J. Oceanol. Liminol.* **2009**, *27*, 578–582. [CrossRef]

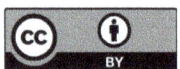 © 2020 by the authors. Licensee MDPI, Basel, Switzerland. This article is an open access article distributed under the terms and conditions of the Creative Commons Attribution (CC BY) license (http://creativecommons.org/licenses/by/4.0/).

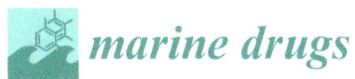

Article

Improvement of Psoriasis by Alteration of the Gut Environment by Oral Administration of Fucoidan from *Cladosiphon Okamuranus*

Masanobu Takahashi [1], Kento Takahashi [1], Sunao Abe [2], Kosuke Yamada [1], Manami Suzuki [1], Mai Masahisa [1], Mari Endo [1], Keiko Abe [3,4], Ryo Inoue [5] and Hiroko Hoshi [1,*]

[1] Department of Biotechnology, Maebashi Institute of Technology, 460-1 kamisadori-machi, maebashi, Gunma 371-0816, Japan; mt1181028@gmail.com (M.T.); kento11240504@gmail.com (K.T.); yg26utumi@gmail.com (K.Y.); manami_bird@yahoo.co.jp (M.S.); collon.mmmf@gmail.com (M.M.); kuoria112@yahoo.co.jp (M.E.)
[2] Marine Products Kimuraya Co., Ltd., 3307 Watari-cho, Sakaiminato, Tottori 684-8790, Japan; abe@mozuku-1ban.jp
[3] Graduate School of Agricultural and Life Science, The University of Tokyo, 1-1-1 Yayoi, Bunkyo-ku, Tokyo 113-8657, Japan; aka7308@mail.ecc.u-tokyo.ac.jp
[4] Group of Food Functionality Assessment, Kanagawa Institute of Industrial Science and Technology, Kawasaki-ku, Kawasaki, Kanagawa 213-0012, Japan
[5] Department of Agriculture and Life science, Kyoto Prefectural University, 1-5 Shimogamohangi-cho, Sakyo-ku, Kyoto 606-8522, Japan; r-inoue@kpu.ac.jp
* Correspondence: hihoshi@maebashi-it.ac.jp; Tel.: +81-27-265-7373

Received: 1 February 2020; Accepted: 5 March 2020; Published: 10 March 2020

Abstract: Psoriasis is a chronic autoimmune inflammatory disease for which there is no cure; it results in skin lesions and has a strong negative impact on patients' quality of life. Fucoidan from *Cladosiphon okamuranus* is a dietary seaweed fiber with immunostimulatory effects. The present study reports that the administration of fucoidan provided symptomatic relief of facial itching and altered the gut environment in the TNF receptor-associated factor 3-interacting protein 2 (*Traf3ip2*) mutant mice (m-*Traf3ip2* mice); the *Traf3ip2* mutation was responsible for psoriasis in the mouse model used in this study. A fucoidan diet ameliorated symptoms of psoriasis and decreased facial scratching. In fecal microbiota analysis, the fucoidan diet drastically altered the presence of major intestinal opportunistic microbiota. At the same time, the fucoidan diet increased mucin volume in ileum and feces, and IgA contents in cecum. These results suggest that dietary fucoidan may play a significant role in the prevention of dysfunctional immune diseases by improving the intestinal environment and increasing the production of substances that protect the immune system.

Keywords: fucoidan; psoriasis; *Traf3ip2*; microbiota; mucin; IgA

1. Introduction

Psoriasis is a chronic autoimmune inflammatory disease characterized by skin lesions and abnormal keratinocyte proliferation. The number of cases of psoriasis vulgaris is increasing worldwide [1]. The etiology of psoriasis remains unclear, although there is evidence for genetic predisposition. The TNF receptor-associated factor 3-interacting protein 2 (*TRAF3IP2*) gene was identified in 2010 as a new susceptibility locus containing the psoriasis vulgaris disease gene in European genome-wide association studies [2]. The *TRAF3IP2* gene encodes a protein involved in IL-17 signaling, which interacts with members of the nuclear factor-kappa-B transcription factor family. Recently, an important genetic influence of the polymorphism in *TRAF3IP2* on the susceptibility to psoriasis, but not to atopic dermatitis, was reported in a Japanese population [3,4]. Matsushima et al. [5] also reported that a genetic mutation in *Traf3ip2* mice caused an atopic dermatitis-like skin disease with hyper-IgE-emia.

The gut microbiota observed in patients with psoriatic was less diverse when compared to that of healthy controls [6]. The gut microbiota profile in the gut environment has been found to significantly influence autoimmune diseases such as multiple sclerosis [7,8]. Recently, however, adults with psoriasis and/or psoriatic arthritis have learned to supplement their standard medical therapies with dietary interventions to reduce disease severity [9]. There are many reports about the relationship between immunostimulatory effects and dietary components of microbiota [10]. Polysaccharides are considered a dietary fiber, and work as prebiotics which are beneficial for the intestinal environment [11]. Fructo-oligosaccharides maintain intestinal barrier function, as does immunoglobulin A (IgA), in a methionine–choline-deficient mouse model of nonalcoholic steatohepatitis [12]. Secreted IgA cells in colonic tissue generate mucus that is secreted into the outermost intestinal cecal patch; the secreted mucus entraps bacteria and prevents their translocation into the tissue [13].

This study was focused on fucoidan, which is found in the cell wall matrix of brown algae. Fucoidan is a high-molecular weight (over 200,000 Daltons) sulfated polysaccharide; it consists mostly, i.e., 13% or more, of sulfated fucose and glucuronic acid [14,15]. Many reports have reported that fucoidans from various brown algae have some biological activities, such as antitumor, anticoagulant, and apoptosis induction, along with other antiallergic and immunologic activities [16–18]. Fucoidan supplementation improved fecal microbiota composition and repaired intestinal barrier function; moreover, fucoidan is an intestinal flora modulator for the potential prevention of breast cancer [19]. However, it has not been reported whether fucoidan in the diet affects psoriasis or changes the intestinal environment components of the intestinal environment such as mucin, IgA, and bacterial flora.

The present study demonstrated that fucoidan affects psoriasis symptoms; it ameliorated the effect of phenotype and altered the intestinal microbiota and the quality of secreted IgA and mucin in m-*Traf3ip2* mutant mice.

2. Results

2.1. Fucoidan Diet Rescued Psoriasis Symptoms on m-Traf3ip2 Mouse Faces and Reduced Scratching

Psoriasis is a chronic immunological inflammatory disease of the skin characterized by dry silvery scales with eruptions. In this study, the severity of symptoms on the faces of *m-Traf3ip2* mice was graded by phenotype using a scoring system based on clinical Psoriasis Area and Severity Index (PASI) and an ethological method as a scratch test. For this study, 1% fucoidan or 1% cellulose was administered by adding it to the AIN-93G diet, which is a normal diet. *m-Traf3ip2* mice facial skin showed significant differences in symptoms between the fucoidan and normal diet groups. *m-Traf3ip2* mice which were on the normal diet showed severe symptoms of psoriasis on their faces, whereas the mice on the fucoidan diet showed improved facial symptoms after 21 days and tended to enter remission in the following weeks (Figure 1A). The normal diet group exhibited increased scratching within a certain time frame, whereas the fucoidan diet group showed significantly decreased facial scratching from 1 week until after 56 days (Figure 1B). In the normal diet group, the mice with the highest PASI scores showed the most serious symptoms and the most severe scratch test results. On the other hand, the symptoms of the fucoidan diet mice group decreased from 21 days until after 63 days, and were significantly lower than in those of the control group (Figure 1C). Histological sections of the facial skin of mice that had high PASI scores showed thickening of both the epithelium and keratin layer of the epidermis by hematoxylin-eosin (HE) staining (Figure 1D).

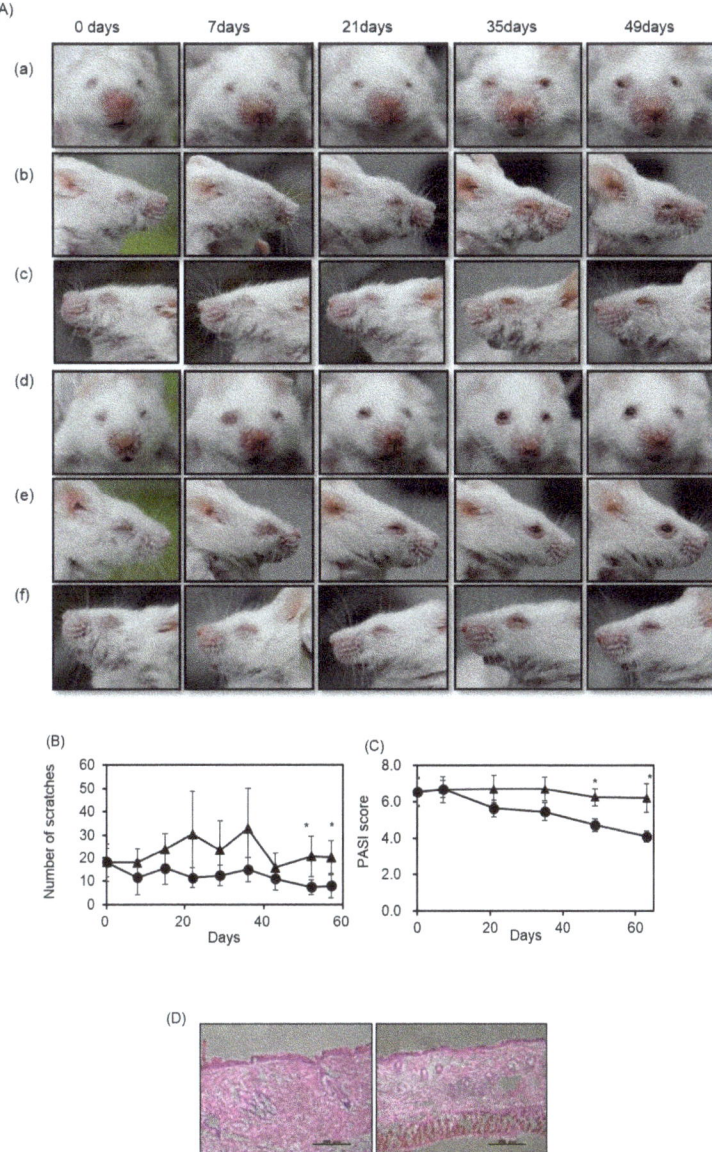

Figure 1. Effects of fucoidan diet on *m-Traf3ip2* mouse faces by PASI score analysis and scratching actions. (**A**) Aspects of *m-Traf3ip2* typical mouse face over time. (a), (b), (c) Sections are normal diet mice and (d), (e), (f) sections are fucoidan diet mice. (**B**) Scratching behavior of individual mice. Closed triangle shows normal diet group and closed circle shows fucoidan diet group. PASI test scored 5 persons and each value. The calculated values for the in vitro experiments are mean ± SD (fucoidan diet group $n = 14$ and normal diet group $n = 9$). (**C**) The severity of the psoriasis-like skin condition. (**D**) Histological analysis by HE staining of faces. Normal diet mice and fucoidan diet mice epidermal sections are shown on left and right, respectively. Bars show 0.2 mm. Asterisk (*) shows significant difference ($p < 0.05$).

These results suggested that fucoidan improved psoriasis symptoms on the faces of *m-Traf3ip2* mice.

2.2. Fucoidan Drastically Changed Microbiota in the Small Intestines of m-Traf3ip2 Mice

Dietary fiber is a prebiotic, which is useful in the intestinal environment [11,12]. In the present study, 16S rRNA from intestinal microorganisms in fecal samples was analyzed using next-generation genome sequences. In phylum analysis, fecal microflora in the fucoidan diet group showed significantly increasing relative abundance of the *Bacteroidetes* and *Proteobacteria* phyla during each time course (i.e., 6, 28, and 56 days) compared to mice fed the normal diet, whereas the relative abundance of the *Firmicutes* and *TM7* phyla significantly decreased in the fucoidan diet group after 6 days and remained at a low level until the end of the experiment (Figure 2A) compared to the fecal microorganisms of the normal diet fed mice. Table 1 shows the changes in phylum levels in fecal microflora of *m-Traf3ip2* fucoidan diet and normal diet mice over time. The relative abundance of *Deferribacteres* and *Actinobacteria* phyla, which were the lowest of all the phyla, were higher in the fucoidan diet group than in the normal diet group. The differences between the fucoidan and normal diet samples were then analyzed by taxonomy, class, order, family, and genus. After 56 days, levels of fecal microbiota belonging to the *Bacteroidaceae* and *Paraprevotellaceae* families in the *Bacteroidetes* phylum in fucoidan diet group were significantly higher than those of normal diet group. On the other hand, the fecal microbiota of fucoidan diet group in the family of *F16* in the phylum of *TM-7*, and those in the family of *Odoribacteraceae* in the phylum *Bacteroidetes*, showed decreased levels of the same kinds of microflora after 56 days (Figure 2B,C) compared to the microbiota of normal diet mice group. In the genus analysis, fecal microflora of fucoidan diet group showed significantly increased relative abundance of unclassified *Paraprevotellaceae* genera and *Bacteroides* genera in the family of *Bacteroidetes* compared to fecal microflora of the normal diet group (Figure 2D,E).

Table 1. Changes in phylum levels in fecal microbiota of *m-Traf3ip2* fucoidan diet group and normal diet group. Significant difference between fucoidan and normal diets. ($p < 0.01$ (c), $p < 0.05$ (d)). Significant difference from before to after same diet administration. ($p < 0.01$ (a), $p < 0.05$ (b)).

Administration Days (D)	0 D		6 D		28 D		56 D	
Diet	Norml	Fucoidan	Normal	Fucoidan	Normal	Fucoidan	Normal	Fucoidan
	Relative abundance (%)							
Actinobacteria	0.43 ± 0.15	0.48 ± 0.15	0.38 ± 0.04	0.25 ± 0.05 (b, d)	0.70 ± 0.19	1.88 ± 1.52 (b, c)	0.45 ± 0.15	0.83 ± 0.72
Bacteroidetes	60.0 ± 7.69	65.4 ± 5.57	60.2 ± 2.90	79.2 ± 1.74 (c, a)	59.1 ± 4.18	77.4 ± 2.78	59.4 ± 9.69	78.2 ± 6.42 (b, d)
Deferribacteres	0.10 ± 0.07	0.08 ± 0.04	0.25 ± 0.11	0.33 ± 0.33	0.05 ± 0.05	0.10 ± 0.00 (a, c)	0.20 ± 0.12	0.40 ± 0.31
Firmicutes	36.3 ± 8.56	29.2 ± 4.43	33.1 ± 2.18	16.3 ± 2.25 (b, c)	30.8 ± 2.27	15.2 ± 1.9 (a, c)	34.3 ± 9.05	16.3 ± 4.98 (b, d)
Proteobacteria	1.35 ± 0.27	1.10 ± 0.16	1.95 ± 0.30	3.03 ± 0.33 (c, a)	1.40 ± 0.27	3.50 ± 0.87 (a, c)	1.73 ± 0.53	3.05 ± 0.62 (a, d)
TM7	3.75 ± 1.51	3.58 ± 1.29	3.73 ± 0.62	0.98 ± 0.26 (b, c)	7.78 ± 1.92	1.98 ± 0.19 (c)	3.80 ± 0.24	1.23 ± 0.11 (b, c)

Microorganisms of the *Desulfovibrionaceae* family were found at slightly higher levels in the fecal microbiota of the fucoidan diet group compared to that of the normal diet group. The fecal microbiota of fucoidan diet group showed significantly lower populations of the genera *Prevotella* and *Odoribacter*, as well as of an unclassified *S24-7* family in the *Bacteroidetes* phylum, than in the normal diet group after 56 days. In the *Firmicutes* phylum, the genera of *Coprococcus*, unclassified members of the *Ruminococcaceae* family, and unclassified members of the order *Clostridiales* were lower in fecal microbiota of the fucoidan diet group compared to those of the normal diet group. The normal diet group showed significant increase in the fecal microbiota of *F16* family compared to those of the fucoidan diet group.

These results suggested that the fucoidan diet altered the taxonomic compositions of many microbiota in *m-Traf3ip2* mice 6 days after feeding, and thereafter, the microbiota conditions were continuously maintained.

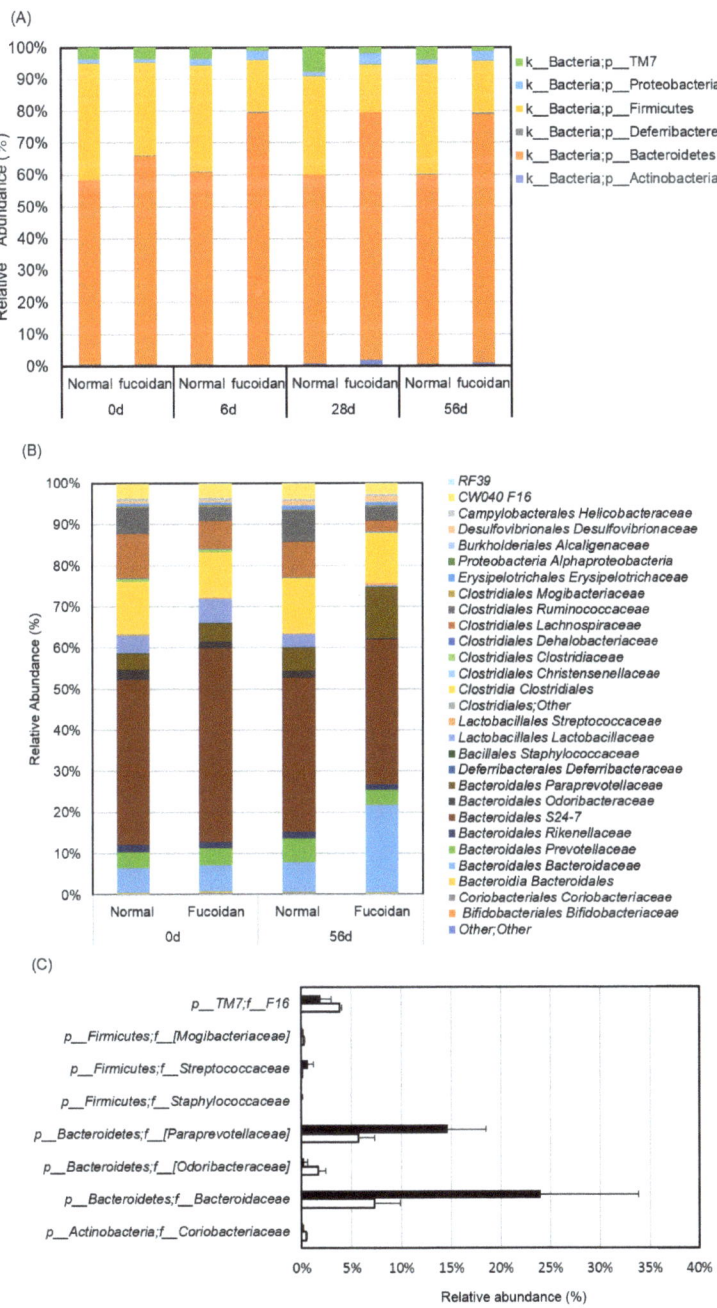

Figure 2. *Cont.*

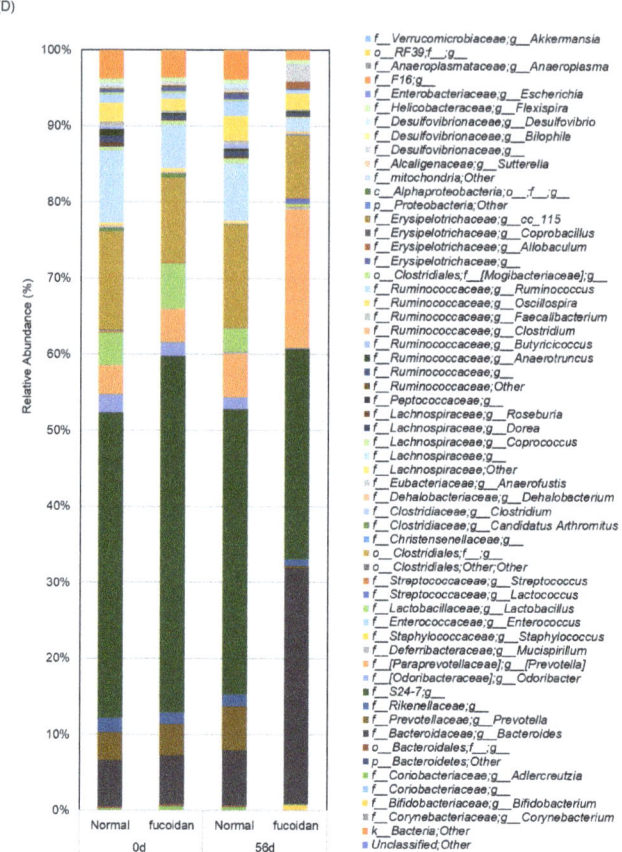

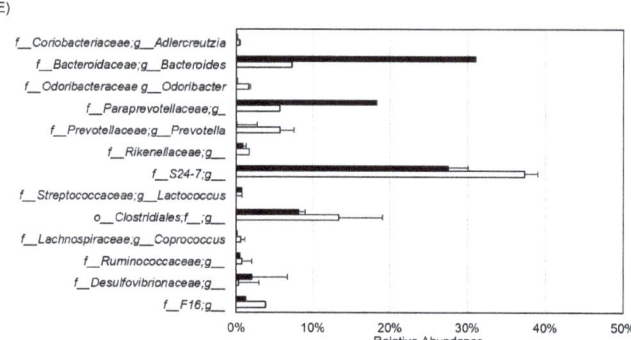

Figure 2. Fecal microbiota analysis. 16S rRNA genome-wide screening analysis. Time dependence of fecal microbiota analyses were performed on the phylum (**A**), family (**B**), (**C**), and genus (**D**), (**E**), levels of normal diet group (left) and fucoidan diet group (right). White bar shows normal diet group and black bar shows fucoidan group. The calculated values for the *in vitro* experiments are means ± SD (n =5).

2.3. Fucoidan Diet Promoted Fecal Mucin Production

Mucin, which is produced by mucous/goblet cells, is a major component of mucosal fluid. Alterations in gastrointestinal mucin induced by dietary fiber may affect nutrient bioavailability, cytoprotection of the mucosa, or other aspects of gastrointestinal function [20,21]. In this study, mucin production in feces by mucous goblet cells was measured. Fluorescence labeling was used to measure terminal N-acetylgalactosamine in mucin components in feces. In *m-Traf3ip2* mice, the fucoidan diet group showed increased mucin production, especially from 21 days after the diet had begun, whereas the normal diet group showed little change (Figure 3A). Similarly, wild-type, not mutated gene of *Traf3ip2* BALB/c mice, fed a fucoidan diet showed significantly increasing mucin secretion compared to the group of a normal diet mice (Figure 3B). These results suggested that fucoidan promoted mucin production and created a better intestinal environment.

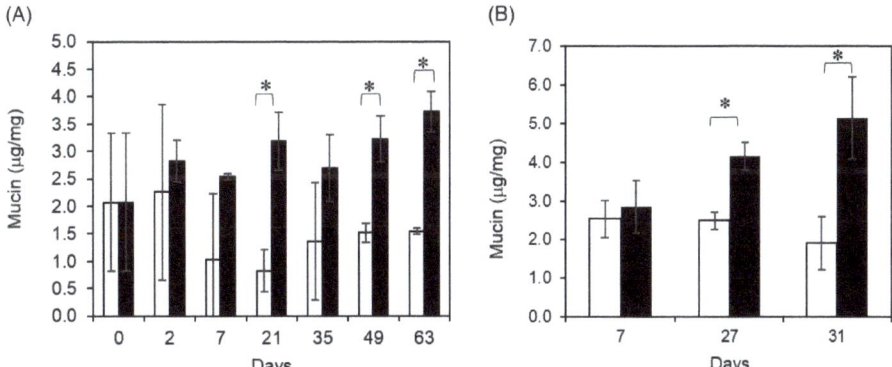

Figure 3. Quantification of mouse fecal mucin. Volume concentrations of (**A**) *m-Traf3ip2* and (**B**) wild type mouse in fecal mucin. White bar shows normal diet group and black bar shows fucoidan group from fecal. The calculated values for the in vitro experiments are mean ± SD ($n = 5$). Asterisk (*) shows significant difference ($p < 0.05$).

2.4. Production of IgA in Feces and Cecum

Secreted of IgA in the gut mucosal layer plays important roles in intestinal immune function, e.g., prevention of bacterial and viral invasion. IgA suppresses the expression of bad bacteria and maintains a healthy balance of gut microbiota. Enzyme-linked immunosorbent assay (ELISA) was used to evaluate IgA expression in feces and cecum of *m-Traf3ip2* mice fed on fucoidan with or without diet for 63 days. The assay showed that secreted IgA was not present, or was present at levels below detection, in fecal samples from both groups. It was reported that the cecum produces IgA [22]. Our study detected total IgA in the cecum of both groups in the samples obtained at 63 days. Total IgA volume was obviously higher in the ceca of the fucoidan fed mice group compared to those of the normal diet mice group (Figure 4A). Wild type mice fed a fucoidan diet also showed higher total IgA compared to the normal diet group of wild type mice (Figure 4B).

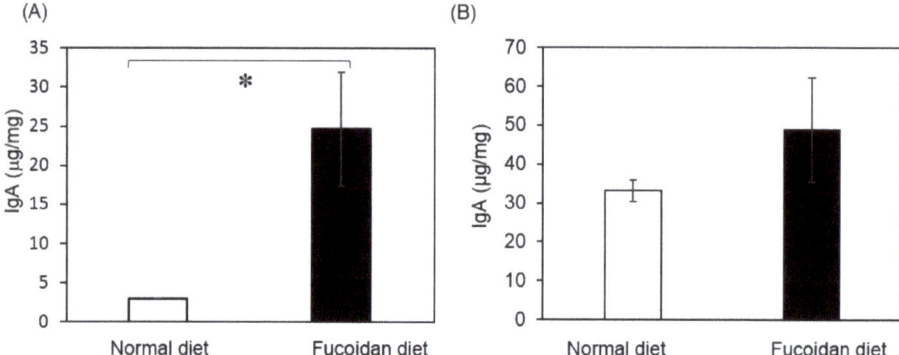

Figure 4. Quantification of total IgA in cecal contents of fucoidan diet group and normal diet group. Volume concentrations of (**A**) *m-Traf3ip2* and (**B**) wild type mouse total IgA were quantified from 63 days and 31 days, respectively, in cecum contents by ELISA. White bar shows normal diet group and black bar shows fucoidan diet group from cecum. The absorbance of reaction products was determined at 450 nm, and the production was quantified. The calculated values for the in vitro experiments are expressed as mean ± SD ($n = 5$). Asterisk (*) shows significant difference ($p < 0.05$).

This result indicated that fucoidan promotes the secretion of IgA in the cecum and improves the intestinal immunity.

3. Discussion

The present study showed that the administration of the sulfated polysaccharide fucoidan improves the symptoms of psoriasis, an immune disorder disease, changes the composition of intestinal microbiota to include high relative abundance of *Bacteroidetes*, and improves the gut environment by increasing the volumes of mucin and IgA.

First, the administration of the fucoidan diet to psoriasis model mice with the *m-Traf3ip2* mutation gradually improved symptoms, and especially significantly improved phenotypes, scratch test scores, and PASI scores, beginning at 21 days until after 56 days. However, *m-Traf3ip2* mice did not show a preference for the fucoidan diet, and mice in the two dietary groups showed no weight difference. In the same period, we showed the alteration of microflora and the production of mucin at the lamina propria of the mucous membrane and of IgA in cecum. *Bacteroidetes* and *Firmicutes*, which comprise more than 90% of all phylogenetic types, are the two dominant bacterial phyla in the human, mouse [23–25], and pig [26] gut. An analysis of fecal microbiota by genome sequences revealed that feeding of fucoidan to *m-Traf3ip2* mice significantly increased relative abundance of the phylum *Bacteroidetes* for all bacteria beginning at 6 days and continuing beyond 56 days compared to the relative abundance in the normal diet mice.

In a comparison between two phylum groups, *Bacteroidetes* and *Firmicutes*, for all bacteria, *Firmicutes* levels decreased from 2 days after the beginning of the experiments and remained low after 56 days; the analysis was performed using quantitative PCR. These results showed that feed intake of fucoidan by *m-Traf3ip2* mice increased the relative abundance of the *Bacteroidetes* phylum and decreased those of the *Firmicutes* phylum. However, the family S24-7 in the phylum *Bacteroidetes* was decreased in the fucoidan diet group. It was reported that S24-7 is related to bowel inflammation [27]. A fucoidan diet changes fecal microbiota and may also have anti-inflammatory effects. On the other hand, the fucoidan diet group showed drastically decreased the relative abundance of the phylum *Firmicutes*. *Firmicutes* was reported to have a wide range of both beneficial and harmful effects on autoimmune disorders. The feces of fucoidan diet group showed a significantly lower relative abundance of the phylum *Firmicutes* compared with the growth rate of control diet group. In this study, levels of two *Clostridiales* families, *Lachnospiraceae* and *Ruminococcaceae*, were decreased in the intestinal microflora of the fucoidan diet group. Especially, fucoidan administration decreased the presence of *Ruminococcaceae Oscillospira* species in the intestinal microbiota. Our results corresponded with those of another microbiota analysis: soluble dextrin fibers altered the intestinal microbiota and reduced proinflammatory cytokine secretion in male IL-10-deficient mice [28]. Some unidentified members of the *Clostridiales* family may be related to the induction of Th17 cells in the small intestine and aid in protection against pathogens. Th17 cell induction is harmful in patients with an autoimmune disorder [29].

The relative abundance of the phylum *Proteobacteria*, family *Desulfovibrionaceae*, was also higher in the fucoidan diet group than in the control group. Glycomacropeptide is a prebiotic that reduces *Desulfovibrio* bacteria, increases cecal short-chain fatty acids, and has an anti-inflammatory effect in mice [30]. In the present study, fucoidan was a possible source of *Desulfovibrionaceae* consumption as a source of nutrition. The increased relative abundance of the family *Desulfovibrionaceae* may be related to some improvement in the symptoms of psoriasis in the present study. The analysis suggested that the fecal microbiota of *Bacteroidetes acidifaciens* were drastically increased in fucoidan diet group in this study (data not shown). Species of *B. acidifaciens* promote the expression of secreted IgA in the large intestine [13,31], and members of the genus *Rikenellaceae* are often found in the gastrointestinal tracts of a number of animals [32]. The species of *B. acidifaciens* may be related to the improvement of symptoms of psoriasis. Additionally, levels of the *Bacteroidetes* species *Parabacteroides* was increased in the fecal microbiota of the fucoidan diet group. Intestinal microbiota of the genus *Bacteroides*, as well as those of *Porphyromonadaceae Parabacteroides*, produce antagonistic substances in ecological niches, preventing the colonization and invasion of exogenous bacteria, and might be one of the mechanisms underlying such prevention [33]. In the present study, drastic increase in the volumes of cecal IgA and ileal mucin was observed in the intestines of fucoidan fed *m-Traf3ip2* mice. Interestingly, these increases coincided with the increase in the *Bacteroidetes* population. β-glucans also have distinctive immunomodulatory characteristics [11,34,35]. In children with chronic respiratory problems, short-term oral application of β-glucan affects mucosal immunity by stabilizing secreted IgA levels [36]. The present results suggest that fucoidan administration induces the production of IgA and mucin, rearranging the intestinal environment to regulate immune response [37]. In pigs, a laminarin diet affects immune function by increasing genes that encode mucin expression, namely, *MUC2*, *MUC4*, IL-6, and IL-8 in the ileum [11]. Laminarin also binds to mammalian non-Toll-like pattern-recognition receptors, such as, dectin-1, complement receptor-3, lactosylceramide, and scavenger, thereby stimulating innate immunity through the activation of macrophages, dendritic cells, neutrophils, natural killer cells, and helper T-cells [35]. Our study did not elucidate the relation of administration of fucoidan and its molecular action in psoriasis model mice. It will be necessary to elucidate the mechanism underlying the effect of fucoidan on the remission of psoriasis.

In conclusion, fucoidan as a dietary supplement could modulate the fecal microbiota composition and repair intestinal barrier function. This study suggested that fucoidan can be used to improve the symptoms of psoriasis.

4. Materials and Methods

4.1. Reagents

All reagents used in the enzyme assays were obtained from Wako Pure Chemical Industries (Tokyo, Japan). Fucoidan from *Cladosiphon Okamuranus* was provided by Marine Products Kimuraya Co., Ltd. (Tottori, Japan). The average molecular weight of fucoidan is 300,000 Dalton as analyzed by size exclusion chromatography. The fucose content is about 60%, and sulfated fucose is 14.3% in total fucoidan. Food entrainment, i.e., AIN-93G, was purchased from CREA Japan Inc. (Tokyo, Japan).

4.2. Animals and Diets

m-Traf3ip2 and BALB/c mice were previously generated as described in prior studies [5] and purchased from Japan SLC, Inc. (Shizuoka, Japan). SPF-grade animals were maintained under conventional conditions in animal facilities certified by the Animal Care and Use Committee of the Maebashi Institute of Technology. The experimental procedures were all in accordance with the National Institutes of Health guidelines for the care of experimental animals, and the experimental protocol was approved by the Institutional Animal Care and Use Committee of Maebashi Institute of Technology (16-001). The animals were housed individually in plastic cages, allowing for the separation and collection of feces, at 21 °C with a relative humidity of 55% under a 12:12 h light:dark cycle. 6-week-old mice were housed as 5 mice per cage in a controlled environment. After 1 week of acclimatization, the mice were randomly divided into two groups, and thereafter, were fed the experimental/normal or fucoidan diets with free access to drinking water. The animals were fed Rodent Diet AIN-93G (CLEA Japan, Tokyo, Japan). Two groups of 14 or 9 Traf3ip2 mutant mice were fed a diet containing 1.0% w/w fucoidan or crystalline cellulose, respectively. Each group was fed for 9 weeks. Two groups of five wild type, BALB/c mice, were fed a diet containing 1.0% w/w fucoidan or crystalline cellulose, respectively. Each group was fed for 31days.

4.3. Analysis of Phenotype and Scratch Test

The face of each mouse was photographed from three angles: front, left side, and right side. To score the severity of skin inflammation, the severity of the psoriasis-like skin condition in the facial area of m-Traf3ip2 mice was monitored and graded every 7 days. The scoring system was based on the clinical PASI [38]. The modified PASI score was based on three parameters, namely, erythema, scaling, and thickening. Each parameter score was assigned independently on a scale of 0 to 4 as follows: 0, none; 1, slight; 2, moderate; 3, marked; and 4, very marked. A scoring table with red taints was used to score the level of erythema. The cumulative score (erythema, desquamation, swelling, and scaling area) denoted the severity of inflammation (scale 0–100%). The modified PASI test was applied to each mouse by five persons. Accurate scratching behavior of individual mice was assessed by counting the scratches. Scratching behavior was monitored and the number of scratching movements was counted during a 10-minute period each week.

4.4. Histochemical Analysis of Facial Skin Dissection

After shaving the faces of mice, their facial skin was fixed with 4% paraformaldehyde and then OTC-embedded punch biopsies were sectioned longitudinally into 7–8 μm thick sections. The sections were stained using HE for histological evaluation and for the evaluation of the microarchitecture of thickened epithelium and the keratinocyte layer. Experiments were conducted in triplicate; the data were averaged to evaluate inflammation and epithelial and keratinocyte changes.

4.5. Microbiota Analysis in Feces

DNA was extracted from fecal samples for microflora analyses using 16S rRNA high-throughput sequencing. For DNA extraction, the fecal microbiomes were analyzed from 20 mg fecal samples obtained from each animal in the normal as well as fucoidan diet group. For each mouse in either group, total DNA was extracted from a 100 mg fecal sample using QIAamp DNA Stool Mini Kit (Qiagen, Venlo, Netherlands) according to the manufacturer's instructions. The DNA concentration was determined using a NanoDrop (Scrum, Tokyo, Japan). Extracted fecal DNA was examined using 16S rDNA gene sequencing by MiSeq (Illumina, Tokyo, Japan). Library preparation, deep sequence, and data analysis were carried out using methods described by Inoue et al [39]. Data analysis was performed by Bio-Linux, a Linux computing platform customized for bioinformatics research [40].

4.6. Quantification of Fecal Mucin and Cecum IgA

Mucin was extracted from each 100 mg fecal sample. Fecal mucin contents were determined using a fecal mucin assay kit (Mucin Assay Kit, Cosmo Bio, Co., Ltd., Tokyo, Japan). A fluorometric assay discriminated O-linked glycoproteins (mucins) from N-linked glycoproteins. Fluorescence was measured using a SoftMax® Pro spectrometer (Molecular Devices, CA, USA). Total IgA was extracted from 50 mg of cecum samples and quantified using a mouse IgA ELISA quantitation kit (Immundiagnostik, Bensheim, Germany) as specified in the manufacturer's instructions. The reaction products were determined from absorbance at 450 nm using XFluor4 (Tecan, Zurich Switzerland), and IgA was qualified.

4.7. Statistical Analysis

The calculated values for the in vitro and in vivo experiments are expressed as mean ± SD. Student's *t* test was used for statistical analysis.

Author Contributions: Conceptualization, H.H.; Data curation, M.T., K.T., M.S., K.Y. and M.M.; Formal analysis, K.T., M.E. and R.I.; Investigation, S.A.; Resources, S.A.; Supervision, K.A.; Writing—original draft, H.H. All authors have read and agreed to the published version of the manuscript.

Funding: This research received no external funding.

Acknowledgments: The authors thank Y. Matsushima and T. Taira for discussing this study with them.

Conflicts of Interest: Authors do not have any conflicts of interest.

References

1. World Health Organization. Global Report on Psoriasis. Available online: https://apps.who.int/iris/bitstream/handle/10665/204417/9789241565189_eng.pdf.psoriasis;jsessionid=54912784D28C9F36ECCD45471AC5775B?sequence=1 (accessed on 10 March 2020).
2. Genetic Analysis of Psoriasis Consortium & the Wellcome Trust Case Control Consortium; Strange, A.; Capon, F.; Spencer, C.C.A.; Knight, J.; Weale, M.E.; Allen, M.H.; Barton, A.; Band, G.; Bellenguez, C.; et al. A genome-wide association study identifies new psoriasis susceptibility loci and an interaction between HLA-C and ERAP1. *Nat. Genet.* **2010**, *42*, 985–990. [PubMed]
3. Hayashi, M.; Hirota, T.; Saeki, H.; Nakagawa, H.; Ishiuji, Y.; Matsuzaki, H.; Tsunemi, Y.; Kato, T.; Shibata, S.; Sugaya, M.; et al. Genetic polymorphism in the TRAF3IP2 gene is associated with psoriasis vulgaris in a Japanese population. *J. Dermatol. Sci.* **2014**, *73*, 264–265. [CrossRef] [PubMed]
4. Hüffmeier, U.; Uebe, S.; Ekici, A.B.; Bowes, J.; Giardina, E.; Korendowych, E.; Juneblad, K.; Apel, M.; McManus, R.; Ho, P.; et al. Common variants at TRAF3IP2 are associated with susceptibility to psoriatic arthritis and psoriasis. *Nat. Genet.* **2010**, *42*, 996–999. [CrossRef] [PubMed]
5. Matsushima, Y.; Kikkawa, Y.; Takada, T.; Matsuoka, K.; Seki, Y.; Yonekawa, H.; Minegishi, Y.; Karsuyama, H.; Yonekawa, H. An atopic dermatitis-like skin disease with hyper-IgE-emia develops in mice carrying a spontaneous recessive point mutation in the Traf3ip2 (Act1/CIKS) gene. *J. Immunol.* **2010**, *185*, 2340–2349. [CrossRef]
6. Scher, J.U.; Ubeda, C.; Artacho, A.; M, A.; Isaac, S.; Reddy, S.M.; Marmon, S.; Neimann, A.; Brusca, S.; Patel, T.; et al. Decreased bacterial diversity characterizes the altered gut microbiota in patients with psoriatic arthritis, resembling dysbiosis in inflammatory bowel disease. *Arthritis Rheumatol.* **2015**, *67*, 128–139. [CrossRef]
7. Becattini, S.; Taur, Y.; Pamer, E.G. Antibiotic-Induced Changes in the Intestinal Microbiota and Disease. *Trends Mol. Med.* **2016**, *22*, 458–478. [CrossRef]
8. Chiodini, R.J.; Dowd, S.E.; Chamberlin, W.M.; Galandiuk, S.; Davis, B.; Glassing, A. Microbial Population Differentials between Mucosal and Submucosal Intestinal Tissues in Advanced Crohn's Disease of the Ileum. *PLoS ONE* **2015**, *10*, e0134382. [CrossRef]
9. Ford, A.; Siegel, M.; Bagel, J.; Cordoro, K.; Garg, A.; Gottlieb, A.B.; Green, L.J.; Gudjonsson, J.E.; Koo, J.; Lebwohl, M.; et al. Dietary Recommendations for Adults With Psoriasis or Psoriatic Arthritis From the Medical Board of the National Psoriasis Foundation. *JAMA Dermatol.* **2018**, *154*, 934–950. [CrossRef]

10. Szabó-Fodor, J.; Bónai, A.; Bóta, B.; Egyed, L.S.; Lakatos, F.; Pápai, G.; Zsolnai, A.; Glávits, R.; Horvatovich, K.; Kovács, M. Physiological Effects of Whey- and Milk-Based Probiotic Yogurt in Rats. *Pol. J. Microbiol.* **2017**, *66*, 483–490. [CrossRef]
11. O'Shea, C.J.; O'Doherty, J.V.; Callanan, J.J.; Doyle, D.; Thornton, K.; Sweeney, T. The effect of algal polysaccharides laminarin and fucoidan on colonic pathology, cytokine gene expression and Enterobacteriaceae in a dextran sodium sulfate-challenged porcine model. *J. Nutr. Sci.* **2016**, *5*, 15. [CrossRef]
12. Matsumoto, K.; Ichimura, M.; Tsuneyama, K.; Moritoki, Y.; Tsunashima, H.; Omagari, K.; Hara, M.; Yasuda, I.; Miyakawa, H.; Kikuchi, K. Fructo-oligosaccharides and intestinal barrier function in a methionine-choline-deficient mouse model of nonalcoholic steatohepatitis. *PLoS ONE* **2017**, *12*, e0175406. [CrossRef] [PubMed]
13. Masahata, K.; Umemoto, E.; Kayama, H.; Kotani, M.; Takeda, K.; Kurakawa, T.; Kikuta, J.; Gotoh, K.; Motooka, D.; Sato, S.; et al. Generation of colonic IgA-secreting cells in the cecal patch. *Nat. Commun.* **2014**, *5*, 3704. [CrossRef] [PubMed]
14. Cumashi, A.; Ushakova, N.A.; Preobrazhenskaya, M.E.; D'Incecco, A.; Piccoli, A.; Totani, L.; Tinari, N.; Morozevich, G.E.; Berman, A.E.; Bilan, M.I.; et al. A comparative study of the anti-inflammatory, anticoagulant, antiangiogenic, and antiadhesive activities of nine different fucoidans from brown seaweeds. *Glycobiology* **2007**, *17*, 541–552. [CrossRef] [PubMed]
15. Teruya, T.; Tatemoto, H.; Konishi, T.; Tako, M. Structural characteristics and in vitro macrophage activation of acetyl fucoidan from Cladosiphon okamuranus. *Glycoconj. J.* **2009**, *26*, 1019–1028. [CrossRef] [PubMed]
16. Fukahori, S.; Yano, H.; Akiba, J.; Ogasawara, S.; Momosaki, S.; Sanada, S.; Kuratomi, K.; Ishizaki, Y.; Moriya, F.; Yagi, M.; et al. Fucoidan, a major component of brown seaweed, prohibits the growth of human cancer cell lines in vitro. *Mol. Med. Rep.* **2011**, *1*, 537–542. [CrossRef]
17. Mori, N.; Nakasone, K.; Tomimori, K.; Ishikawa, C. Beneficial effects of fucoidan in patients with chronic hepatitis C virus infection. *World J. Gastroenterol.* **2012**, *18*, 2225–2230. [CrossRef]
18. Yang, J.-H. Topical Application of Fucoidan Improves Atopic Dermatitis Symptoms in NC/Nga Mice. *Phytother. Res.* **2012**, *26*, 1898–1903. [CrossRef]
19. Xue, M.; Ji, X.; Liang, H.; Liu, Y.; Wang, B.; Sun, L.; Li, W. The effect of fucoidan on intestinal flora and intestinal barrier function in rats with breast cancer. *Food Funct.* **2018**, *9*, 1214–1223. [CrossRef]
20. Gill, S.R.; Pop, M.; DeBoy, R.T.; Eckburg, P.B.; Turnbaugh, P.J.; Samuel, B.; Gordon, J.I.; Relman, D.A.; Fraser, C.M.; Nelson, K.E. Metagenomic Analysis of the Human Distal Gut Microbiome. *Science* **2006**, *312*, 1355–1359. [CrossRef]
21. Satchithanandam, S.; Vargofcak-Apker, M.; Calvert, R.J.; Leeds, A.R.; Cassidy, M.M. Alteration of Gastrointestinal Mucin by Fiber Feeding in Rats. *J. Nutr.* **1990**, *120*, 1179–1184. [CrossRef]
22. Shi, H.; Zheng, R.; Wu, J.; Zuo, T.; Xue, C.; Tang, Q.J. The Preventative Effect of Dietary Apostichopus japonicus on Intestinal Microflora Dysregulation in Immunosuppressive Mice Induced by Cyclophosphamide. *J. Biosci. Med.* **2016**, *4*, 24–35.
23. Bäckhed, F. Host-Bacterial Mutualism in the Human Intestine. *Science* **2005**, *307*, 1915–1920. [CrossRef] [PubMed]
24. Ley, R.E.; Turnbaugh, P.J.; Klein, S.; Gordon, J.I. Human gut microbes associated with obesity. *Nature* **2006**, *444*, 1022–1023. [CrossRef] [PubMed]
25. Shang, Q.; Shan, X.; Cai, C.; Hao, J.; Li, G.; Yu, G. Dietary fucoidan modulates the gut microbiota in mice by increasing the abundance ofLactobacillusandRuminococcaceae. *Food Funct.* **2016**, *7*, 3224–3232. [CrossRef]
26. Guevarra, R.B.; Hong, S.H.; Cho, J.H.; Kim, B.-R.; Shin, J.; Lee, J.H.; Na Kang, B.; Kim, Y.H.; Wattanaphansak, S.; Isaacson, R.; et al. The dynamics of the piglet gut microbiome during the weaning transition in association with health and nutrition. *J. Anim. Sci. Biotechnol.* **2018**, *9*, 54. [CrossRef]
27. Palm, N.W.; De Zoete, M.R.; Cullen, T.W.; Barry, N.A.; Stefanowski, J.; Hao, L.; Degnan, P.H.; Hu, J.; Peter, I.; Zhang, W.; et al. Immunoglobulin A coating identifies colitogenic bacteria in inflammatory bowel disease. *Cell* **2014**, *158*, 1000–1010. [CrossRef]
28. Duan, M.; Sun, X.; Ma, N.; Liu, Y.; Luo, T.; Song, S.; Xu, Y. Polysaccharides from Laminaria japonica alleviated metabolic syndrome in BALB/c mice by normalizing the gut microbiota. *Int. J. Boil. Macromol.* **2019**, *121*, 996–1004. [CrossRef]
29. Tanoue, T.; Honda, K. Regulation of intestinal Th17 and Treg cells by gut microbiota. *Inflamm. Regen.* **2015**, *35*, 99–105. [CrossRef]

30. Sawin, E.A.; De Wolfe, T.J.; Aktas, B.; Stroup, B.M.; Murali, S.G.; Steele, J.L.; Ney, D.M. Glycomacropeptide is a prebiotic that reduces Desulfovibrio bacteria, increases cecal short-chain fatty acids, and is anti-inflammatory in mice. *Am. J. Physiol. Liver Physiol.* **2015**, *309*, G590–G601. [CrossRef]
31. Yanagibashi, T.; Hosono, A.; Oyama, A.; Tsuda, M.; Suzuki, A.; Hachimura, S.; Takahashi, Y.; Momose, Y.; Itoh, K.; Hirayama, K.; et al. IgA production in the large intestine is modulated by a different mechanism than in the small intestine: Bacteroides acidifaciens promotes IgA production in the large intestine by inducing germinal center formation and increasing the number of IgA+ B cells. *Immunobiology* **2013**, *218*, 645–651. [CrossRef]
32. Graf, J. The Family Rikenellaceae. In *The Prokaryotes*; Springer: Berlin/Heidelberg, Germany, 2014; pp. 857–859.
33. Nakano, V. Intestinal Bacteroides and Parabacteroides Species Producing Antagonistic Substances. Current Trends in Microbiology. Available online: http://www.icb.usp.br/~{}bmm/mariojac/arquivos/nakano%20et%20al.%202013.pdf (accessed on 10 March 2020).
34. Soltanian, S.; Stuyven, E.; Cox, E.; Sorgeloos, P.; Bossier, P. Beta-glucans as immunostimulant in vertebrates and invertebrates. *Crit. Rev. Microbiol.* **2009**, *35*, 109–138. [CrossRef] [PubMed]
35. Goodridge, H.S.; Wolf, A.J.; Underhill, D.M. β-Glucan recognition by the innate immune system. *Immunol. Rev.* **2009**, *230*, 38–50. [CrossRef] [PubMed]
36. Richter, J.; Svozil, V.; Král, V.; Dobiášová, L.R.; Vetvicka, V. β-glucan affects mucosal immunity in children with chronic respiratory problems under physical stress: Clinical trials. *Ann. Transl. Med.* **2015**, *3*, 2305–5839.
37. Malin, E.V.J.; Gunnar, C.H. Immunological aspects of intestinal mucus and mucins. *Nat. Rev. Immunol.* **2016**, *16*, 639–649.
38. Fredriksson, T.; Pettersson, U. Severe Psoriasis—Oral Therapy with a New Retinoid. *Dermatologica* **1978**, *157*, 238–244. [CrossRef]
39. Inoue, R.; Ohue-Kitano, R.; Tsukahara, T.; Tanaka, M.; Masuda, S.; Inoue, T.; Yamakage, H.; Kusakabe, T.; Hasegawa, K.; Shimatsu, A.; et al. Prediction of functional profiles of gut microbiota from 16S rRNA metagenomic data provides a more robust evaluation of gut dysbiosis occurring in Japanease type 2 diabitic patients. *J. Clin. Biochem. Nutr.* **2017**, *61*, 217–221. [CrossRef]
40. Krampis, K.; Booth, T.; Chapman, B.; Tiwari, B.; Bicak, M.; Field, D.; Nelson, K.E. Cloud BioLinux: Pre-configured and on-demand bioinformatics computing for the genomics community. *BMC Bioinform.* **2012**, *13*, 42. [CrossRef]

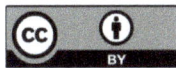

© 2020 by the authors. Licensee MDPI, Basel, Switzerland. This article is an open access article distributed under the terms and conditions of the Creative Commons Attribution (CC BY) license (http://creativecommons.org/licenses/by/4.0/).

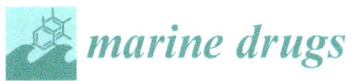

Review

Fucoidans: Downstream Processes and Recent Applications

Ahmed Zayed [1,2] and Roland Ulber [1,*]

[1] Institute of Bioprocess Engineering, Technical University of Kaiserslautern, Gottlieb-Daimler-Straße 49, 67663 Kaiserslautern, Germany; ahmed.zayed1@pharm.tanta.edu.eg
[2] Department of Pharmacognosy, Tanta University, College of Pharmacy, El Guish Street, Tanta 31527, Egypt
* Correspondence: ulber@mv.uni-kl.de; Tel.: +49-0631-205-4043; Fax: +49-6312-05-4312

Received: 6 February 2020; Accepted: 15 March 2020; Published: 18 March 2020

Abstract: Fucoidans are multifunctional marine macromolecules that are subjected to numerous and various downstream processes during their production. These processes were considered the most important abiotic factors affecting fucoidan chemical skeletons, quality, physicochemical properties, biological properties and industrial applications. Since a universal protocol for fucoidans production has not been established yet, all the currently used processes were presented and justified. The current article complements our previous articles in the fucoidans field, provides an updated overview regarding the different downstream processes, including pre-treatment, extraction, purification and enzymatic modification processes, and shows the recent non-traditional applications of fucoidans in relation to their characters.

Keywords: fucoidans; extraction; brown algae; production; bioactivities

---

1. Introduction

Polysaccharides, nucleic acids, and peptides are considered the main three types of bioactive polymeric macromolecules [1]. Among these, polysaccharides serve various roles in living cells including structural functions, where cellulose and chitin represent the major components of the different cell wall matrices [2,3], energy storage (e.g., starch and glycogen) [4,5], and hydration and signaling functions (e.g., mucilage and alginic acid) [6,7].

Particularly, marine homo- and heteropolysaccharides are derived from marine organisms, which represent a large part of global biodiversity [8]. Among these are the algal polysaccharides, such as fucoidan and alginate in brown seaweeds, carrageenan in red seaweeds and ulvan in green seaweeds. These were reported to have interesting nutraceutical, biomedical, pharmaceutical and cosmeceutical applications, including dietary fibers; anti-inflammatory, anti-tumor, anti-oxidant, hepatoprotective and anti-coagulant properties; and drug carrier functionality. Therefore, they have been extensively investigated during the last few decades [9–13], especially after the emergence of glycobiology and glycomics [14–17].

Polysaccharides such as dietary fibers of brown algae are abundant and diverse (e.g., alginates, cellulose, fucoidans and laminarins) constituting the major components (up to 75%) of the dried thallus weight (% DW) [18–20]. Previous work investigated their abundance in different species, reporting *Fucus*, *Ascophyllum*, *Saccharina*, and *Sargassum* to contain 65.7, 69.6, 57.8 and 67.8 % DW, respectively [21,22]. Specifically, fucoidans are found in the cell walls and extracellular matrices of brown algae in addition to more than 265 genera and 2040 species of marine invertebrates (e.g., sea cucumbers), where they perform vital structural functions [23–26]. Fucoidans are assumed to act as cross-linkers between the major threads of cellulose and hemicellulose, promoting cellular integrity and maintaining cellular hydration (especially during drought seasons) [27]. They also act in other reproductive, immune and cell-to-cell communicative roles [23]. As recommended by the International

Union of Pure and Applied Chemistry (IUPAC), fucoidans is a general term used to describe sulfated L-fucose-based polymers including sulfated fucans cited by the Swedish scholar Kylin, as well as other fucose-rich sulfated heteropolysaccharides [23,28]. Their chemical structures, in terms of monomeric composition and branching, are quite simple in marine invertebrates compared to their analogues in brown algae [13,29].

Hundreds of articles have thoroughly discussed and reviewed the biological, pharmacological and pharmaceutical applications of fucoidans [30–33], including nanomedicine, [34] which has made it a hot topic in the last few decades [35–37]. All these studies tried to investigate fucoidans molecular mechanisms in relation to their chemical structure and physicochemical properties. Therefore, different hypotheses were suggested for each activity, such as anti-tumor [31,38–40], anti-coagulant [41,42], anti-viral [43,44] and anti-inflammatory activity[45,46]. These investigations revealed that various factors are relevant, such as molecular weight, sulfation pattern, sulfate content and monomeric composition [47–49]. For example, different fractions were produced with different physicochemical properties in our previous experiments; sulfation pattern and sulfate content were highly related to anti-viral and cytotoxic activities against HSV-1 and Caco-2 cell lines, respectively, while molecular weight and sugar composition were potential factors in anti-coagulation activity [41,50]. In addition, degree of purity was reported as an influential factor [32], where co-extracted contaminants (e.g., phlorotannins or polyphenols) could lead to significant interference in anti-oxidant activity and, consequently, cosmetic applications [51,52].

Therefore, several key production challenges regarding fucoidans were discussed in our last review article in order to obtain a product that follows the universal good manufactured practice (GMP) guidelines. The article discussed sources of heterogeneity in extracted fucoidans, including the different biotic (e.g., biogenic, geographical and seasonal factors) and abiotic (e.g., downstream processes) factors affecting the fucoidans physicochemical and chemical properties [53]. Others patented production techniques that have assisted in the marketing of several commercial fucoidans by well-known companies (e.g., Sigma-Aldrich®, Algues and Mer and Marinova®) derived from *Fucus vesiculosus* and other brown algae species [54–56].

Furthermore, the improvement of fucoidans activity was investigated, targeting several points. Among these was the modification of the chemical structure of the native fucoidans scaffolding, including depolymerization [57,58] and over-sulfation [59]. These modifications could be attempted chemically [60], enzymatically [35,61] or physically [62]. Predetermined synthesis of oligomers [63,64] and low molecular weight polymers with defined monomeric units [65] is also involved. Additionally, fractionation of fucoidans is a common approach during extraction and purifications steps by applying different extraction and purification conditions (e.g., pH, time, molarity of NaCl) [49,55].

The current article aimed at complementing our previously published article discussing the reasons for heterogeneity of fucoidans [53]. It reviewed and evaluated the different downstream processes used in production as the most important abiotic factors affecting the fucoidans quality and structural features; it then addressed recent uncommon applications and prospective bioproduction of fucoidans. In addition, the updated status of enzymatic structural modifications of fucoidans, especially by fucoidanases, were presented.

2. Global Market and Cultivation of Brown Algae

Marine hydrocolloids (e.g., agar, carrageenan and alginate) are of particular industrial interest, with worldwide annual production of approx. 100,000 tons and a value above US $1.1 billion [66]. Based on FAO periodical reports (FAO, 2014, 2016), among the top seven most-cultivated seaweeds, three taxa are mainly used for hydrocolloids production; these include Rhodophyta (e.g., *Eucheuma* sp. and *Kappaphycus alvarezii*) for carrageenan production and *Gracilaria* sp. for agar production [67]. These data encouraged the global marine market to escalate the production yield by finding alternative, eco-friendly seaweed cultivation techniques, such as sea farming or aquaculture and biotechnology [53]. In 2014, the annual production of cultivated seaweeds reached 27.3 million tons [68], representing 27%

of the total marine aquaculture production, while the global market of marine biotechnology (blue biotechnology) for industrial applications has been expected to achieve US $4.8 billion in 2020 and grow to US $6.4 billion by 2025 [69].

Species of brown macroalgae (Phaeophyceae) are distributed among the orders Fucales and Laminariales, which are the major commercial sources of the algal sulfated polysaccharides, in addition to Chordariales, Dictyotales, Dictyosiphonales, Ectocarpales, and Scytosiphonales. Moreover, phylogenetic analysis showed that Fucales are one of the largest and most diversified orders within Phaeophyceae, having eight families (41 genera and 485 species), named Ascoseiraceae, Cystoseiraceae, Durvillaeaceae, Fucaceae, Hormosiraceae, Himanthaliaceae, Sargassaceae, and Seirococcaceae [70]. Figure 1 illustrates the distribution of several examples of well-known brown algae species which are considered potential sources of sulfated polysaccharides dominating tropical to temperate marine forests and intertidal regions. The data were based on Wahl, et al. [71].

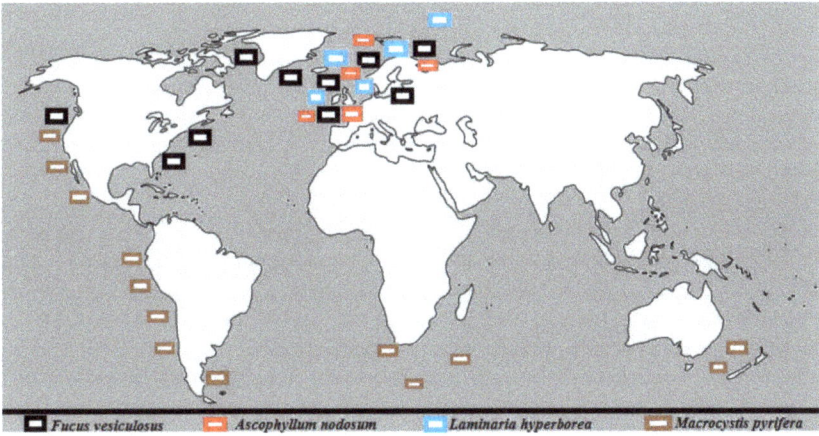

Figure 1. Global distribution of the major brown seaweeds' species. They dominate tropical to temperate marine forests and intertidal regions.

Furthermore, like terrestrial plant tissue culture (PTC), several biotechnological attempts were performed to cultivate and/or regenerate thallus from different species of brown seaweeds using seaweeds tissue culture [72]. They include micropropagation, callus induction and protoplast isolation [69,73–75]. They are very promising techniques as it may not only help to overcome the previously mentioned fucoidans production heterogeneity challenges [53] but also provide a sustainable supply [76]. However, compared to PTC, STC is still not well-enough established to be used for production of hydrocolloids and fucoidans [77] or cultivation in closed, well-controlled bioreactors, as in case of the red algae organism *Agardhiella subulata* [78].

3. Downstream Processes

Fucoidans are anionic polymers occurring in highly complicated matrices in cell walls and intercellular spaces along with other carbohydrate polymers (e.g., alginate, cellulose and laminarin), polyphenols and proteins [79]. Additionally, due to the sulfate ester groups, fucoidans are water soluble polysaccharide polymers [80] exhibiting high affinity to other cell wall components, especially polyphenols [81]. Therefore, various and complicated downstream processes are required to remove such extraneous substances before and after precipitation with ethanol or cationic surfactants to obtain high-purity fucoidans [82,83]. The processes always include pre-treatment, extraction and purification stages as shown in Figure 2.

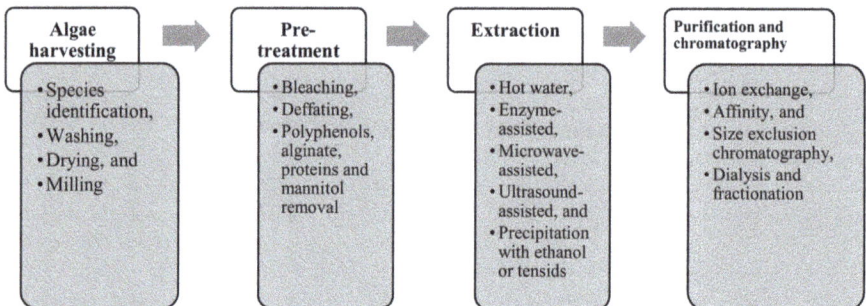

Figure 2. Required downstream processes including steps in each process for fucoidans production.

3.1. Pre-Treatment

After harvesting algal biomass from beaches, the biomass should be washed thoroughly with tap water to remove sands and epiphytes, then dried and milled to increase the area-to-mass ratio. Several pre-treatment steps are performed before the extraction step to release fucoidans from intercalating components, ease the following extraction process, improve the extraction yield, and decrease the possible interferences from co-extracted components in purification and biological investigations.

Previous experiments tried to remove pigments (e.g., chlorophyll, flavins and carotenoids) and lipids in specific bleaching and defatting steps with acetone, toluene, charcoal or 80%–85% (v/v) ethanol [34,84,85]. Since fucoidans are negatively charged molecules, they remained unaffected by incubation with organic solvents (e.g., acetone, toluene or hexane:isopropanol (3:2) mixture) during pre-treatment of the dried algal biomass. Such extracts were further treated to obtain carotenoids, represented by fucoxanthin in brown algae [86], lipids and fatty acid metabolites (especially essential polyunsaturated fatty acids (PUFA) and fucosterol), adding to nutraceutical applications of brown algae [87,88]. In contrast, activated carbon materials, such as charcoal, adsorb the target fucoidans molecules, adversely affecting the final production yield [79].

Other studies tried to exclude the tightly non-covalently bound polyphenolic compounds represented by phloroglucinol-type phlorotannins [89], which contribute to the light to dark brown color of the crude fucoidans extract (along with fucoxanthin) [41,81]. They reported comparatively high phlorotannins content, reaching approximately one fifth of the brown algae dry weight [25]. Phlorotannins perform major structural and physiological functions, like tannins found in plants, including defense against biotic and abiotic stresses [90,91]. Despite of the great pharmacological importance of phlorotannins [92,93], their presence in high-quality fucoidans is not acceptable because of the possibility of interference with the anti-oxidant [25,52,94] and anti-tumor activities of fucoidans [95]. Therefore, the natural phenolics content of fucoidans should be determined before the measurement of their biological activities [96]. Therefore, nearly all pre-extraction protocols for fucoidans involved strategies to remove such contaminants, e.g., incubation with EtOH:H_2O:HCHO (16:3:1) (v/v/v) at pH 2. Under such conditions, formaldehyde enhances the crosslinking and polymerization of such polyphenolic contaminants and the high volume of ethanol results in protein denaturation [41,60,97,98]. However, the toxicity of formaldehyde limits its utilization in pre-treatment protocols [51].

Furthermore, pre-treatment steps are performed to remove other carbohydrates such as alginate, the major hydrocolloids in brown algae [99]. This is commonly removed by formation of water-insoluble calcium complex either before [60] or during the extraction procedure using 1%–4% (w/v) $CaCl_2$ followed by a filtration or centrifugation step to remove the formed precipitate [58,98,100,101]. These previously mentioned procedures were optimized using successive incubation, centrifugation or filtration, washing and drying for the main extraction step of the dried, milled algal biomass, as described in Figure 3. The application of such an optimized protocol resulted in a dried, pre-treated powder representing 71% (*w/w*) of the starting material [98]. Despite these results, downstream processing of fucoidans, except with enzymatic modification, starts with a small scale (e.g., 5–10 g of the dried algal biomass) to optimize parameters like dried biomass to solvent ratio, temperatures, pH, and incubation time, based on preliminary quality and yield of crude fucoidans measured by infra-red spectroscopy (IR), simple sugar tests and elemental analysis. After this, transfer to large scale production could be accomplished using larger biomass quantities (e.g., 500–1000 g).

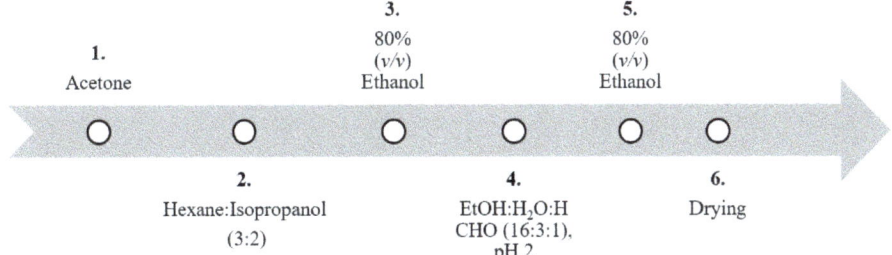

Figure 3. Overview of optimized pre-treatment steps of the dried algae biomass before fucoidans extraction. All steps were performed at 25 °C overnight and the ratio between dried algal biomass to solvent was 1:10, except for the acetone step, which was 1:20 (modified after [98,102]).

Due to several complicated pre-treatment steps, general protocols always employ a single incubation step using the ternary mixture composed of $CH_3OH:CH_3Cl:H_2O$ (4:2:1) (v/v/v) [103], binary mixture of $CH_2Cl_2:EtOH$ (94.2:5.8, *v/v*) [104], or aqueous ethanol (e.g., 95% *v/v*) [105,106] to remove pigments [107], polyphenols [51,103] and lipids [108]. Nevertheless, pre-treatment steps may be insufficient for complete removal or prevention of some residual co-extraction.

Notably, all these procedures were carried out at room temperature in organic solvents and high volumes of ethanol, in which fucoidans are insoluble. Theoretically, the native structural backbone should not be affected. However, similar polymeric carbohydrates such as laminarin may still be present, contaminating the extract after these steps.

Recently, in order to decrease pollution of organic toxic solvents, compressional-puffing pre-treatment was applied for *Sargassum hemiphyllum* and *S. glaucescens* fucoidans. The pre-treatment method was based on mechanical pressure at higher temperatures that loosen the cell wall matrix before the step of extraction. Such methods succeeded in increasing the production yield, but they affected the molecular features of the fucoidans, including molecular weight [109,110].

3.2. Extraction

As previously mentioned, fucoidans are principally anionic water-soluble macromolecules. Therefore, they can be extracted from the pre-treated biomass using a simple hot- or cold-water incubation. Afterwards, the extracted fucoidans can be precipitated by high volumes of solvents with a low dielectric constant (e.g., >70% (*v/v*), > 2.5 volume ethanol [111,112], <2 volume acetone [113]) or cationic surfactants (e.g., hexadecyltrimethylammonium bromide (Cetavlon®) 10% (*v/v*)) [55] via an affinity complex formation at low temperatures (4 °C) to remove the undesired salts from the sulfated polysaccharides [52]. This specific precipitation reaction between fucoidans and Cetavlon® is applied in screening tests of microorganisms for putative fucoidanase activity [114].

Ale et al. published comprehensive articles discussing the history of extraction, including the different classical extraction methods of fucoidans, and reported that extraction procedures significantly affect the polymers monomeric composition, even for the same organism [60,115]. Beyond simple hot water extraction [58,116], attempts were made to increase the selectivity and extraction yields, including extraction in acidic [117], alkaline [118], and buffered [41,119] aqueous solutions. However, a neutralization step is required, using Na_2CO_3 or $(NH_4)_2CO_3$ directly after extraction to guard against the non-specific acidic hydrolysis of the polymer [101,115]. Such drastic pH changes affect the chemical and physicochemical properties of fucoidans during the extraction step.

Currently, besides the previously discussed classical extraction methods based on thermal energy, extraction protocols based on vibrational energy have been developed. These protocols are based on microwave-assisted (MAE) [120,121] or ultrasound-assisted (UAE) [94,122] extraction steps to elicit cell wall degradation which improves the polymer release into aqueous solvent. These protocols were optimized either using an approach that modified one factor at a time or a multiple factorial design, setting the polymers production yield, monomeric composition and biological activities as the measured responses.

Recently, combined sulfated polysaccharides extraction protocols were optimized from different brown algae species using hydrothermal-assisted extraction (HAE) followed by sequential ultrasound and thermal technologies [123]. Similarly, subcritical water extraction was applied to increase the production yield of fucoidans from *Nizamuddinia zanardinii* [124]; such mild conditions may be advantageous to preserve the native chemical backbone and physicochemical characters of fucoidans.

Recently, as a trial to reduce such undesirable effects, enzyme-aided or assisted extraction (EAE) protocols are being developed using enzymes instead of harsh chemicals and high extraction temperatures during extraction. These include cellulase, papain, laminarinase, alginate lyase, and protease, which are present in products of Novozymes [79,125–128]. In addition, other cost-effective and time-saving techniques are reported, like those for terrestrial plant polysaccharides, such as extraction under vacuum to lower the boiling point of water and hence avoid possible heat-induced fucoidans degradation [129]. Alternatively, 0.5% (*w/v*) ethylenediaminetetraacetic acid (EDTA) was applied at 70 °C for simultaneous extraction of *Laminaria japonica* fucoidans and removal of pigments [130].

3.3. Separation Physical Methods

Filtration, dialysis and centrifugation, either for the algal biomass or precipitates, are also among the downstream processes after pre-treatment and extraction steps [131–133]. Cross-flow filtration and dialysis against water are usually performed using different molecular weight cut-off (MWCO) membranes for isolation of fucoidans from smaller compounds depending on the high molecular weight of fucoidans [134] and also for fractionation purposes, where low molecular weight fucoidans (LMWF) can be separated from high molecular weight analogues (HMWF) [49].

In addition, filtration, concentration, and fractionation are simultaneously performed using centrifugal concentrators (Vivaspin®) equipped with membranes with certain MWCO, like in protein purification. However, in some cases, especially in the presence of bulk masses or high concentrations of salts and small contaminants, the use of centrifugal concentrators becomes practically and economically unsuitable for fucoidans purification. In such cases, bulky contaminants result in membrane clogging leading to its deterioration and increasing the production cost.

3.4. Purification

Despite the previously mentioned purification steps, residuals of co-extracted contaminants are still present, and resulting fucoidans are still crude-type. [27]. Therefore, further selective purification steps are needed to obtain a high-quality product for reproducible and accurate biological investigations. Some researches adopted simple, non-chromatographic steps, such as bleaching of the crude fucoidans (NaClO$_2$ in dilute HCl) followed by precipitation with cetyltrimethylammonium bromide [135] or by cold overnight incubation in aqueous buffered solution of calcium acetate (20 mM, pH = 6.5 -7.5) followed by dialysis [136]. In addition, membrane filtration was reported to produce fucoidans fractions of different molecular weight [137].

However, other chromatographic purification techniques were discussed in our previous publications [41,53,98,102]. Almost all the chromatographic techniques are based on the permanent negatively charged sulfate ester groups distributed on the polymer backbone which allow selective fucoidans capture. However, carboxylated (e.g., alginate) and phosphorylated (e.g., nucleic acids) compounds might interfere [138,139]. Therefore, the pH value of the applied solvents is critical during chromatographic purification. One option for this uses anionic exchange resins (e.g., diethylaminoethyl cellulose or DEAE-cellulose), which was performed at pH 7.2 using 0.1 M sodium phosphate buffer [140]. An alternative is cationic dyes (e.g., toluidine blue- or perylene diimide derivative), modified resins or chitosan functioning in buffered solutions [27,102]. Both anion exchange and dye affinity chromatography involve the use of highly concentrated NaCl elution solvents. As a result, a subsequent purification step using chromatographic gel permeation [141] or dialysis [140] is required to remove salts, increasing the production costs. Other methods based on the use of biological macromolecules, such as lectins and anti-thrombin III, were also reported [53].

Novel innovative purification techniques were recently developed, such as selective solid phase extraction for purifying fucoidans and other complex seaweeds polymers by molecularly imprinted polymers (MIP) [142,143] or MIP modified by deep eutectic solvents [142,143]. Abdella et al., developed a green and time-saving purification protocol using genipin cross-linked toluidine blue immobilized-chitosan beads employing fucoidans affinity to cationic thiazine dyes [102].

4. Recent Uncommon Applications

In addition to the classical therapeutic applications of fucoidans, including anti-coagulant [41,144], anti-viral [145,146], anti-inflammatory [46,147] and selective cytotoxic and anti-tumor uses [39,50], uncommon bioactivities, including cosmeceutical, pharmaceutical, diagnostic, and synergistic therapeutic applications were recently reported [32]. Recent fucoidans uses included therapeutic treatment of major blindness diseases [148]. It has also been used as a drug carrier, especially for anti-cancer treatments and anti-biotics. Additionally, fucoidans have been shown to improve drug bioavailability and efficacy in pharmaceutical formulations, including in nanoparticles, liposomes, microparticles, and semisolid formulations [28,149,150]. Table 1 summarizes some of the recent and uncommon fucoidans applications based on in-vitro or in-vivo studies, in addition to biogenic resources and physicochemical features.

Table 1. Some selected recent therapeutic, diagnostic and pharmaceutical applications of fucoidans including the biogenic sources.

Application	Biogenic Source	Quality Grade/Purification Method	Structural Features	Involved Mechanism	Ref.
Therapeutic					
Anti-viral (IAV)	*Kjellmaniella crassifolia* (Laminariales)	*		Inhibition of the viral neuraminidase (NA) Interference with the cellular EGFR pathway	[43]
Anti-metabolic syndrome	*Fucus vesiculosus* (Fucales)	Dialysis of crude alginate-free fucoidans	Alternating $\alpha(1\rightarrow3)/\alpha(1\rightarrow4)$ linked fucose, Mw > 7.0×10^3 g/mol	Regulation of jnk, akt, and ampk signaling Alleviation of insulin resistance Regulation of lipid metabolism	[151]
Anti-leishmaniasis		Commercial product purchased from Sigma-Aldrich®	Polymer of α-$(1\rightarrow3)$ linked fucose	Activation of the mitogen-activated protein kinase (MAPK)/NF-κB pathway against *Leishmania donovani*-infected macrophages	[152]
				Enhancement of dendritic cells maturation, production of pro-inflammatory cytokines, and down-regulation of anti-inflammatory cytokines	[153,154]
Immunostimulant	*Nizamuddinia zanardinii* (Fucales)	A fraction of DEAE Sepharose Fast Flow column	Highly branched polymer Mw: 953.6×10^3 g/mol	Stimulation of RAW264.7 murine macrophage and NK cells	[155]
Anti-metastasis	*Undaria pinnatifida* (Laminariales)	DEAE-cellulose, and Sephadex G-100 column chromatography (purity>90%)	Mw: of 10.4356×10^4 g/mol	- Suppression of Hca-F cell growth, adhesion, invasion, and metastasis capabilities, - Inactivation of the NF-κB pathway	[156]
Gastrointestinal tract protective		Purity ≥ 95% (Commercial product purchased from Sigma-Aldrich®)		Protection against H_2O_2-induced damage via activation of the NRF2 signaling pathway	[157]
Anti-malaria		- Partial purification by cetylpyridinium chloride Fractionation by DEAE-Sephadex A-25 column	Sugar monomers, and uronic acid, M.wt: approx. 15×10^3 g/mol	In-vitro and in-vivo inhibition of erythrocytes invasion by *P. falciparum* merozoites	[158]
Renal protective	*Laminaria japonica* (Laminariales)		LMWF (Mw: 7×10^3 g/mol)	Inhibition of overexpression of pro-inflammatory and pro-fibrotic factors, oxidative stress and apoptosis	[159,160]
Cardio-, hepatic- and renal protective		Commercial product purchased from Absunutrix Lyfetrition®		Reduction of oxidative stress, pro-inflammatory effects and injuries to the cardiac, hepatic, and renal tissues	[161]
Inhibition of tumor angiogenesis	*Sargassum hemiphyllum* (Fucales)	Hydrolyzed crude extract	LMWF; 760 g/mol	Suppression of HIF-1/VEGF-regulated signaling pathway	[162]
Pro-angiogenic	*Ascophyllum nodosum* (Fucales)	Fractionated with dialysis commercial crude fucoidan (ASPHY)	LMWF (<4.9×10^3 g/mol)	Increase of the vascular network formation regulated via Erk1/2 and PI3K/AKT cell signaling pathways	[163]
Alleviation of diabetic complications	*S. Fusiforme* (Fucales)	Crude extract	Mw: 205.89×10^3 g/mol, high sulfate content	- Suppression of oxidative stress - Alteration of the gut microbiota - Attenuation of the pathological changes in heart and liver	[164]

Table 1. Cont.

Application	Biogenic Source	Quality Grade/Purification Method	Structural Features	Involved Mechanism	Ref.
Diagnostic					
Imaging of cardiovascular diseases	*Ascophyllum nodosum* (Fucales)	An oxidative-reductive degraded crude extract (purchased from Algues and Mer, Ascophyscient®)	GMP-grade LMWF (7.1×10^3 g/mol)	Synthesis of technetium-99m-fucoidan radiotracer for detection of P-selectin	[56]
		Commercial product from Algues and Mer		Synthesis of polycyanoacrylate-fucoidan microcapsules (Fuco-MCs) for detection of P-selectin	[165]
Cosmeceutical					
Anti-Photoaging	*Ecklonia cava* (Laminariales)	Enzymatic degradation of a commercial HMWF	LMWF (Mw: 8×10^3 g/mol)	Anti-oxidant, anti-apoptotic, and MMP-9-inhibiting effects	[166]
Skin brightening and age spot reduction	*F. vesiculosus* (Fucales)	Crude extracts purchased from Marinova® Pty Ltd.	58.6% fucoidans, 33.7% polyphenol	Increase of Sirtuin 1 (*SIRT1*) expression in vitro	[167,168]
Skin immunity, soothing and protection	*U. pinnatifida* (Laminariales)		89.6% fucoidans, <2% polyphenol		
Reconstruction of skin	*F. vesiculosus* (Fucales)	Commercial product from Sigma-Aldrich® (not determined the degree of purity)		Increase of proliferating cell nuclear antigen (PCNA) p63 and α6-integrin expression	[169]
Pharmaceutical technology					
As vehicle for drug delivery	*F. vesiculosus* (Fucales)	Commercial product purchased from Sigma-Aldrich®	Mw: 57.26×10^3 g/mol	- Chitosan-fucoidans-based nanoparticles for delivery of anti-cancers (e.g., curcumin-loaded NPs) - Nanoencapsulation of poly L-lysine	[170,171]
				Piperlongumine (PL)-loaded chitosan-fucoidan nanoparticles (PL-CS-F NPs)	[172]
				Synthesis of fucoidan/trimethylchitosan nanoparticles (FUC-TMC-NPs) as adjuvant in anthrax vaccine adsorbed	[173]
Green synthesis of silver nanoparticles				Synthesis of chitosan-fucoidan complex-coated AgNPs	[174]

*: Not specified.

5. Enzymatic Modification of Native Fucoidans

Owing to their high molecular weight, therapeutic applications of native fucoidans face many challenges including structure elucidation, solubility, manufacturing, and handling [63,116], in addition to safety as a food supplement [175]. Structure elucidation and quantitation of native fucoidans is highly complicated and requires advanced or hyphenated spectroscopic techniques such as HPLC-MS/MS as it applied in Sea Cucumbers fucoidans [176,177]. Also, these techniques must be applied after a step of enzymatic or acid hydrolysis to transform the fucoidans polymers to oligomers. According to their molecular weight, fucoidans are classified into three classes: LMWF (<10 kDa), medium molecular weight fucoidan (MMWF) (10–10000 kDa), and HMWF (>10000 kDa) [31]. LMWF demonstrated better bioavailability and bioactivities than HMWF [178,179]. As a consequence, several articles reported physical, chemical and enzymatic modification of the native HMWF to get LMWF of higher biological activity [62]. Specifically, enzymatic modification of macroalgal polysaccharides, including fucoidans by either fucoidanases or sulfatases, is characterized by regioselectivity and stereospecificity. This new trend is considered crucial and highly promising for current and future applications of polysaccharides [180].

Nevertheless, our publications in 2009 particularly reviewed the specific enzymatic degradation of fucoidans induced by fucoidanases (EC 3.2.1.44) and α-L-fucosidases (EC 3.2.1.51), mainly those isolated from marine bacteria [35]. Cumashi, et al. studied the chemical structures of different fucoidans isolated from a number of brown algal species [181]. Their proposed models, which were highly appreciated and recommended by many researchers [60], showed the backbone of fucoidans to be mainly an alternating α-(1-4) and α-(1-3) linked L-fucopyranoside. Regarding the sulfation pattern, C-2 is usually substituted with sulfate ester groups in addition to alternating C-3 or C-4 in L-fucopyranose residue, according to the glycosidic linkages. In addition, branched chain polymers were also found as in *F. serratus*. Other minor sugar units (e.g., mannose, galactose, glucose and xylose) occur as well in fucoidans structure; however, their distribution pattern and positions are still unknown [60,181]. Now, the mechanism of enzymatic degradation can be described in relation to fucoidans chemical structures.

Despite the increasing number of publications investigating fucoidanase activity of different marine species cell extracts, few of these enzymes have been isolated and characterized. Moreover, genome sequences encoding few fucoidanases have been published, including Ffa2 and FFA1 from *Formosa algae* KMM 3553^T [182,183], FcnA from *Mariniflexili fucanivorans* SW5T [184]. Therefore, specificity of fucoidanases, type of cleaved glycoside bond, structure-activity relationship studies and enzyme stability are still poorly described. It was only observed that identified microbial fucoidanses act only on fucoidans isolated from their respective symbionts [185]. In fact, fucoidanases have not actually been fully utilized yet as a powerful tool either for the structural studies of fucoidans or production of defined and well-characterized bioactive fragments of extracted fucoidans, as shown in Table 2.

Similarly, recent advances in bioinformatics and genome sequencing of microbial species have resulted in a continual increase of novel genome sequences. These genomes demonstrated various potential genes encoding for enzymes with biopolymer-degrading capabilities, such as *Shewanella violacea* DSS12 (NC_014012.1), *Formosa algae* KMM 3553 (NZ_LMAK01000014.1) [182], *Formosa haliotis* MA1 (NZ_BDEL01000001.1) [198], *Wenyingzhuangia fucanilytica* CZ1127 (NZ_CP014224.1) [199] and *Pseudoalteromonas* sp. strain A601 (MXQF01000000) [200]. Moreover, production of stabilized fucoidanases has been achieved by targeted truncation of the C-terminal of FcnA2, Fda1 and Fda2. This recently developed method may help with enzymatic production of defined degrees of polymerization and more bioactive products from native fucoidan substrates [201].

Table 2. Source of fucoidans as a substrate and mode of action of some fucoidanases.

Biogenic Source of Fucoidans	Fucoidanase Source	Mode of Action	Ref.
F. evanescens	Formosa algae KMM 3553	Endo α-1→4	[61,182]
	Pseudoalteromonas citrea strains KMM 3296, KMM 3297, KMM 3298	Endo α-1→3	[186]
F. vesiculosus	Dendryphiella. arenaria TM94	Endo n.d. *	[187]
Kjellmaniella crassifolia	Fucobacter marina SA-0082	Endo β-1→4	[188]
Cladosiphon okamuranus	Fucophilus fucoidanolyticus SI-1234	Endo α-1→3	[189]
	Flavobacterium sp. F-31	Endo n.d.	[190]
F. distichus	Littorina kurila	Endo α-1→3	[191]
Pelvetia canaliculata	Mariniflexile fucanivorans SW5^T	Endo α-1→4	[184]
Undara pinnatifida	Sphingomonas paucimobilis PF-1	Endo n.d.	[192,193]
Saccharina cichorioides	Pseudoalteromonas citrea strains KMM 3296, KMM 3297, KMM 3298	Endo α-1→3	[186]
Nemacystus decipiens	Mizuhopecten yessoensis	Endo n.d.	[194]
Ascophyllum nodosum	Pecten maximus	Exo n.d.	[195,196]
Thelenota ananas (Wild sea cucumber)	Wenyingzhuangia Fucanilytica	Endo n.d.	[197]

* n.d.: not determined.

6. Conclusion and Future Prospective

As multifunctional molecules, fucoidans have received special interest based on their proven efficacy in different fields. The current article reviewed many aspects related to fucoidans' production, mainly from brown algae. Biogenic source and downstream processes were shown as major factors determining their application, which is affected by molecular weight and quality grade of fucoidans. Therefore, the alteration of fucoidans' native structure was recommended, especially as performed by fucoidanases. Their production in nanoform or in combination with other polymers can improve or modify their potential uses, allowing their expanded potential as therapeutic agents, e.g., in anti-cancer applications [202].

Production of high-quality purified fucoidans is urgently required to clarify the relationships between chemical structure and the various bioactivities attributed to fucoidans, eliminating any interference from contaminants. However, it was observed in some cases that crude extracts and presence of co-extracted contaminants, especially polyphenolic phlorotannins, have advantageous cosmeceutical effects due to their powerful anti-oxidant activity [203,204].

Novel techniques, either in cultivation or downstream processes, have been established, increasing the global production yields and reducing ecological and economic problems. A new advance toward achieving such goals was established by optimization of water extraction via measurement of kinetic parameters [205]. In addition to this, it is expected that most future trends in marine biotechnology research will focus on the cell wall and extracellular matrix components of brown algae, including fucoidans' biosynthetic genes and production regulators [23,53,63,206–208]. Such trials may enable the scientific community to produce more bioactive molecules of fucoidans with defined characteristics, including degree of polymerization, sulfate content and pattern, in reproducible manners.

Author Contributions: R.U. planned the manuscript's topics and is the corresponding author, while A.Z. collected the data and wrote the article. All authors have read and agreed to the published version of the manuscript.

Acknowledgments: The research is funded by the „Deutsche Forschungsgemeinschaft (DFG, German Research Foundation)-Project-ID 172116086-SFB 926". The authors would like also to thank Mrs. Aya Abdella and Ms. Gabrielle Phillips for helpful comments and English editing of the manuscript.

Conflicts of Interest: The authors declare no conflicts of interests.

References

1. Munoz-Bonilla, A.; Echeverria, C.; Sonseca, A.; Arrieta, M.P.; Fernandez-Garcia, M. Bio-based polymers with antimicrobial properties towards sustainable development. *Materials* **2019**, *12*, 641. [CrossRef] [PubMed]
2. Amos, R.A.; Mohnen, D. Critical review of plant cell wall matrix polysaccharide glycosyltransferase activities verified by heterologous protein expression. *Front. Plant Sci.* **2019**, *10*, 915. [CrossRef]
3. Lampugnani, E.R.; Flores-Sandoval, E.; Tan, Q.W.; Mutwil, M.; Bowman, J.L.; Persson, S. Cellulose synthesis—central components and their evolutionary relationships. *Trends Plant Sci.* **2019**, *24*, 402–412. [CrossRef] [PubMed]
4. Helle, S.; Bray, F.; Verbeke, J.; Devassine, S.; Courseaux, A.; Facon, M.; Tokarski, C.; Rolando, C.; Szydlowski, N. Proteome analysis of potato starch reveals the presence of new starch metabolic proteins as well as multiple protease inhibitors. *Front. Plant Sci.* **2018**, *9*, 746. [CrossRef] [PubMed]
5. Ball, S.; Colleoni, C.; Cenci, U.; Raj, J.N.; Tirtiaux, C. The evolution of glycogen and starch metabolism in eukaryotes gives molecular clues to understand the establishment of plastid endosymbiosis. *J. Exp. Bot.* **2011**, *62*, 1775–1801. [CrossRef] [PubMed]
6. Edmond Ghanem, M.; Han, R.-M.; Classen, B.; Quetin-Leclerq, J.; Mahy, G.; Ruan, C.-J.; Qin, P.; Pérez-Alfocea, F.; Lutts, S. Mucilage and Polysaccharides in the Halophyte plant species Kosteletzkya virginica: Localization and composition in relation to salt stress. *J. Plant Physiol.* **2010**, *167*, 382–392. [CrossRef]
7. Shukla, P.S.; Mantin, E.G.; Adil, M.; Bajpai, S.; Critchley, A.T.; Prithiviraj, B. *Ascophyllum nodosum*-based biostimulants: sustainable applications in agriculture for the stimulation of plant growth, stress tolerance, and disease management. *Front. Plant Sci.* **2019**, *10*, 655. [CrossRef]
8. Hamed, I.; Özogul, F.; Özogul, Y.; Regenstein, J.M. Marine bioactive compounds and their health benefits: A review. *Compr. Rev. Food Sci. Food Saf.* **2015**, *14*, 446–465. [CrossRef]
9. Lee, Y.-E.; Kim, H.; Seo, C.; Park, T.; Lee, K.B.; Yoo, S.Y.; Hong, S.C.; Kim, J.T.; Lee, J. Marine polysaccharides: therapeutic efficacy and biomedical applications. *Arch. Pharmacal Res.* **2017**, *40*, 1006–1020. [CrossRef]
10. Ruocco, N.; Costantini, S.; Guariniello, S.; Costantini, M. Polysaccharides from the marine environment with pharmacological, cosmeceutical and nutraceutical potential. *Molecules* **2016**, *21*, 551. [CrossRef]
11. Laurienzo, P. Marine Polysaccharides in Pharmaceutical Applications: An Overview. *Mar. Drugs* **2010**, *8*, 2435–2465. [CrossRef] [PubMed]
12. Meenakshi, S.; Umayaparvathi, S.; Saravanan, R.; Manivasagam, T.; Balasubramanian, T. Hepatoprotective effect of fucoidan isolated from the seaweed turbinaria decurrens in ethanol intoxicated rats. *Int. J. Biol. Macromol.* **2014**, *67*, 367–372. [CrossRef] [PubMed]
13. Cunha, L.; Grenha, A. Sulfated seaweed polysaccharides as multifunctional materials in drug delivery applications. *Mar. Drugs* **2016**, *14*, 42. [CrossRef] [PubMed]
14. Hudak, J.E.; Bertozzi, C.R. Glycotherapy: New advances inspire a reemergence of glycans in medicine. *Chem. Biol.* **2014**, *21*, 16–37. [CrossRef] [PubMed]
15. Novotny, M.V.; Alley, W.R., Jr. Recent trends in analytical and structural glycobiology. *Curr. Opin. Chem. Biol.* **2013**, *17*, 832–840. [CrossRef] [PubMed]
16. Caldwell, G.S.; Pagett, H.E. Marine glycobiology: Current status and future perspectives. *Mar. Biotechnol.* **2010**, *12*, 241–252. [CrossRef]

17. Pomin, V.H. Marine medicinal Gglycomics. *Front. Cell. Infect. Microbiol.* **2014**, *4*, 5. [CrossRef]
18. De Jesus Raposo, M.F.; de Morais, A.M.B.; de Morais, R.M.S.C. Marine polysaccharides from algae with potential biomedical applications. *Mar. Drugs* **2015**, *13*, 2967–3028. [CrossRef]
19. Gobet, A.; Barbeyron, T.; Matard-Mann, M.; Magdelenat, G.; Vallenet, D.; Duchaud, E.; Michel, G. Evolutionary evidence of algal polysaccharide degradation acquisition by *Pseudoalteromonas carrageenovora* 9^T to adapt to macroalgal niches. *Front. Microbiol.* **2018**, *9*, 2740. [CrossRef]
20. Maneein, S.; Milledge, J.J.; Nielsen, B.V.; Harvey, P.J. A Review of seaweed pre-treatment methods for enhanced biofuel production by anaerobic digestion or fermentation. *Fermentation* **2018**, *4*, 100. [CrossRef]
21. Afonso, N.C.; Catarino, M.D.; Silva, A.M.S.; Cardoso, S.M. Brown macroalgae as valuable food ingredients. *Antioxidants* **2019**, *8*, 365. [CrossRef]
22. Catarino, M.D.; Silva, A.M.S.; Cardoso, S.M. Phycochemical constituents and biological activities of *Fucus* spp. *Mar. Drugs* **2018**, *16*, 249. [CrossRef]
23. Deniaud-Bouët, E.; Hardouin, K.; Potin, P.; Kloareg, B.; Hervé, C. A review about brown algal cell walls and fucose-containing sulfated polysaccharides: Cell wall context, biomedical properties and key research challenges. *Carbohydr. Polym.* **2017**, *175*, 395–408. [CrossRef] [PubMed]
24. Deniaud-Bouët, E.; Kervarec, N.; Michel, G.; Tonon, T.; Kloareg, B.; Hervé, C. Chemical and enzymatic fractionation of cell walls from Fucales: Insights into the structure of the extracellular matrix of brown algae. *Ann. Bot.* **2014**, *114*, 1203–1216. [CrossRef] [PubMed]
25. Generalić Mekinić, I.; Skroza, D.; Šimat, V.; Hamed, I.; Čagalj, M.; Popović Perković, Z. Phenolic content of brown algae (Pheophyceae) species: Extraction, identification, and quantification. *Biomolecules* **2019**, *9*, 244. [CrossRef] [PubMed]
26. Chang, Y.; Xue, C.; Tang, Q.; Li, D.; Wu, X.; Wang, J. Isolation and characterization of a sea cucumber fucoidan-utilizing marine bacterium. *Lett. Appl. Microbiol.* **2010**, *50*, 301–307. [CrossRef]
27. Zayed, A.; Dienemann, C.; Giese, C.; Krämer, R.; Ulber, R. An immobilized perylene diimide derivative for fucoidan purification from a crude brown algae extract. *Process Biochem.* **2018**, *65*, 233–238. [CrossRef]
28. Citkowska, A.; Szekalska, M.; Winnicka, K. Possibilities of fucoidan utilization in the development of pharmaceutical dosage forms. *Mar. Drugs* **2019**, *17*, 458. [CrossRef]
29. Li, S.; Li, J.; Zhi, Z.; Hu, Y.; Ge, J.; Ye, X.; Tian, D.; Linhardt, R.J.; Chen, S. 4-*O*-sulfation in sea cucumber fucodians contribute to reversing dyslipidiaemia caused by HFD. *Int. J. Biol. Macromol.* **2017**, *99*, 96–104. [CrossRef]
30. Fitton, J.H.; Stringer, D.S.; Park, A.Y.; Karpiniec, S.N. Therapies from fucoidan: new developments. *Mar. Drugs* **2019**, *17*, 571. [CrossRef]
31. Van Weelden, G.; Bobinski, M.; Okla, K.; van Weelden, W.J.; Romano, A.; Pijnenborg, J.M.A. Fucoidan structure and activity in relation to anti-cancer mechanisms. *Mar. Drugs* **2019**, *17*, 32. [CrossRef] [PubMed]
32. Wang, Y.; Xing, M.; Cao, Q.; Ji, A.; Liang, H.; Song, S. Biological activities of fucoidan and the factors mediating its therapeutic effects: A review of recent studies. *Mar. Drugs* **2019**, *17*, 183. [CrossRef] [PubMed]
33. Luthuli, S.; Wu, S.; Cheng, Y.; Zheng, X.; Wu, M.; Tong, H. Therapeutic effects of fucoidan: A review on recent studies. *Mar. Drugs* **2019**, *17*, 487. [CrossRef] [PubMed]
34. Chollet, L.; Saboural, P.; Chauvierre, C.; Villemin, J.N.; Letourneur, D.; Chaubet, F. Fucoidans in nanomedicine. *Mar. Drugs* **2016**, *14*, 145. [CrossRef] [PubMed]
35. Holtkamp, A.D.; Kelly, S.; Ulber, R.; Lang, S. Fucoidans and fucoidanases-focus on techniques for molecular structure elucidation and modification of marine polysaccharides. *Appl. Microbiol. Biotechnol.* **2009**, *82*, 1–11. [CrossRef] [PubMed]
36. Ustyuzhanina, N.E.; Bilan, M.I.; Ushakova, N.A.; Usov, A.I.; Kiselevskiy, M.V.; Nifantiev, N.E. Fucoidans: Pro- or antiangiogenic agents? *Glycobiology* **2014**, *24*, 1265–1274. [CrossRef]
37. Zhao, Y.; Zheng, Y.; Wang, J.; Ma, S.; Yu, Y.; White, W.L.; Yang, S.; Yang, F.; Lu, J. Fucoidan extracted from *Undaria pinnatifida*: Source for nutraceuticals/functional foods. *Mar. Drugs* **2018**, *16*, 321. [CrossRef]
38. Arumugam, P.; Arunkumar, K.; Sivakumar, L.; Murugan, M.; Murugan, K. Anticancer effect of fucoidan on cell proliferation, cell cycle progression, genetic damage and apoptotic cell death in HepG2 cancer cells. *Toxicol. Rep.* **2019**, *6*, 556–563.
39. Atashrazm, F.; Lowenthal, R.M.; Woods, G.M.; Holloway, A.F.; Dickinson, J.L. Fucoidan and cancer: A multifunctional molecule with anti-tumor potential. *Mar. Drugs* **2015**, *13*, 2327–2346. [CrossRef]

40. Chen, L.-M.; Liu, P.-Y.; Chen, Y.-A.; Tseng, H.-Y.; Shen, P.-C.; Hwang, P.-A.; Hsu, H.-L. Oligo-fucoidan prevents IL-6 and CCL2 production and cooperates with p53 to suppress ATM signaling and tumor progression. *Sci. Rep.* **2017**, *7*, 11864. [CrossRef]
41. Zayed, A.; Muffler, K.; Hahn, T.; Rupp, S.; Finkelmeier, D.; Burger-Kentischer, A.; Ulber, R. Physicochemical and biological characterization of fucoidan from *Fucus vesiculosus* purified by dye affinity chromatography. *Mar. Drugs* **2016**, *14*, 79. [CrossRef] [PubMed]
42. Zhao, X.; Dong, S.; Wang, J.; Li, F.; Chen, A.; Li, B. A comparative study of antithrombotic and antiplatelet activities of different fucoidans from *Laminaria japonica*. *Thromb. Res.* **2012**, *129*, 771–778. [CrossRef] [PubMed]
43. Wang, W.; Wu, J.; Zhang, X.; Hao, C.; Zhao, X.; Jiao, G.; Shan, X.; Tai, W.; Yu, G. Inhibition of influenza A virus infection by fucoidan targeting viral neuraminidase and cellular EGFR pathway. *Sci. Rep.* **2017**, *7*, 40760. [CrossRef] [PubMed]
44. Prokofjeva, M.M.; Imbs, T.I.; Shevchenko, N.M.; Spirin, P.V.; Horn, S.; Fehse, B.; Zvyagintseva, T.N.; Prassolov, V.S. Fucoidans as potential inhibitors of HIV-1. *Mar. Drugs* **2013**, *11*, 3000–3014. [CrossRef] [PubMed]
45. Takahashi, H.; Kawaguchi, M.; Kitamura, K.; Narumiya, S.; Kawamura, M.; Tengan, I.; Nishimoto, S.; Hanamure, Y.; Majima, Y.; Tsubura, S.; et al. An exploratory study on the anti-inflammatory effects of fucoidan in relation to quality of life in advanced cancer patients. *Integr. Cancer Ther.* **2018**, *17*, 282–291. [CrossRef]
46. Park, H.Y.; Han, M.H.; Park, C.; Jin, C.-Y.; Kim, G.-Y.; Choi, I.-W.; Kim, N.D.; Nam, T.-J.; Kwon, T.K.; Choi, Y.H. Anti-inflammatory effects of fucoidan through inhibition of NF-κB, MAPK and Akt activation in lipopolysaccharide-induced BV$_2$ microglia cells. *Food Chem. Toxicol.* **2011**, *49*, 1745–1752. [CrossRef]
47. Li, B.; Lu, F.; Wei, X.; Zhao, R. Fucoidan: Structure and bioactivity. *Molecules* **2008**, *13*, 1671–1695. [CrossRef]
48. Lu, J.; Shi, K.K.; Chen, S.; Wang, J.; Hassouna, A.; White, L.N.; Merien, F.; Xie, M.; Kong, Q.; Li, J.; et al. Fucoidan extracted from the New Zealand *Undaria pinnatifida*-Physicochemical comparison against five other fucoidans: Unique low molecular weight fraction bioactivity in breast cancer cell lines. *Mar. Drugs* **2018**, *16*, 461. [CrossRef]
49. Yoo, H.J.; You, D.-J.; Lee, K.-W. Characterization and immunomodulatory effects of high molecular weight fucoidan fraction from the sporophyll of *Undaria pinnatifida* in cyclophosphamide-induced immunosuppressed mice. *Mar. Drugs* **2019**, *17*, 447. [CrossRef]
50. Zayed, A.; Hahn, T.; Finkelmeier, D.; Burger-Kentischer, A.; Rupp, S.; Krämer, R.; Ulber, R. Phenomenological investigation of the cytotoxic activity of fucoidan isolated from *Fucus vesiculosus*. *Process Biochem.* **2019**, *81*, 182–187. [CrossRef]
51. Imbs, T.I.; Skriptsova, A.V.; Zvyagintseva, T.N. Antioxidant activity of fucose-containing sulfated polysaccharides obtained from Fucus evanescens by different extraction methods. *J. Appl. Phycol.* **2015**, *27*, 545–553. [CrossRef]
52. Hifney, A.F.; Fawzy, M.A.; Abdel-Gawad, K.M.; Gomaa, M. Industrial optimization of fucoidan extraction from *Sargassum* sp. and its potential antioxidant and emulsifying activities. *Food Hydrocoll.* **2016**, *54*, 77–88. [CrossRef]
53. Zayed, A.; Ulber, R. Fucoidan Production: Approval Key Challenges and Opportunities. *Carbohydr. Polym.* **2019**, *211*, 289–297. [CrossRef] [PubMed]
54. Fitton, J.H.; Stringer, D.N.; Karpiniec, S.S. Therapies from fucoidan: An update. *Mar. Drugs* **2015**, *13*, 5920–5946. [CrossRef]
55. Mak, W.; Wang, S.K.; Liu, T.; Hamid, N.; Li, Y.; Lu, J.; White, W.L. Anti-proliferation potential and content of fucoidan extracted from sporophyll of New Zealand *Undaria pinnatifida*. *Front. Nutr.* **2014**, *1*, 9. [CrossRef]
56. Chauvierre, C.; Aid-Launais, R.; Aerts, J.; Chaubet, F.; Maire, M.; Chollet, L.; Rolland, L.; Bonafe, R.; Rossi, S.; Bussi, S.; et al. Pharmaceutical development and safety evaluation of a GMP-grade fucoidan for molecular diagnosis of cardiovascular diseases. *Mar. Drugs* **2019**, *17*, 699. [CrossRef]
57. Torres, M.D.; Flórez-Fernández, N.; Simón-Vázquez, R.; Giménez-Abián, J.F.; Díaz, J.F.; González-Fernández, Á.; Domínguez, H. Fucoidans: The importance of processing on their anti-tumoral properties. *Algal Res.* **2020**, *45*, 101748. [CrossRef]

58. Borazjani, N.J.; Tabarsa, M.; You, S.; Rezaei, M. Improved immunomodulatory and antioxidant properties of unrefined fucoidans from *Sargassum angustifolium* by hydrolysis. *J. Food Sci. Technol.* **2017**, *54*, 4016–4025. [CrossRef]
59. Koyanagi, S.; Tanigawa, N.; Nakagawa, H.; Soeda, S.; Shimeno, H. Oversulfation of fucoidan enhances its anti-angiogenic and antitumor activities. *Biochem. Pharmacol.* **2003**, *65*, 173–179. [CrossRef]
60. Ale, M.T.; Mikkelsen, J.D.; Meyer, A.S. Important determinants for fucoidan bioactivity: A critical review of structure-function relations and extraction methods for fucose-containing sulfated polysaccharides from brown seaweeds. *Mar. Drugs* **2011**, *9*, 2106–2130. [CrossRef]
61. Silchenko, A.S.; Rasin, A.B.; Kusaykin, M.I.; Malyarenko, O.S.; Shevchenko, N.M.; Zueva, A.O.; Kalinovsky, A.I.; Zvyagintseva, T.N.; Ermakova, S.P. Modification of native fucoidan from fucus evanescens by recombinant fucoidanase from marine bacteria *Formosa algae*. *Carbohydr. Polym.* **2018**, *193*, 189–195. [CrossRef] [PubMed]
62. Jiao, G.; Yu, G.; Zhang, J.; Ewart, H.S. Chemical structures and bioactivities of sulfated polysaccharides from marine algae. *Mar. Drugs* **2011**, *9*, 196–223. [CrossRef] [PubMed]
63. Suprunchuk, V.E. Low-molecular-weight fucoidan: Chemical modification, synthesis of its oligomeric fragments and mimetics. *Carbohydr. Res.* **2019**, *485*, 107806. [CrossRef] [PubMed]
64. Kardeby, C.; Fälker, K.; Haining, E.J.; Criel, M.; Lindkvist, M.; Barroso, R.; Påhlsson, P.; Ljungberg, L.U.; Tengdelius, M.; Rainger, G.E.; et al. Synthetic glycopolymers and natural fucoidans cause human platelet aggregation via PEAR1 and GPIbα. *Blood Adv.* **2019**, *3*, 275–287. [CrossRef]
65. Kasai, A.; Arafuka, S.; Koshiba, N.; Takahashi, D.; Toshima, K. Systematic synthesis of low-molecular weight fucoidan derivatives and their effect on cancer cells. *Org. Biomol. Chem.* **2015**, *13*, 10556–10568. [CrossRef]
66. Rhein-Knudsen, N.; Ale, M.T.; Meyer, A.S. Seaweed hydrocolloid production: An update on enzyme assisted extraction and modification technologies. *Mar. Drugs* **2015**, *13*, 3340–3359. [CrossRef]
67. Buschmann, A.H.; Camus, C.; Infante, J.; Neori, A.; Israel, Á.; Hernández-González, M.C.; Pereda, S.V.; Gomez-Pinchetti, J.L.; Golberg, A.; Tadmor-Shalev, N.; et al. Seaweed production: Overview of the global state of exploitation, farming and emerging research activity. *Eur. J. Phycol.* **2017**, *52*, 391–406. [CrossRef]
68. Duarte, C.M.; Wu, J.; Xiao, X.; Bruhn, A.; Krause-Jensen, D. Can seaweed farming play a role in climate change mitigation and adaptation? *Front. Mar. Sci.* **2017**, *4*, 100.
69. Zayed, A.; Kovacheva, M.; Muffler, K.; Breiner, H.-W.; Stoeck, T.; Ulber, R. Induction and genetic identification of a callus-like growth developed in the brown alga *Fucus vesiculosus*. *Eng. Life Sci.* **2019**, *19*, 363–369. [CrossRef]
70. Cho, G.Y.; Rousseau, F.; de Reviers, B.; Boo, S.M. Phylogenetic relationships within the fucales (Phaeophyceae) assessed by the photosystem I coding psaa sequences. *Phycologia* **2006**, *45*, 512–519. [CrossRef]
71. Wahl, M.; Molis, M.; Hobday, A.J.; Dudgeon, S.; Neumann, R.; Steinberg, P.; Campbell, A.H.; Marzinelli, E.; Connell, S. The responses of brown macroalgae to environmental change from local to global scales: Direct versus ecologically mediated effects. *Perspect. Phycol.* **2015**, *2*, 11–29. [CrossRef]
72. Crous, P.W.; Wingfield, M.J.; Burgess, T.I.; Hardy, G.S.J.; Gené, J.; Guarro, J.; Baseia, I.G.; García, D.; Gusmão, L.F.P.; Souza-Motta, C.M.; et al. Fungal planet description sheets: 716–784. *Persoonia* **2018**, *40*, 240–393. [CrossRef] [PubMed]
73. Kumar, G.R.; Reddy, C.R.K.; Jha, B. Callus induction and thallus regeneration from callus of phycocolloid yielding seaweeds from the Indian coast. *J. Appl. Phycol.* **2007**, *19*, 15–25. [CrossRef]
74. Muhamad, S.N.S.; Ling, A.P.-K.; Wong, C.-L. Effect of plant growth regulators on direct regeneration and callus induction from *Sargassum polycystum* C. Agardh. *J. Appl. Phycol.* **2018**, *30*, 3299–3310. [CrossRef]
75. Avila-Peltroche, J.; Won, B.Y.; Cho, T.O. Protoplast isolation and regeneration from *Hecatonema terminale* (Ectocarpales, Phaeophyceae) using a simple mixture of commercial enzymes. *J. Appl. Phycol.* **2019**, *31*, 1873–1881. [CrossRef]
76. Luiten, E.E.; Akkerman, I.; Koulman, A.; Kamermans, P.; Reith, H.; Barbosa, M.J.; Sipkema, D.; Wijffels, R.H. Realizing the promises of marine biotechnology. *Biomol. Eng.* **2003**, *20*, 429–439. [CrossRef]
77. Baweja, P.; Sahoo, D.; García-Jiménez, P.; Robaina, R.R. Review: Seaweed tissue culture as applied to biotechnology: Problems, achievements and prospects. *Phycol. Res.* **2009**, *57*, 45–58. [CrossRef]
78. Huang, Y.M.; Rorrer, G.L. Cultivation of microplantlets derived from the marine red alga Agardhiella subulata in a stirred tank photobioreactor. *Biotechnol. Prog.* **2003**, *19*, 418–427. [CrossRef]

79. Hahn, T.; Lang, S.; Ulber, R.; Muffler, K. Novel procedures for the extraction of fucoidan from brown algae. *Process Biochem.* **2012**, *47*, 1691–1698. [CrossRef]
80. Thinh, P.D.; Menshova, R.V.; Ermakova, S.P.; Anastyuk, S.D.; Ly, B.M.; Zvyagintseva, T.N. Structural characteristics and anticancer activity of fucoidan from the brown alga *Sargassum mcclurei*. *Mar. Drugs* **2013**, *11*, 1456–1476. [CrossRef]
81. De Reviers, B. Fucans and alginates without phenolic compounds. *J. Appl. Phycol.* **1989**, *1*, 75–76. [CrossRef]
82. Yang, W.N.; Chen, P.W.; Huang, C.Y. Compositional characteristics and in vitro evaluations of antioxidant and neuroprotective properties of crude extracts of fucoidan prepared from compressional puffing-pretreated *Sargassum crassifolium*. *Mar. Drugs* **2017**, *15*, 183. [CrossRef] [PubMed]
83. Zhang, R.; Zhang, X.; Tang, Y.; Mao, J. Composition, isolation, purification and biological activities of *Sargassum fusiforme* polysaccharides: A review. *Carbohydr. Polym.* **2020**, *228*, 115381. [CrossRef] [PubMed]
84. Spicer, S.E.; Adams, J.M.M.; Thomas, D.S.; Gallagher, J.A.; Winters, A.L. Novel rapid method for the characterisation of polymeric sugars from macroalgae. *J. Appl. Phycol.* **2017**, *29*, 1507–1513. [CrossRef]
85. Zou, P.; Lu, X.; Zhao, H.; Yuan, Y.; Meng, L.; Zhang, C.; Li, Y. Polysaccharides derived from the brown algae *Lessonia nigrescens* enhance salt stress tolerance to wheat seedlings by enhancing the antioxidant system and modulating intracellular ion concentration. *Front. Plant Sci.* **2019**, *10*, 48. [CrossRef]
86. Peng, J.; Yuan, J.-P.; Wu, C.-F.; Wang, J.-H. Fucoxanthin, a marine carotenoid present in brown seaweeds and diatoms: Metabolism and bioactivities relevant to human health. *Mar. Drugs* **2011**, *9*, 1806–1828. [CrossRef]
87. Da Costa, E.; Domingues, P.; Melo, T.; Coelho, E.; Pereira, R.; Calado, R.; Abreu, M.H.; Domingues, M.R. Lipidomic signatures reveal seasonal shifts on the relative abundance of high-valued lipids from the brown algae *Fucus vesiculosus*. *Mar. Drugs* **2019**, *17*, 335. [CrossRef]
88. Terasaki, M.; Hirose, A.; Narayan, B.; Baba, Y.; Kawagoe, C.; Yasui, H.; Saga, N.; Hosokawa, M.; Miyashita, K. Evaluation of recoverable functional lipid components of several brown seaweeds (Phaeophyta) from Japan with special reference to fucoxanthin and fucosterol contents. *J. Phycol.* **2009**, *45*, 974–980. [CrossRef]
89. Zhu, F. Interactions between cell wall polysaccharides and polyphenols. *Crit. Rev. Food Sci. Nutr.* **2018**, *58*, 1808–1831. [CrossRef]
90. Li, Y.; Fu, X.; Duan, D.; Liu, X.; Xu, J.; Gao, X. Extraction and Identification of Phlorotannins from the Brown Alga, Sargassum fusiforme (Harvey) Setchell. *Mar. Drugs* **2017**, *15*, 49. [CrossRef]
91. Bertoni, G. A key step in phlorotannin biosynthesis revealed. *Plant Cell* **2013**, *25*, 2770. [CrossRef] [PubMed]
92. Catarino, M.D.; Silva, A.M.S.; Cardoso, S.M. Fucaceae: A source of bioactive phlorotannins. *Int. J. Mol. Sci.* **2017**, *18*, 1327. [CrossRef] [PubMed]
93. Thomas, N.V.; Kim, S.K. Potential pharmacological applications of polyphenolic derivatives from marine brown algae. *Environ. Toxicol. Pharmacol.* **2011**, *32*, 325–335. [CrossRef] [PubMed]
94. Agregán, R.; Munekata, P.E.S.; Franco, D.; Carballo, J.; Barba, F.J.; Lorenzo, J.M. Antioxidant potential of extracts obtained from macro- (*Ascophyllum nodosum*, *Fucus vesiculosus* and *Bifurcaria bifurcata*) and micro-Algae (*Chlorella vulgaris* and *Spirulina platensis*) assisted by ultrasound. *Medicines* **2018**, *5*, 33.
95. Zhang, M.Y.; Guo, J.; Hu, X.M.; Zhao, S.Q.; Li, S.L.; Wang, J. An in vivo anti-tumor effect of eckol from marine brown algae by improving the immune response. *Food Funct.* **2019**, *10*, 4361–4371. [CrossRef]
96. Gall, E.A.; Lelchat, F.; Hupel, M.; Jégou, C.; Stiger-Pouvreau, V. Extraction and purification of phlorotannins from brown algae. In *Natural Products from Marine Algae: Methods and Protocols*; Stengel, D.B., Connan, S., Eds.; Springer: New York, NY, USA, 2015; pp. 131–143.
97. Brzonova, I.; Kozliak, E.I.; Andrianova, A.A.; LaVallie, A.; Kubátová, A.; Ji, Y. Production of lignin based insoluble polymers (anionic hydrogels) by *C. versicolor*. *Sci. Rep.* **2017**, *7*, 17507. [CrossRef]
98. Hahn, T.; Zayed, A.; Kovacheva, M.; Stadtmüller, R.; Lang, S.; Muffler, K.; Ulber, R. Dye affinity chromatography for fast and simple purification of fucoidan from marine brown algae. *Eng. Life Sci.* **2016**, *16*, 78–87. [CrossRef]
99. Chades, T.; Scully, S.M.; Ingvadottir, E.M.; Orlygsson, J. Fermentation of mannitol extracts from brown macro algae by *Thermophilic clostridia*. *Front. Microbiol.* **2018**, *9*, 1931. [CrossRef]
100. Balboa, E.M.; Rivas, S.; Moure, A.; Dominguez, H.; Parajo, J.C. Simultaneous extraction and depolymerization of fucoidan from *Sargassum muticum* in aqueous media. *Mar. Drugs* **2013**, *11*, 4612–4627. [CrossRef]
101. Descamps, V.; Colin, S.; Lahaye, M.; Jam, M.; Richard, C.; Potin, P.; Barbeyron, T.; Yvin, J.-C.; Kloareg, B. Isolation and culture of a marine bacterium degrading the sulfated fucans from marine brown algae. *Mar. Biotechnol.* **2006**, *8*, 27–39. [CrossRef]

102. Abdella, A.A.; Ulber, R.; Zayed, A. Chitosan-toluidine blue beads for purification of fucoidans. *Carbohydr. Polym.* **2020**, *231*, 115686. [CrossRef] [PubMed]
103. Kadam, S.U.; Tiwari, B.K.; O'Donnell, C.P. Application of novel extraction technologies for bioactives from marine algae. *J. Agric. Food Chem.* **2013**, *61*, 4667–4675. [CrossRef]
104. Pozharitskaya, O.N.; Shikov, A.N.; Faustova, N.M.; Obluchinskaya, E.D.; Kosman, V.M.; Vuorela, H.; Makarov, V.G. Pharmacokinetic and tissue distribution of fucoidan from *Fucus vesiculosus* after oral administration to rats. *Mar. Drugs* **2018**, *16*, 132. [CrossRef] [PubMed]
105. Hadj Ammar, H.; Lajili, S.; Ben Said, R.; Le Cerf, D.; Bouraoui, A.; Majdoub, H. Physico-chemical characterization and pharmacological evaluation of sulfated polysaccharides from three species of Mediterranean brown algae of the genus Cystoseira. *DARU J. Pharm. Sci.* **2015**, *23*, 1. [CrossRef] [PubMed]
106. Zhang, Y.; Xu, M.; Hu, C.; Liu, A.; Chen, J.; Gu, C.; Zhang, X.; You, C.; Tong, H.; Wu, M.; et al. *Sargassum fusiforme* fucoidan SP2 extends the lifespan of *Drosophila melanogaster* by upregulating the Nrf2-mediated antioxidant signaling pathway. *Oxidative Med. Cell. Longev.* **2019**, *2019*, 8918914. [CrossRef]
107. Saepudin, E.; Sinurat, E.; Suryabrata, I.A. Depigmentation and characterization of fucoidan from brown seaweed *Sargassum binderi* Sonder. *IOP Conference Series: Mater. Sci. Eng.* **2018**, *299*, 012027. [CrossRef]
108. Patel, A.; Mikes, F.; Matsakas, L. An overview of current pretreatment methods used to improve lipid extraction from Oleaginous micro-organisms. *Molecules* **2018**, *23*, 1562. [CrossRef]
109. Huang, C.-Y.; Kuo, C.-H.; Chen, P.-W. Compressional-puffing pretreatment enhances neuroprotective effects of fucoidans from the brown seaweed *Sargassum hemiphyllum* on 6-hydroxydopamine-induced apoptosis in SH-SY5Y cells. *Molecules* **2017**, *23*, 78. [CrossRef]
110. Huang, C.-Y.; Wu, S.-J.; Yang, W.-N.; Kuan, A.-W.; Chen, C.-Y. Antioxidant activities of crude extracts of fucoidan extracted from *Sargassum glaucescens* by a compressional-puffing-hydrothermal extraction process. *Food Chem.* **2016**, *197*, 1121–1129. [CrossRef]
111. Kordjazi, M.; Shabanpour, B.; Zabihi, E.; Faramarzi, M.A.; Feizi, F.; Ahmadi Gavlighi, H.; Feghhi, M.A.; Hosseini, S.A. Sulfated polysaccharides purified from two species of Padina improve collagen and epidermis formation in the rat. *Int. J. Mol. Cell. Med.* **2013**, *2*, 156–163.
112. Cho, M.L.; Lee, B.-Y.; You, S.G. Relationship between oversulfation and conformation of low and high molecular weight fucoidans and evaluation of their in vitro anticancer activity. *Molecules* **2010**, *16*, 291–297. [CrossRef] [PubMed]
113. Oliveira, R.M.; Câmara, R.B.G.; Monte, J.F.S.; Viana, R.L.S.; Melo, K.R.T.; Queiroz, M.F.; Filgueira, L.G.A.; Oyama, L.M.; Rocha, H.A.O. Commercial fucoidans from *Fucus vesiculosus* can be grouped into antiadipogenic and adipogenic agents. *Mar. Drugs* **2018**, *16*, 193. [CrossRef] [PubMed]
114. Kusaykin, M.I.; Silchenko, A.S.; Zakharenko, A.M.; Zvyagintseva, T.N. Fucoidanases. *Glycobiology* **2015**, *26*, 3–12. [CrossRef] [PubMed]
115. Ale, M.T.; Meyer, A.S. Fucoidans from brown seaweeds: An update on structures, extraction techniques and use of enzymes as tools for structural elucidation. *RSC Adv.* **2013**, *3*, 8131–8141. [CrossRef]
116. Huang, C.-Y.; Kuo, C.-H.; Lee, C.-H. Antibacterial and antioxidant capacities and attenuation of lipid accumulation in 3T3-L1 adipocytes by low-molecular-weight fucoidans prepared from compressional-puffing-pretreated *Sargassum crassifolium*. *Mar. Drugs* **2018**, *16*, 24. [CrossRef] [PubMed]
117. Imbs, T.I.; Shevchenko, N.M.; Sukhoverkhov, S.V.; Semenova, T.L.; Skriptsova, A.V.; Zvyagintseva, T.N. Seasonal variations of the composition and structural characteristics of polysaccharides from the brown alga *Costaria costata*. *Chem. Nat. Compd.* **2009**, *45*, 786–791. [CrossRef]
118. Fidelis, G.P.; Silva, C.H.F.; Nobre, L.; Medeiros, V.P.; Rocha, H.A.O.; Costa, L.S. Antioxidant fucoidans obtained from tropical seaweed protect pre-osteoblastic cells from hydrogen peroxide-induced damage. *Mar. Drugs* **2019**, *17*, 506. [CrossRef]
119. Rohwer, K.; Neupane, S.; Bittkau, K.S.; Galarza Perez, M.; Dorschmann, P.; Roider, J.; Alban, S.; Klettner, A. Effects of Crude Fucus distichus Subspecies evanescens Fucoidan Extract on Retinal Pigment Epithelium Cells-Implications for Use in Age-Related Macular Degeneration. *Mar. Drugs* **2019**, *17*, 538. [CrossRef]
120. Rodriguez-Jasso, R.M.; Mussatto, S.I.; Pastrana, L.; Aguilar, C.N.; Teixeira, J.A. Microwave-assisted extraction of sulfated polysaccharides (fucoidan) from brown seaweed. *Carbohydr. Polym.* **2011**, *86*, 1137–1144. [CrossRef]

121. Mussatto, S.I. Microwave-assisted extraction of fucoidan from marine algae. In *Natural Products from Marine Algae: Methods and Protocols*; Stengel, D.B., Connan, S., Eds.; Springer: New York, NY, USA, 2015; pp. 151–157.
122. Alboofetileh, M.; Rezaei, M.; Tabarsa, M.; You, S. Ultrasound-assisted extraction of sulfated polysaccharide from *Nizamuddinia zanardinii*: Process optimization, structural characterization, and biological properties. *J. Food Process Eng.* **2019**, *42*, e12979. [CrossRef]
123. Garcia-Vaquero, M.; O'Doherty, J.V.; Tiwari, B.K.; Sweeney, T.; Rajauria, G. Enhancing the extraction of polysaccharides and antioxidants from macroalgae using sequential hydrothermal-assisted extraction followed by ultrasound and thermal technologies. *Mar. Drugs* **2019**, *17*, 457. [CrossRef] [PubMed]
124. Alboofetileh, M.; Rezaei, M.; Tabarsa, M.; You, S.; Mariatti, F.; Cravotto, G. Subcritical water extraction as an efficient technique to isolate biologically-active fucoidans from *Nizamuddinia zanardinii*. *Int. J. Biol. Macromol.* **2019**, *128*, 244–253. [CrossRef] [PubMed]
125. Qin, Y.; Yuan, Q.; Zhang, Y.; Li, J.; Zhu, X.; Zhao, L.; Wen, J.; Liu, J.; Zhao, L.; Zhao, J. Enzyme-assisted extraction optimization, characterization and antioxidant activity of polysaccharides from sea cucumber *Phyllophorus proteus*. *Molecules* **2018**, *23*, 590. [CrossRef]
126. Wijesinghe, W.A.; Jeon, Y.J. Enzyme-assistant extraction (EAE) of bioactive components: A useful approach for recovery of industrially important metabolites from seaweeds: A review. *Fitoterapia* **2012**, *83*, 6–12. [CrossRef]
127. Ahn, G.; Lee, W.; Kim, K.-N.; Lee, J.-H.; Heo, S.-J.; Kang, N.; Lee, S.-H.; Ahn, C.-B.; Jeon, Y.-J. A sulfated polysaccharide of *Ecklonia cava* inhibits the growth of colon cancer cells by inducing apoptosis. *EXCLI J.* **2015**, *14*, 294–306.
128. Badrinathan, S.; Shiju, T.M.; Sharon Christa, A.S.; Arya, R.; Pragasam, V. Purification and structural characterization of sulfated polysaccharide from *Sargassum myriocystum* and its efficacy in scavenging free radicals. *Indian J. Pharm. Sci.* **2012**, *74*, 549–555. [PubMed]
129. Liu, Y.; Huang, G. Extraction and derivatisation of active polysaccharides. *J. Enzym. Inhib. Med. Chem.* **2019**, *34*, 1690–1696. [CrossRef]
130. Zhao, D.; Xu, J.; Xu, X. Bioactivity of fucoidan extracted from *Laminaria japonica* using a novel procedure with high yield. *Food Chem.* **2018**, *245*, 911–918. [CrossRef]
131. Xing, R.; Liu, S.; Yu, H.; Chen, X.; Qin, Y.; Li, K.; Li, P. Extraction and separation of fucoidan from *Laminaria japonica* with chitosan as extractant. *BioMed Res. Int.* **2013**, *2013*, 193689. [CrossRef]
132. Ertani, A.; Francioso, O.; Tinti, A.; Schiavon, M.; Pizzeghello, D.; Nardi, S. Evaluation of seaweed extracts from *Laminaria* and *Ascophyllum nodosum* spp. as biostimulants in *Zea mays* L. using a combination of chemical, biochemical and morphological approaches. *Front. Plant Sci.* **2018**, *9*, 428. [CrossRef]
133. Lee, J.M.; Oh, S.Y.; Johnston, T.V.; Ku, S.; Ji, G.E. Biocatalysis of fucodian in *Undaria pinnatifida* sporophyll using *Bifidobacterium longum* RD47 for production of prebiotic fucosylated oligosaccharide. *Mar. Drugs* **2019**, *17*, 117. [CrossRef] [PubMed]
134. Somasundaram, S.N.; Shanmugam, S.; Subramanian, B.; Jaganathan, R. Cytotoxic effect of fucoidan extracted from *Sargassum cinereum* on colon cancer cell line HCT-15. *Int. J. Biol. Macromol.* **2016**, *91*. [CrossRef] [PubMed]
135. Ustyuzhanina, N.E.; Ushakova, N.A.; Zyuzina, K.A.; Bilan, M.I.; Elizarova, A.L.; Somonova, O.V.; Madzhuga, A.V.; Krylov, V.B.; Preobrazhenskaya, M.E.; Usov, A.I.; et al. Influence of fucoidans on hemostatic system. *Mar. Drugs* **2013**, *11*, 2444–2458. [CrossRef] [PubMed]
136. Saboural, P.; Chaubet, F.; Rouzet, F.; Al-Shoukr, F.; Azzouna, R.B.; Bouchemal, N.; Picton, L.; Louedec, L.; Maire, M.; Rolland, L.; et al. Purification of a low molecular weight fucoidan for SPECT molecular imaging of myocardial infarction. *Mar. Drugs* **2014**, *12*, 4851–4867. [CrossRef] [PubMed]
137. Garcia-Vaquero, M.; Rajauria, G.; O'Doherty, J.V.; Sweeney, T. Polysaccharides from macroalgae: Recent advances, innovative technologies and challenges in extraction and purification. *Food Res. Int.* **2017**, *99*, 1011–1020. [CrossRef]
138. Hahn, T.; Schulz, M.; Stadtmüller, R.; Zayed, A.; Muffler, K.; Lang, S.; Ulber, R. Cationic dye for the specific determination of sulfated polysaccharides. *Anal. Lett.* **2016**, *49*, 1948–1962. [CrossRef]
139. Lee, J.M.; Shin, Z.U.; Mavlonov, G.T.; Abdurakhmonov, I.Y.; Yi, T.-H. Solid-phase colorimetric method for the quantification of fucoidan. *Appl. Biochem. Biotechnol.* **2012**, *168*, 1019–1024. [CrossRef] [PubMed]

140. Palanisamy, S.; Vinosha, M.; Manikandakrishnan, M.; Anjali, R.; Rajasekar, P.; Marudhupandi, T.; Manikandan, R.; Vaseeharan, B.; Prabhu, N.M. Investigation of antioxidant and anticancer potential of fucoidan from Sargassum polycystum. *Int. J. Biol. Macromol.* **2018**, *116*, 151–161. [CrossRef]
141. Cong, Q.; Chen, H.; Liao, W.; Xiao, F.; Wang, P.; Qin, Y.; Dong, Q.; Ding, K. Structural characterization and effect on anti-angiogenic activity of a fucoidan from Sargassum fusiforme. *Carbohydr. Polym.* **2016**, *136*, 899–907. [CrossRef]
142. Li, G.; Row, K.H. Magnetic molecularly imprinted polymers for recognition and enrichment of polysaccharides from seaweed. *J. Sep. Sci.* **2017**, *40*, 4765–4772. [CrossRef]
143. Guthrie, L.; Wolfson, S.; Kelly, L. The human gut chemical landscape predicts microbe-mediated biotransformation of foods and drugs. *eLife* **2019**, *8*, e42866. [CrossRef] [PubMed]
144. Wang, J.; Zhang, Q.; Zhang, Z.; Song, H.; Li, P. Potential antioxidant and anticoagulant capacity of low molecular weight fucoidan fractions extracted from *Laminaria japonica*. *Int. J. Biol. Macromol.* **2010**, *46*, 6–12. [CrossRef] [PubMed]
145. Lee, J.B.; Hayashi, K.; Hashimoto, M.; Nakano, T.; Hayashi, T. Novel antiviral fucoidan from sporophyll of *Undaria pinnatifida* (Mekabu). *Chem. Pharm. Bull.* **2004**, *52*, 1091–1094. [CrossRef] [PubMed]
146. Elizondo-Gonzalez, R.; Cruz-Suarez, L.E.; Ricque-Marie, D.; Mendoza-Gamboa, E.; Rodriguez-Padilla, C.; Trejo-Avila, L.M. In vitro characterization of the antiviral activity of fucoidan from *Cladosiphon okamuranus* against Newcastle disease virus. *Virol. J.* **2012**, *9*, 307. [CrossRef]
147. Jeong, J.-W.; Hwang, S.J.; Han, M.H.; Lee, D.-S.; Yoo, J.S.; Choi, I.-W.; Cha, H.-J.; Kim, S.; Kim, H.-S.; Kim, G.-Y.; et al. Fucoidan inhibits lipopolysaccharide-induced inflammatory responses in RAW 264.7 macrophages and zebrafish larvae. *Mol. Cell. Toxicol.* **2017**, *13*, 405–417. [CrossRef]
148. Klettner, A. Fucoidan as a potential therapeutic for major blinding diseases - a hypothesis. *Mar. Drugs* **2016**, *14*, 31. [CrossRef]
149. Barbosa, A.I.; Coutinho, A.J.; Costa Lima, S.A.; Reis, S. Marine polysaccharides in pharmaceutical applications: Fucoidan and chitosan as key players in the drug delivery match field. *Mar. Drugs* **2019**, *17*, 654. [CrossRef]
150. Wang, P.; Kankala, R.K.; Fan, J.; Long, R.; Liu, Y.; Wang, S. Poly-L-ornithine/fucoidan-coated calcium carbonate microparticles by layer-by-layer self-assembly technique for cancer theranostics. *J. Mater. Sci. Mater. Med.* **2018**, *29*, 68. [CrossRef]
151. Wang, X.; Shan, X.; Dun, Y.; Cai, C.; Hao, J.; Li, G.; Cui, K.; Yu, G. Anti-metabolic syndrome effects of fucoidan from *Fucus vesiculosus* via reactive oxygen species-mediated regulation of JNK, Akt, and AMPK signaling. *Molecules* **2019**, *24*, 3319. [CrossRef]
152. Sharma, G.; Kar, S.; Basu Ball, W.; Ghosh, K.; Das, P.K. The curative effect of fucoidan on visceral leishmaniasis is mediated by activation of MAP kinases through specific protein kinase C isoforms. *Cell. Mol. Immunol.* **2014**, *11*, 263–274. [CrossRef]
153. Varikuti, S.; Jha, B.K.; Volpedo, G.; Ryan, N.M.; Halsey, G.; Hamza, O.M.; McGwire, B.S.; Satoskar, A.R. Host-directed drug therapies for neglected tropical diseases caused by protozoan parasites. *Front. Microbiol.* **2018**, *9*, 2655. [CrossRef] [PubMed]
154. Jin, J.O.; Zhang, W.; Du, J.Y.; Wong, K.W.; Oda, T.; Yu, Q. Fucoidan can function as an adjuvant in vivo to enhance dendritic cell maturation and function and promote antigen-specific T cell immune responses. *PLoS ONE* **2014**, *9*, e99396. [CrossRef] [PubMed]
155. Tabarsa, M.; Dabaghian, E.H.; You, S.; Yelithao, K.; Cao, R.; Rezaei, M.; Alboofetileh, M.; Bita, S. The activation of NF-κB and MAPKs signaling pathways of RAW264.7 murine macrophages and natural killer cells by fucoidan from Nizamuddinia zanardinii. *Int. J. Biol. Macromol.* **2020**, *148*, 56–67. [CrossRef] [PubMed]
156. Wang, P.; Liu, Z.; Liu, X.; Teng, H.; Zhang, C.; Hou, L.; Zou, X. Anti-metastasis effect of fucoidan from Undaria pinnatifida sporophylls in mouse hepatocarcinoma Hca-F cells. *PLoS ONE* **2014**, *9*, e106071. [CrossRef] [PubMed]
157. Li, Y.; Zhao, W.; Wang, L.; Chen, Y.; Zhang, H.; Wang, T.; Yang, X.; Xing, F.; Yan, J.; Fang, X. Protective effects of fucoidan against hydrogen peroxide-induced oxidative damage in porcine intestinal epithelial cells. *Animals* **2019**, *9*, 1108. [CrossRef]
158. Chen, J.H.; Lim, J.D.; Sohn, E.H.; Choi, Y.S.; Han, E.T. Growth-inhibitory effect of a fucoidan from brown seaweed Undaria pinnatifida on Plasmodium parasites. *Parasitol. Res.* **2009**, *104*, 245–250. [CrossRef]
159. Jia, Y.; Sun, Y.; Weng, L.; Li, Y.; Zhang, Q.; Zhou, H.; Yang, B. Low molecular weight fucoidan protects renal tubular cells from injury induced by albumin overload. *Sci. Rep.* **2016**, *6*, 31759. [CrossRef]

160. Chen, C.-H.; Sue, Y.-M.; Cheng, C.-Y.; Chen, Y.-C.; Liu, C.-T.; Hsu, Y.-H.; Hwang, P.-A.; Huang, N.-J.; Chen, T.-H. Oligo-fucoidan prevents renal tubulointerstitial fibrosis by inhibiting the CD44 signal pathway. *Sci. Rep.* **2017**, *7*, 40183. [CrossRef]
161. Abdel-Daim, M.M.; Abushouk, A.I.; Bahbah, E.I.; Bungău, S.G.; Alyousif, M.S.; Aleya, L.; Alkahtani, S. Fucoidan protects against subacute diazinon-induced oxidative damage in cardiac, hepatic, and renal tissues. *Environ. Sci. Pollut. Res.* **2020**. Online ahead of print. [CrossRef]
162. Chen, M.-C.; Hsu, W.-L.; Hwang, P.-A.; Chou, T.-C. Low molecular weight fucoidan inhibits tumor angiogenesis through downregulation of HIF-1/VEGF signaling under hypoxia. *Mar. Drugs* **2015**, *13*, 4436–4451. [CrossRef]
163. Marinval, N.; Saboural, P.; Haddad, O.; Maire, M.; Bassand, K.; Geinguenaud, F.; Djaker, N.; Ben Akrout, K.; Lamy de la Chapelle, M.; Robert, R.; et al. Identification of a pro-angiogenic potential and cellular uptake mechanism of a LMW highly sulfated fraction of fucoidan from *Ascophyllum nodosum*. *Mar. Drugs* **2016**, *14*, 185. [CrossRef] [PubMed]
164. Cheng, Y.; Sibusiso, L.; Hou, L.; Jiang, H.; Chen, P.; Zhang, X.; Wu, M.; Tong, H. *Sargassum fusiforme* fucoidan modifies the gut microbiota during alleviation of streptozotocin-induced hyperglycemia in mice. *Int. J. Biol. Macromol.* **2019**, *131*, 1162–1170. [CrossRef] [PubMed]
165. Li, B.; Juenet, M.; Aid-Launais, R.; Maire, M.; Ollivier, V.; Letourneur, D.; Chauvierre, C. Development of polymer microcapsules functionalized with fucoidan to target p-selectin overexpressed in cardiovascular diseases. *Adv. Healthc. Mater.* **2017**, *6*, 1601200. [CrossRef] [PubMed]
166. Kim, Y.-I.; Oh, W.-S.; Song, P.H.; Yun, S.; Kwon, Y.-S.; Lee, Y.J.; Ku, S.-K.; Song, C.-H.; Oh, T.-H. Anti-photoaging effects of low molecular-weight fucoidan on ultraviolet B-irradiated mice. *Mar. Drugs* **2018**, *16*, 286. [CrossRef] [PubMed]
167. Kim, J.H.; Lee, J.-E.; Kim, K.H.; Kang, N.J. Beneficial effects of marine algae-derived carbohydrates for skin health. *Mar. Drugs* **2018**, *16*, 459. [CrossRef]
168. Fitton, J.H.; Dell'Acqua, G.; Gardiner, V.-A.; Karpiniec, S.S.; Stringer, D.N.; Davis, E. Topical benefits of two fucoidan-rich extracts from marine macroalgae. *Cosmetics* **2015**, *2*, 66–81. [CrossRef]
169. Song, Y.S.; Li, H.; Balcos, M.C.; Yun, H.-Y.; Baek, K.J.; Kwon, N.S.; Choi, H.-R.; Park, K.-C.; Kim, D.-S. Fucoidan promotes the reconstruction of skin equivalents. *Korean J. Physiol. Pharmacol.* **2014**, *18*, 327–331. [CrossRef]
170. Venkatesan, J.; Anil, S.; Kim, S.-K.; Shim, M.S. Seaweed polysaccharide-based nanoparticles: Preparation and applications for drug delivery. *Polymers* **2016**, *8*, 30. [CrossRef]
171. Pinheiro, A.C.; Bourbon, A.I.; Cerqueira, M.A.; Maricato, É.; Nunes, C.; Coimbra, M.A.; Vicente, A.A. Chitosan/fucoidan multilayer nanocapsules as a vehicle for controlled release of bioactive compounds. *Carbohydr. Polym.* **2015**, *115*, 1–9. [CrossRef]
172. Choi, D.G.; Venkatesan, J.; Shim, M.S. Selective anticancer therapy using pro-oxidant drug-loaded chitosan-fucoidan nanoparticles. *Int. J. Mol. Sci.* **2019**, *20*, 3220. [CrossRef]
173. Tsai, M.-h.; Chuang, C.-c.; Chen, C.-c.; Yen, H.-j.; Cheng, K.-m.; Chen, X.-a.; Shyu, H.-f.; Lee, C.-y.; Young, J.-j.; Kau, J.-h. Nanoparticles assembled from fucoidan and trimethylchitosan as anthrax vaccine adjuvant: In vitro and in vivo efficacy in comparison to CpG. *Carbohydr. Polym.* **2020**, *236*, 116041. [CrossRef]
174. Venkatesan, J.; Singh, S.K.; Anil, S.; Kim, S.-K.; Shim, M.S. Preparation, characterization and biological applications of biosynthesized silver nanoparticles with chitosan-fucoidan coating. *Molecules* **2018**, *23*, 1429. [CrossRef]
175. Hwang, P.-A.; Yan, M.-D.; Lin, H.-T.V.; Li, K.-L.; Lin, Y.-C. Toxicological evaluation of low molecular weight fucoidan in vitro and in vivo. *Mar. Drugs* **2016**, *14*, 121. [CrossRef] [PubMed]
176. Zhu, Z.; Zhu, B.; Ai, C.; Lu, J.; Wu, S.; Liu, Y.; Wang, L.; Yang, J.; Song, S.; Liu, X. Development and application of a HPLC-MS/MS method for quantitation of fucosylated chondroitin sulfate and fucoidan in sea cucumbers. *Carbohydr. Res.* **2018**, *466*, 11–17. [CrossRef] [PubMed]
177. Yu, L.; Xue, C.; Chang, Y.; Xu, X.; Ge, L.; Liu, G.; Wang, Y. Structure elucidation of fucoidan composed of a novel tetrafucose repeating unit from sea cucumber *Thelenota ananas*. *Food Chem.* **2014**, *146*, 113–119. [CrossRef]
178. Zhao, X.; Guo, F.; Hu, J.; Zhang, L.; Xue, C.; Zhang, Z.; Li, B. Antithrombotic activity of oral administered low molecular weight fucoidan from Laminaria Japonica. *Thromb. Res.* **2016**, *144*, 46–52. [CrossRef]

179. Tsai, H.L.; Tai, C.J.; Huang, C.W.; Chang, F.R.; Wang, J.Y. Efficacy of low-molecular-weight fucoidan as a supplemental therapy in metastatic colorectal cancer patients: A double-blind randomized controlled trial. *Mar. Drugs* **2017**, *15*, 122. [CrossRef]
180. Jonsson, M.; Allahgholi, L.; Sardari, R.R.R.; Hreggviethsson, G.O.; Nordberg Karlsson, E. Extraction and modification of macroalgal polysaccharides for current and next-generation applications. *Molecules* **2020**, *25*, 930. [CrossRef] [PubMed]
181. Cumashi, A.; Ushakova, N.A.; Preobrazhenskaya, M.E.; D'Incecco, A.; Piccoli, A.; Totani, L.; Tinari, N.; Morozevich, G.E.; Berman, A.E.; Bilan, M.I.; et al. A comparative study of the anti-inflammatory, anticoagulant, antiangiogenic, and antiadhesive activities of nine different fucoidans from brown seaweeds. *Glycobiology* **2007**, *17*, 541–552. [CrossRef] [PubMed]
182. Silchenko, A.S.; Ustyuzhanina, N.E.; Kusaykin, M.I.; Krylov, V.B.; Shashkov, A.S.; Dmitrenok, A.S.; Usoltseva, R.V.; Zueva, A.O.; Nifantiev, N.E.; Zvyagintseva, T.N. Expression and biochemical characterization and substrate specificity of the fucoidanase from Formosa algae. *Glycobiology* **2017**, *27*, 254–263.
183. Silchenko, A.S.; Rasin, A.B.; Kusaykin, M.I.; Kalinovsky, A.I.; Miansong, Z.; Changheng, L.; Malyarenko, O.; Zueva, A.O.; Zvyagintseva, T.N.; Ermakova, S.P. Structure, enzymatic transformation, anticancer activity of fucoidan and sulphated fucooligosaccharides from *Sargassum horneri*. *Carbohydr. Polym.* **2017**, *175*, 654–660. [CrossRef] [PubMed]
184. Colin, S.; Deniaud, E.; Jam, M.; Descamps, V.; Chevolot, Y.; Kervarec, N.; Yvin, J.C.; Barbeyron, T.; Michel, G.; Kloareg, B. Cloning and biochemical characterization of the fucanase FcnA: Definition of a novel glycoside hydrolase family specific for sulfated fucans. *Glycobiology* **2006**, *16*, 1021–1032. [CrossRef] [PubMed]
185. Nagao, T.; Arai, Y.; Yamaoka, M.; Komatsu, F.; Yagi, H.; Suzuki, H.; Ohshiro, T. Identification and characterization of the fucoidanase gene from Luteolibacter algae H18. *J. Biosci. Bioeng.* **2018**, *126*, 567–572. [CrossRef] [PubMed]
186. Bakunina, I.; Nedashkovskaia, O.I.; Alekseeva, S.A.; Ivanova, E.P.; Romanenko, L.A.; Gorshkova, N.M.; Isakov, V.V.; Zviagintseva, T.N.; Mikhailov, V.V. Degradation of fucoidan by the marine proteobacterium *Pseudoalteromonas citrea*. *Mikrobiologiia* **2002**, *71*, 49–55. [PubMed]
187. Wu, Q.; Zhang, M.; Wu, K.; Liu, B.; Cai, J.; Pan, R. Purification and characteristics of fucoidanase obtained from Dendryphiella arenaria TM94. *J. Appl. Phycol.* **2011**, *23*, 197–203. [CrossRef]
188. Sakai, T.; Kimura, H.; Kojima, K.; Shimanaka, K.; Ikai, K.; Kato, I. Marine bacterial sulfated fucoglucuronomannan (SFGM) lyase digests brown algal SFGM into trisaccharides. *Mar. Biotechnol.* **2003**, *5*, 70–78. [CrossRef]
189. Sakai, T.; Ishizuka, K.; Shimanaka, K.; Ikai, K.; Kato, I. Structures of oligosaccharides derived from Cladosiphon okamuranus fucoidan by digestion with marine bacterial enzymes. *Mar. Biotechnol.* **2003**, *5*, 536–544.
190. Ohshiro, T.; Ohmoto, Y.; Ono, Y.; Ohkita, R.; Miki, Y.; Kawamoto, H.; Izumi, Y. Isolation and characterization of a novel fucoidan-degrading microorganism. *Biosci. Biotechnol. Biochem.* **2010**, *74*, 1729–1732. [CrossRef]
191. Bilan, M.I.; Kusaykin, M.I.; Grachev, A.A.; Tsvetkova, E.A.; Zvyagintseva, T.N.; Nifantiev, N.E.; Usov, A.I. Effect of enzyme preparation from the marine mollusk *Littorina kurila* on fucoidan from the brown alga *Fucus distichus*. *Biochemistry* **2005**, *70*, 1321–1326. [CrossRef]
192. Kim, W.J.; Kim, S.M.; Lee, Y.H.; Kim, H.G.; Kim, H.K.; Moon, S.H.; Suh, H.H.; Jang, K.H.; Park, Y.I. Isolation and characterization of marine bacterial strain degrading fucoidan from korean *Undaria pinnatifida* Sporophylls. *J. Microbiol. Biotechnol.* **2008**, *18*, 616–623.
193. Kim, W.J.; Park, J.W.; Park, J.K.; Choi, D.J.; Park, Y.I. Purification and characterization of a fucoidanase (FNase S) from a marine bacterium *Sphingomonas paucimobilis* PF-1. *Mar. Drugs* **2015**, *13*, 4398–4417. [CrossRef]
194. Kitamura, K.; Matsuo, M.; Tsuneo, Y. Enzymic degradation of fucoidan by fucoidanase from the hepatopancreas of *Patinopecten yessoensis*. *Biosci. Biotechnol. Biochem.* **1992**, *56*, 490–494. [CrossRef]
195. Daniel, R.; Berteau, O.; Chevolot, L.; Varenne, A.; Gareil, P.; Goasdoue, N. Regioselective desulfation of sulfated l-fucopyranoside by a new sulfoesterase from the marine mollusk Pecten maximus. *Eur. J. Biochem.* **2001**, *268*, 5617–5626. [CrossRef]
196. Berteau, O.; McCort, I.; Goasdouć, N.; Tissot, B.; Daniel, R. Characterization of a new alpha-L-fucosidase isolated from the marine mollusk *Pecten maximus* that catalyzes the hydrolysis of alpha-L-fucose from algal fucoidan (*Ascophyllum nodosum*). *Glycobiology* **2002**, *12*, 273–282. [CrossRef]

197. Dong, S.; Chang, Y.; Shen, J.; Xue, C.; Chen, F. Purification, expression and characterization of a novel α-l-fucosidase from a marine bacteria *Wenyingzhuangia fucanilytica*. *Protein Expr. Purif.* **2017**, *129*, 9–17. [CrossRef]
198. Tanaka, R.; Mizutani, Y.; Shibata, T.; Miyake, H.; Iehata, S.; Mori, T.; Kuroda, K.; Ueda, M. Genome sequence of *Formosa haliotis* strain MA1, a brown alga-degrading bacterium isolated from the gut of Abalone *Haliotis gigantea*. *Genome Announc.* **2016**, *4*, e01312-16. [CrossRef]
199. Chen, F.; Chang, Y.; Dong, S.; Xue, C. *Wenyingzhuangia fucanilytica* sp. nov., a sulfated fucan utilizing bacterium isolated from shallow coastal seawater. *Int. J. Syst. Evol. Microbiol.* **2016**, *66*, 3270–3275. [CrossRef]
200. Li, J.; Cheng, Y.; Wang, D.; Li, J.; Wang, Y.; Han, W.; Li, F. Draft genome sequence of the polysaccharide-degrading marine bacterium Pseudoalteromonas sp. Strain A601. *Genome Announc.* **2017**, *5*, e00590-17. [CrossRef]
201. Cao, H.T.T.; Mikkelsen, M.D.; Lezyk, M.J.; Bui, L.M.; Tran, V.T.T.; Silchenko, A.S.; Kusaykin, M.I.; Pham, T.D.; Truong, B.H.; Holck, J.; et al. Novel enzyme actions for sulphated galactofucan depolymerisation and a new engineering strategy for molecular stabilisation of fucoidan degrading enzymes. *Mar. Drugs* **2018**, *16*, 422. [CrossRef]
202. Tran, P.H.L.; Duan, W.; Tran, T.T.D. Fucoidan-based nanostructures: A focus on its combination with chitosan and the surface functionalization of metallic nanoparticles for drug delivery. *Int. J. Pharm.* **2019**, *575*, 118956. [CrossRef]
203. Jesumani, V.; Du, H.; Pei, P.; Aslam, M.; Huang, N. Comparative study on skin protection activity of polyphenol-rich extract and polysaccharide-rich extract from Sargassum vachellianum. *PLoS ONE* **2020**, *15*, e0227308. [CrossRef] [PubMed]
204. Brunt, E.G.; Burgess, J.G. The promise of marine molecules as cosmetic active ingredients. *Int. J. Cosmet. Sci.* **2018**, *40*, 1–15. [CrossRef] [PubMed]
205. Ferreira, R.M.; Ramalho Ribeiro, A.; Patinha, C.; Silva, A.M.S.; Cardoso, S.M.; Costa, R. Water extraction kinetics of bioactive compounds of *Fucus vesiculosus*. *Molecules* **2019**, *24*, 3408. [CrossRef] [PubMed]
206. Michel, G.; Tonon, T.; Scornet, D.; Cock, J.M.; Kloareg, B. The cell wall polysaccharide metabolism of the brown alga *Ectocarpus siliculosus*. Insights into the evolution of extracellular matrix polysaccharides in eukaryotes. *New Phytol.* **2010**, *188*, 82–97. [CrossRef]
207. Chi, S.; Liu, T.; Wang, X.; Wang, R.; Wang, S.; Wang, G.; Shan, G.; Liu, C. Functional genomics analysis reveals the biosynthesis pathways of important cellular components (alginate and fucoidan) of *Saccharina*. *Curr. Genet.* **2018**, *64*, 259–273. [CrossRef] [PubMed]
208. Shao, Z.; Zhang, P.; Lu, C.; Li, S.; Chen, Z.; Wang, X.; Duan, D. Transcriptome sequencing of *Saccharina Japonica* Sporophytes during whole developmental periods reveals regulatory networks underlying alginate and mannitol biosynthesis. *BMC Genom.* **2019**, *20*, 975. [CrossRef]

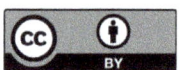

© 2020 by the authors. Licensee MDPI, Basel, Switzerland. This article is an open access article distributed under the terms and conditions of the Creative Commons Attribution (CC BY) license (http://creativecommons.org/licenses/by/4.0/).

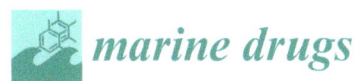

Article

Fucoidan Purified from *Sargassum polycystum* Induces Apoptosis through Mitochondria-Mediated Pathway in HL-60 and MCF-7 Cells

Ilekuttige Priyan Shanura Fernando [1,2], Kalu Kapuge Asanka Sanjeewa [2], Hyo Geun Lee [2], Hyun-Soo Kim [3], Andaravaas Patabadige Jude Prasanna Vaas [4,5], Hondamuni Ireshika Chathurani De Silva [4], Chandrika Malkanthi Nanayakkara [6], Dampegamage Thusitha Udayangani Abeytunga [4], Dae-Sung Lee [7], Jung-Suck Lee [8],* and You-Jin Jeon [2,9],*

1. Department of Marine Bio-Food Sciences, Chonnam National University, Yeosu 59626, Korea; shanurabru@gmail.com
2. Department of Marine Life Science, Jeju National University, Jeju 690-756, Korea; asanka.sanjeewa001@gmail.com (K.K.A.S.); hyogeunlee92@gmail.com (H.G.L.)
3. National Marine Biodiversity Institute of Korea, 75, Jangsan-ro 101-gil, Janghang-eup, Seocheon 33662, Korea; gustn783@mabik.re.kr
4. Department of Chemistry, University of Colombo, Colombo 3, Colombo 00700, Sri Lanka; prasannarokx@gmail.com (A.P.J.P.V.); hicdesilva@gmail.com (H.I.C.D.S.); abeytunga@gmail.com (D.T.U.A.)
5. School of Natural Sciences, University of Tasmania, Private Bag 75, Hobart, Tasmania 7001, Australia
6. Department of Plant Sciences, University of Colombo, Colombo 3, Colombo 00700, Sri Lanka; hewa_nana@yahoo.com
7. Department of Applied Research, National Marine Biodiversity Institute of Korea, 75, Jangsan-ro 101-gil, Janghang-eup, Seocheon 33662, Korea; daesung@mabik.re.kr
8. Research Center for Industrial Development of Seafood, Gyeongsang National University, Tongyeong 53064, Korea
9. Marine Science Institute, Jeju National University, Jeju Self-Governing Province 63333, Korea
* Correspondence: jungsucklee@hanmail.net (J.-S.L.); youjin2014@gmail.com (Y.-J.J.); Tel.: +82-10-9799-2238 (J.-S.L.); +82-64-754-3475 (Y.-J.J.)

Received: 21 March 2020; Accepted: 6 April 2020; Published: 8 April 2020

Abstract: Fucoidans are biocompatible, heterogeneous, and fucose rich sulfated polysaccharides biosynthesized in brown algae, which are renowned for their broad-spectrum biofunctional properties. As a continuation of our preliminary screening studies, the present work was undertaken to extract polysaccharides from the edible brown algae *Sargassum polycystum* by a modified enzyme assisted extraction process using Celluclast, a food-grade cellulase, and to purify fucoidan by DEAE-cellulose anion exchange chromatography. The apoptotic and antiproliferative properties of the purified fucoidan (F5) were evaluated on HL-60 and MCF-7 cells. Structural features were characterized by FTIR and NMR analysis. F5 indicated profound antiproliferative effects on HL-60 leukemia and MCF-7 breast cancer cells with IC_{50} values of 84.63 ± 0.08 µg mL^{-1} and 93.62 ± 3.53 µg mL^{-1} respectively. Further, F5 treatment increased the apoptotic body formation, DNA damage, and accumulation of HL-60 and MCF-7 cells in the Sub-G_1 phase of the cell cycle. The effects were found to proceed via the mitochondria-mediated apoptosis pathway. The Celluclast assisted extraction is a cost-efficient method of yielding fucoidan. With further studies in place, purified fucoidan of *S. polycystum* could be applied as functional ingredients in food and pharmaceuticals.

Keywords: Sri Lankan algae; anticancer; sulfated polysaccharide; fucoidan; Celluclast; sargassum

1. Introduction

Fucoidans found in brown algae are documented for their broad spectrum of bioactive properties, including anticancer, anticoagulant, antioxidant, anti-inflammatory, and immunomodulatory activities beneficial for the pharmaceutical, cosmeceutical, nutraceutical, and functional food industries [1]. The structure of fucoidan comprises of alternating units of L-fucose with mannose, glucose, galactose, and xylose monosaccharides with substituted sulfate groups. The primary linkage between α-l-fucopyranosyl residues is the (1→3) and (1→4) with sulfate groups substituted at either C2, C4, or both positions [1,2]. However, differences in fucoidan structure have been observed in different brown algae and remain ambiguous for their structures are highly heterogeneous. Typically, the structural characterization of fucoidan is accomplished by analyzing the monosaccharides composition, their connectivity, and substituted functional groups (methylation analysis, FTIR, and NMR) [3]. The publication by Bilan et al. (2013) reveals some significant findings regarding the fucoidan structure of S. polycystum harvested from Vietnam, which is comprised of 3-linked α-l-fucopyranose 4-sulfate residues [4]. Apart from the species specificity, fucoidan structure could vary depending on environmental factors and stress conditions. The structure of fucoidan (molecular weight, monosaccharide composition, and their sequence, degree, and substitution of sulfate groups) is a critical factor that determines its biofunctional properties. Li et al. (2008) provide a detailed review of up to date understanding regarding the structure-activity relationship of fucoidans [5]. By far, the anticancer properties of fucoidan have been found to increase with the increasing degree of sulfation and with reduction of molecular weight up to a certain limit.

Cancer has become a burden and a leading cause of death throughout the world. The number of cancer incidents in 2012 reached approximately 14.1 million, among which 8.2 million deaths have been reported [6]. The rapid growth of cancer incidents is predicted to be due to the increasing population and modernizing lifestyle patterns. Consumption of foods with artificial coloring, flavoring, and preservatives, use of tobacco, physical inactivity, exposure to ionizing radiation, and carcinogenic substances are among the major factors that contribute to the development of cancer [7]. Though a vast number of anticancer drugs are available, continuing the search for new cancer medicine is a prevailing task as many available anticancer agents cause serious side effects on normal tissues. The lack of selectivity is one of the major drawbacks in many of these drugs except for a limited number of anticancer medications such as "vemurafenib" that show their effects on melanoma cells with V600E BRAF mutation and monoclonal antibodies that specifically target cancer antigens [8]. The heterogeneous nature of cancers and multidrug resistance causes the development of anticancer drugs a challenging task [9]. Fucoidans, by far, have been recognized as a biocompatible substance that indicates positive biological responses. A recent study by Silchenko et al. (2017) describes the anticancer activity of fucoidan and sulfated fucooligosaccharides from *Sargassum horneri*, whereas the fucoidans are reported to suppress the colony formation of DLD-1 (colorectal adenocarcinoma) cells [10]. Fucoidans mediate anticancer functions not only by regulating intracellular mechanisms of cancer cells such as apoptosis, but also the activity of immune cells such as lymphocytes and natural killer cells [8,11]. Apart from the direct chemotherapeutic effects, fucoidan rich polysaccharides have shown radioprotective effects that make them a useful substance in cancer-radiotherapy [12]. The objective of the current study was to explore the anticancer activity of fucoidan rich polysaccharides of untapped *S. polycystum* harvested from the tropical island, Sri Lanka, and to explore its structural properties. Recently Palanisamy et al. (2017) have reported the anticancer potential of a fucoidan extract from *S. polycystum* on MCF-7 cells [13]. The present study so far is the first to report modified enzyme assisted extraction of fucoidan enriched polysaccharides from *S. polycystum*, anion exchange chromatographic purification, and detailed information of their anticancer properties.

2. Results

2.1. Yields and Chemical Composition of the Polysaccharide Extracts and Fractions

Based on the compositional analysis (AOAC methods) *S. polycystum* indicated 2.75 ± 0.08% moisture, 17.62 ± 0.16% ash, 52.46 ± 0.52% carbohydrate, 17.36 ± 0.04% protein, and 1.85 ± 0.06% lipids on a dry basis. The yield of ethanol precipitate was 6.88 ± 0.52%. The ash content of the ethanol precipitate was 0.08 ± 0.01% (relative to the dry weight of raw material).

2.2. Purification of Polysaccharides Molecular Weight Distribution and Monosaccharide Composition

As indicated in Figure 1a, anion exchange purification resolved the polysaccharide precipitate into five fractions (F1–F5). The recovery yield of F1 and F5 was higher than other fractions. The molecular weight distribution of fractions (F1–F5) indicated a decreasing trend and was estimated to be centered on 77.0, 65.5, 59.5, 60.0, and 39.5 kDa, respectively (Figure 1b). The monosaccharide composition of each fraction is given in Table 1. F1 had a higher galactose and mannose content, whereas the other successive fractions indicated increasing amounts of fucose. Fucose content was highest in F5 (Figure 1c) with galactose and a minor amount of glucose.

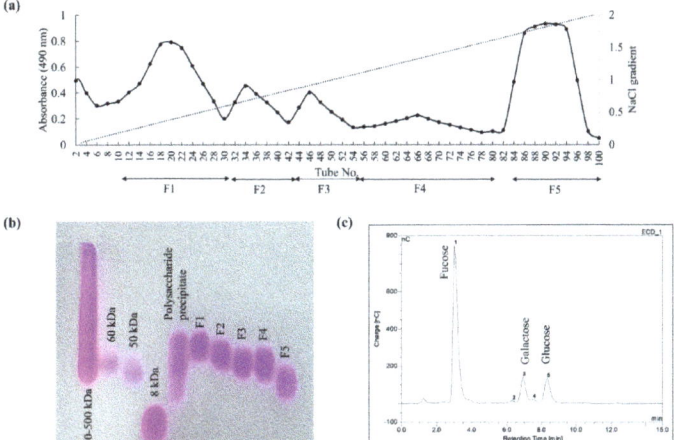

Figure 1. Purification of precipitated polysaccharides by DEAE-cellulose anion exchange chromatography. (**a**) Separating the collected column eluates into five fractions based on their polysaccharide content, (**b**) molecular weight distribution of the eluted column fractions (F1–F5), and (**c**) the monosaccharide composition analysis of the fraction F5.

Table 1. The composition of column fractions.

		F1	F2	F3	F4	F5
	Yield (%)	32.52 ± 0.17	12.24 ± 0.14	9.36 ± 0.09	11.78 ± 0.07	34.09 ± 0.14
Chemical composition (%)	Polysaccharide	81.42 ± 0.09	75.66 ± 0.11	70.25 ± 0.26	64.82 ± 0.24	59.36 ± 0.03
	Sulfate	12.42 ± 0.30	18.75 ± 0.00	23.12 ± 0.29	28.61 ± 0.22	33.56 ± 0.07
	Protein	0.36 ± 0.02	0.28 ± 0.01	0.25 ± 0.02	0.33 ± 0.03	0.28 ± 0.00
	Polyphenol	0.52 ± 0.02	0.55 ± 0.00	0.48 ± 0.04	0.39 ± 0.01	0.27 ± 0.02
Monosaccharide composition (%)	Fucose	20.06	33.20	49.06	63.84	71.96
	Rhamnose	1.72	1.45	0.89	0.60	N.D.
	Arabinose	2.52	2.39	1.15	0.62	N.D.
	Galactose	33.32	27.64	22.64	17.39	12.31
	Glucose	7.48	5.81	3.74	1.46	1.41
	Mannose	32.67	26.29	N.D.	N.D.	N.D.
	Others	2.22	3.22	22.52	16.09	14.32

Chemical composition was calculated based on triplicate determinations. Results are given as the means ± SD.

2.3. Characterization of Polysaccharide Structure (FTIR and NMR Analysis)

Wavenumber range 400–2000 cm^{-1} of FTIR spectra covering the fingerprint region of polysaccharides were used to characterize the structural properties of polysaccharides. All FTIR spectra, including column fractions and the commercial fucoidan standard, indicated prominent peaks at 845, 1035, 1616 cm^{-1}, and a broad peak between 1220–1270 cm^{-1}. A clear difference was seen for the intensity of 1220–1270 cm^{-1} peak between each spectrum, although the intensity of the peak at 1035 cm^{-1} was similar between all. The peak at 1733 cm^{-1} was absent in the commercial fucoidan, whereas a minor peak was recorded for F5. However, 1733 cm^{-1} peak was prominent in all other fractions (F1–F4). ^{1}H and ^{13}C NMR spectra of deuterium exchanged F5 fraction are presented in Figure 2b,C. In the ^{1}H spectrum, solvent peaks were observed at 2.50 ppm for dimethyl sulfoxide and 4.80 ppm for deuterium oxide. Unresolved peaks between 5.1–5.4 ppm could be assigned to protons of α-L-fucopyranosyl units. Prominent peaks observed at 4.46, 3.90, and 3.71 ppm were respectively assigned to H-1, H-5, and H-3 of D-galactons. The two overlapping peaks at 1.15, and 1.4 ppm were assigned to methyl groups in fucose [1,2]. In the ^{13}C spectrum, prominent peak 101.6 and peaks between 65–80 are arising from the (1–6)-β-D-linked galactons [2].

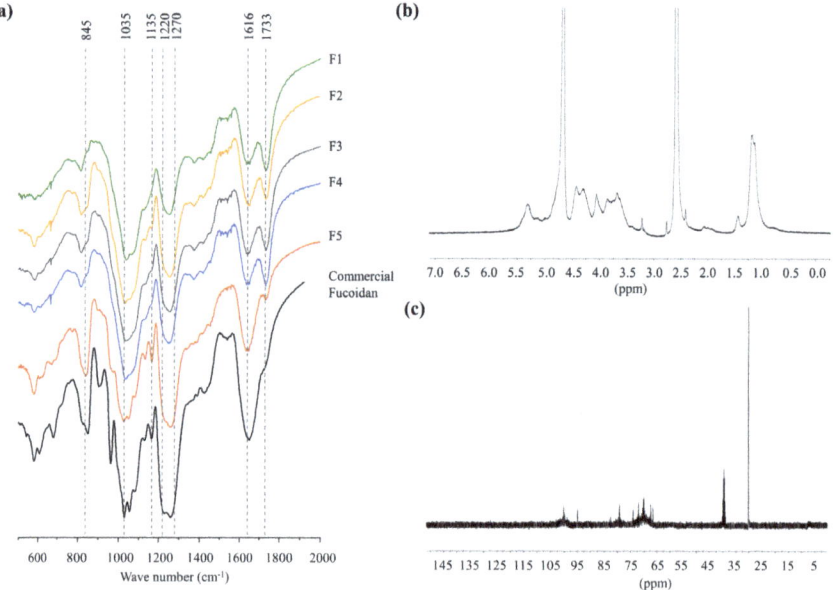

Figure 2. Structural characterization of polysaccharide fractions. (**a**) FTIR spectra of the fractions (F1–F5) provided in comparison to the commercial fucoidan, (**b**) ^{1}H NMR spectrum of F5, and (**c**) ^{13}C NMR spectrum of F5. The NMR spectra were obtained for the deuterium exchanged polysaccharides.

2.4. Variation of Antiproliferative Activity of the Column Fractions

As shown in Figure 3, F4 and F5 promptly reduced the viability of both HL-60 and MCF-7 cells compared to other fractions. The antiproliferative effects of F5 were stronger than F4. The IC$_{50}$ values related to F5 treatment was 84.63 ± 0.08 µg mL^{-1} and 93.62 ± 3.53 µg mL^{-1} respectively on HL-60 and MCF-7 cells. The viability of Vero cells (Figure 3c) was simultaneously evaluated to compare the cytotoxic effects of these polysaccharides on non-cancerous cells. The viability of Vero cells was 89.83 ± 1.76% at 100 µg mL^{-1} concentration.

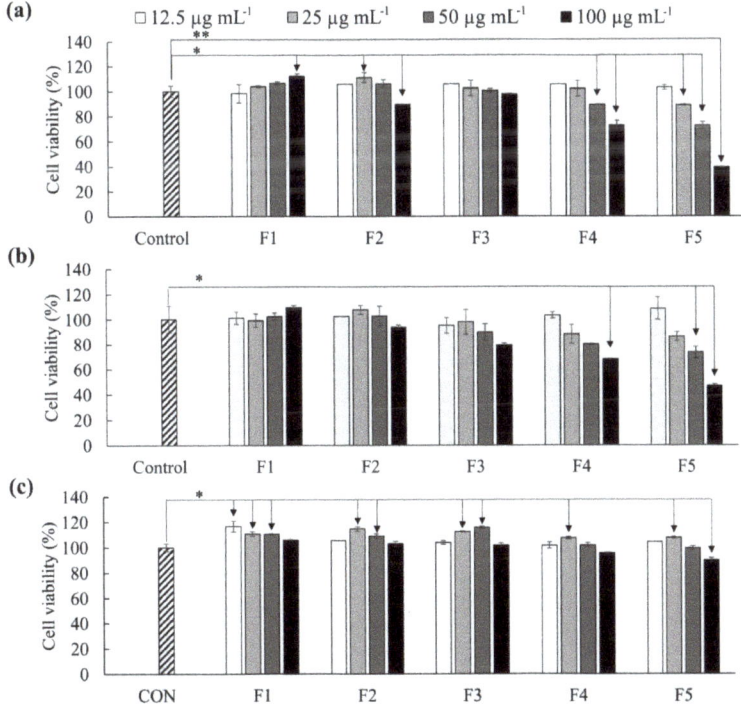

Figure 3. Antiproliferative activity of polysaccharide fractions as a measure of cell viability. (**a**) HL-60, (**b**) MCF-7, and (**c**) Vero cells. Cells were pre-seeded in 96 well plates for 24 h and incubated with samples for another 24 h. Cell viability was measured by MTT assay. Results are given as the means ± SD (n = 3). Significant differences from the control were identified at * $p < 0.05$ and ** $p < 0.001$.

2.5. Effect of F5 upon Apoptotic Body Formation in HL-60 and MCF-7 Cells and Pathway Studies by Western Blot Analysis

As shown in Figure 4a, under the Hoechst 33342 staining, HL-60 and MCF-7 cells indicated increased nuclear fragmentation and condensation (intensified spots) for increasing F5 concentrations. Nuclear double staining method (Figure 4c) assists in distinguishing early and late apoptosis or necrosis. Green fragmented nuclei (early apoptosis) were seen under 25 μg mL^{-1} of F5 treatment after a 24 h incubation period, which increased with increasing F5 concentrations. The presence of orange color spots together with green color fragmented nuclei (late apoptosis) were detected under 50 μg mL^{-1} concentration. Increased late apoptosis events were observed with 100 μg mL^{-1} of F5 concentration, whereas a few necrotic HL-60 cells were also detected. Western blot results indicated increased production of Bax, caspases, and p53 (only MCF-7) levels with increasing F5 concentrations together with increased PARP cleavage. Alternatively, reducing levels of Bcl-xL were also detected with increasing F5 concentrations.

2.6. F5 Increased the DNA Damage in HL-60 and MCF-7 Cells and the Population of Sub-G_1 Hyperploid Cells

Comet assay serves as a tool in identifying cellular DNA damage. As depicted in Figure 5a,b, the length of the comet tail increased in both HL-60 and MCF-7 cells with increasing F5 concentrations. Flow cytometric analysis with propidium iodide (PI) is widely employed in identifying the accumulation of cells in different phases of cell cycle based on their DNA content [14]. According to Figure 5c,d, the proportion of Sub-G_1 apoptotic cells increased with increasing F5 concentrations.

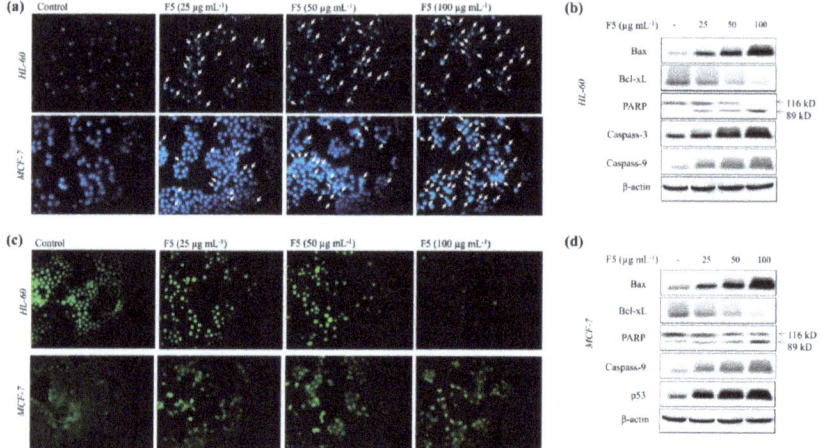

Figure 4. Effects of F5 in inducing apoptotic body formation in HL-60 and MCF-7 cells and analysis of the levels of molecular mediators. (**a**) Cells under Hoechst 33342 staining, (**b**) Western blot analysis of the levels of apoptosis-related molecular mediators in HL-60 cells, (**c**) cells under nuclear double staining, and (**d**) Western blot analysis of the levels of apoptosis-related molecular mediators in MCF-7 cells. Experiments were repeated three times to confirm the reproducibility.

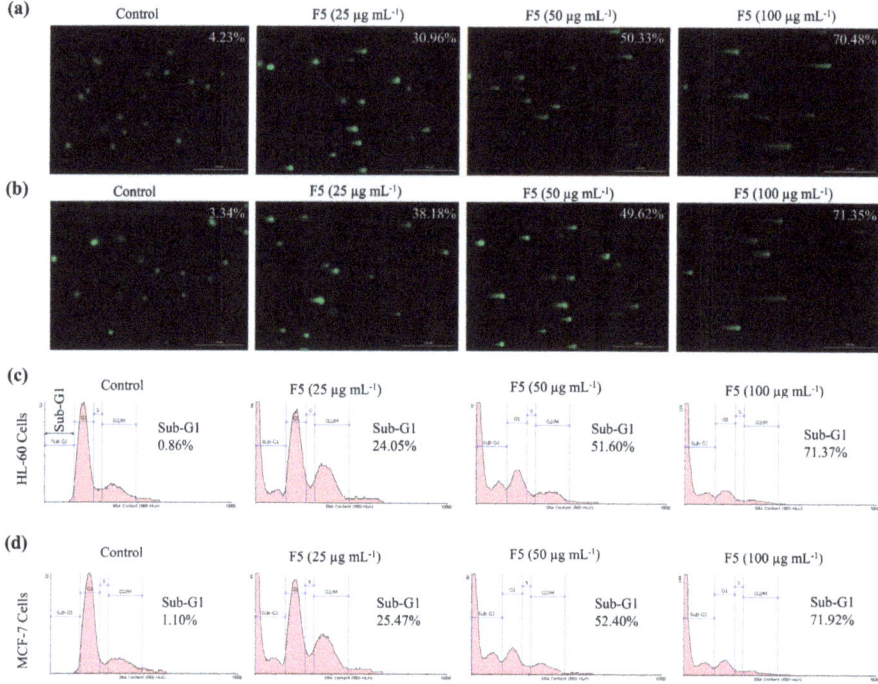

Figure 5. Effects of F5 in inducing single-cell DNA damage in HL-60 and MCF-7 cells and cell cycle analysis. Comet assay (**a**) HL-60 cells, (**b**) MCF-7 cells. Cell cycle analysis of (**c**) HL-60 cells, and (**d**) MCF-7 cells. Pre-seeded cells were exposed to different concentrations of F5 for 24 h. Experiments were repeated three times to confirm the reproducibility.

3. Discussion

Cancer is one of the leading causes of death throughout the world, which is predicted to increase in the future. The need for anticancer agents is an ever-increasing necessity, as many anticancer drugs cause serious side effects related to their inherent toxic effects. The literature suggests that fucoidan from brown algae could be a potential anticancer agent with promising bioactive effects and biocompatible properties [15]. A recent clinical study suggests that the administration of low molecular weight fucoidans to patients undergoing chemotherapy for metastatic colorectal cancer significantly improved the disease control rate compared to the control group [16]. The bioactive properties of fucoidan largely depend upon its structural characteristics. The structure of fucoidan is highly heterogeneous and indicates variation based on its source. In a previous study, fucoidan obtained from *S. polycystum* by hot water extraction has shown moderate antioxidant activity for DPPH scavenging, total antioxidant and reducing power assays, and anticancer activity in MCF-7 cells with an IC_{50} of 50 µg mL^{-1} [13]. Current investigations focus on the evaluation of antiproliferative properties of polysaccharides, and a purified fucoidan fraction from the Celluclast assisted extraction of *S. polycystum*. The selection of enzyme-assisted extraction supposedly gives better extraction yields compared to the conventional water extraction of polysaccharides. Here Celluclast, a food-grade cellulase, assists in hydrolyzing cellulose in cell walls [17]. Hexane washing removes the lipids and nonpolar pigments, whereas ethanol assists in removing un-bound phenolic compounds. Formaldehyde pretreatment causes polymerization of phenolic compounds that remain bound to the polysaccharide matrix and with other polar molecules via strong intermolecular interactions [1]. This prevents the water-based extract from getting contaminated by phenolic compounds. pH value is another factor that determines the solubility of anionic and cationic polysaccharides. Brown algae are rich in anionic polyelectrolyte alginic acid (pKa around 3.4–4.4) unlike other than fucoidan (pKa around 1.0–2.5) [18]. The optimum extraction conditions of Celluclast (pH 4.5) hence minimize the solubility of high molecular weight alginic acid, thus preventing the contamination of intended fucoidan extraction. However, $CaCl_2$ was incorporated into the extract at a later stage to facilitate the complexation and precipitation of any remaining alginic acid as calcium alginate [1]. Proteins are among the compounds soluble in water, which get precipitated with the addition of ethanol. To prevent the contamination of the final ethanol precipitate with proteins, we incorporated a commercial food grade protease (Alcalase) to the extraction mixture to facilitate the hydrolysis of proteins. Finally, ethanol was added to the neutralized and concentrated extraction mixture to lower its dielectric constant and precipitate polysaccharides. Essentially, the above extraction method, except for some minor modifications, was optimized during our previous studies to be efficient in purifying fucoidans [1]. The precipitated polysaccharides were subjected to anion exchange chromatography, where five fractions were obtained. Elution of the DEAE-Sepharose column with increasing Cl$^-$ concentrations enabled the successive elution of less negative to highly negatively charged polysaccharides. The chemical composition of the fractions indicates increasing amounts of sulfate through the successive column fractions agreeable with the increasing negative charge of the polysaccharides. The total polyphenol and protein contents were negligible in the fractions.

The molecular weight of sulfated polysaccharides is a major deterministic factor of its bioactivity [1]. The fractions indicated that different molecular weights ranged between 39–77 kDa. The lowest molecular weight was observed in F5, which indicated the best antiproliferative properties. Similar observations have reported that low molecular weight fucoidans are very effective as antiproliferative agents [5]. The composition of monosaccharides explicated substantial deviation from each other. An increase of the fucose content was observed with successive fractions, the highest being 71.96% in F5 with 12.31% of galactose (a galactofucan). L-fucose is the major monosaccharide constituent in fucoidans, which reports associating with sulfate groups. This agrees with the relatively high sulfate content in F5 compared to other fractions. Much evidence is, therefore, in agreement with F5 being a fucoidan. Crude fucoidan obtained from *S. polycystum* by Palanisamy et al. (2017) reported 46.8% fucose content with 22.35 ± 0.23% sulfate with minor amounts of other monosaccharides, galactose

(14.3%), glucose (11.5%), and xylose (13.2%) [13]. Bilan et al. (2013) have described the purification (anion-exchange chromatography) and structural characterization of two highly sulfated galactofucan fractions from *S. polycystum* following desulfation, methylation analysis, Smith degradation, and partial acid hydrolysis following mass-spectrometric and NMR monitoring [4]. Their fine structure report consists of mainly 3-linked α-l-fucopyranose units with C4-sulfate substitution, which is common to fucoidans and short sequences of above structures interspersed by residues of single 2-linked α-d-galactopyranose with C4 sulfation which is rather an unusual configuration.

Vibrational spectroscopic data were used in the structural characterization of the polysaccharides as they provide information about functional groups. The prominent peaks at 845–1035 cm^{-1} and the broad peak between 1220–1270 cm^{-1} respectively, representing the bending vibration of C-O-S, stretching vibration of glycosidic (C-O-C) bridge (typical to all polysaccharides), and the stretching vibrations of S=O bond in sulfate groups [1]. Interestingly the broadened peak between 1220 and 1270 cm^{-1} indicated a higher intensity in both commercial fucoidan and F5 fraction, suggesting a higher sulfate substitution. The intensity of that peak increased with successive fractions agreeing with the increased sulfate content observed. The intense peak at 1616 cm^{-1} is resulting from the asymmetric carboxylate O-C-O vibration [19].

Based on MTT cell viability assay, F5 indicated cytotoxicity on HL-60 and MCF-7 cancer cells with IC_{50} values of 84.63 ± 0.08 µg mL^{-1} and 93.62 ± 3.53 µg mL^{-1} respectively. Nonmalignant monkey kidney epithelial cells (Vero) were the least sensitive. Previous studies report substantially different IC_{50} values for the anticancer activity of fucoidans. According to Isnansetyo et al. (2017), fucoidans purified (anion exchange chromatography) from three tropical algae *Sargassum cristaefolium*, *Turbinaria conoides*, and *Padina fraseri* have shown substantially different IC_{50} values for cytotoxicity on MCF-7 and WiDr cell lines [19]. Herein *P. fraseri* fucoidan has shown IC_{50} of 144 and 118 µg mL^{-1}, respectively, on MCF-7 and WiDr cells, whereas the IC_{50} has ranged between 461 and 663 µg mL^{-1} for the fucoidans of *S. cristaefolium*, and *T. conoides*.

There could be a number of possibilities for the observed antiproliferative effects such as apoptosis, necrosis, cell cycle arrest, or a combination of two or more of the above effects. Evaluation of nuclear morphology revealed that F5 treatment increased the apoptotic body formation with an increased number of cells in late apoptosis. Further, the accumulation of cells in the Sub-G1 phase of the cell cycle agrees with the observed formation of apoptotic bodies. As evident from comet assay, DNA fragmentation is a characteristic feature observed in cells undergoing apoptosis. Apoptosis is a cellular homeostatic process that eliminates damaged cells without causing damage to neighboring tissues [20]. Hence substances that could induce apoptosis in cancer cells receive greater attention in the discovery of anticancer drugs.

Apoptosis could be triggered by two main pathways, either the mitochondria-mediated intrinsic pathway or cell surface receptor-mediated extrinsic pathway. Sensitivity to a vast number of death stimuli makes mitochondria-mediated apoptosis the most frequently studied death mechanism. This mechanism is inactivated in many cancer cells. Thus, its activation ramifies the therapeutic perspectives of treating several malignant diseases [20]. The mitochondria-mediated apoptotic pathway is controlled via a complex web of signaling cascade. Some of the major signaling molecules involved are Bax, Bcl-xL, PARP, p53, and caspase-9 and -3. The pro-apoptotic protein, Bax and the anti-apoptotic protein, Bcl-xL, belong to Bcl-2 family proteins. The Bax/Bcl-xL ratio is considered a major prognostic factor of apoptosis. Activation of Bax causes disruptions in the voltage-dependent anion channels in mitochondria releasing pro-apoptotic factors and cytochrome c that propagate apoptosis. Bcl-xL, which resides on the outer mitochondrial membrane, inhibits the activation of pro-apoptotic proteins such as Bax, thereby inhibiting the release of pro-apoptotic factors and cytochrome c [21]. In the present study, treatment of F5 increased the levels of Bax while reducing Bcl-xL. Caspases are next in line where their activation is triggered by cytochrome c, initiator caspases such as caspase-8 and -9, or by autocatalytic processes. The activated effector caspases (caspase-3, -6, and -7) catalyze the cleavage of critical regulatory proteins, such as PARP, which is involved in maintaining genomic stability by regulating base-excision DNA repair. F5 markedly increased the levels of caspase-9 in both HL-60 and MCF-7 cells. Although caspase-3 is produced in HL-60 cells, MCF-7 cells cannot synthesize caspase-3 due to a deletion in the CASP-3 gene [22]. However, PARP cleavage was observed in both cell lines suggesting that it could have proceeded via activation of another effector caspase in MCF-7 cells. These evidences conclude that the mitochondria-mediated pathway is a possible route of apoptosis in HL-60 and MCF-7 cells upon treatment with fucoidan purified from *S. polycystum*. While caspases are considered key biomarkers of apoptosis, numerous other apoptogenic molecular mediators, which do not require caspase activation, have been discovered as potential targets for anticancer drugs. Mitogen-activated protein kinases are a major grouping of such proteins involved in mediating apoptosis, which could be targeted by fucoidans [23]. Hence further analysis of F5 could widen its potential use in anticancer drug research. Structure-activity relationships of fucoidan are still a controversy where fucoidan is highly heterogeneous in its structure. A large number of studies on this topic suggest that sulfate content and molecular weight of polymer are major factors related to the antioxidant, anticancer, and immunomodulatory properties of fucoidan [24]. Present evidence suggests that fucoidans from *S. polycystum* could provide health benefits and could be utilized as candidates in cancer chemotherapy.

4. Materials and Methods

4.1. Materials

Celluclast was purchased from Novozyme (Nordisk, Bagsvaerd, Denmark). Dulbecco's Modified Eagle Medium (DMEM), fetal bovine serum (FBS), and penicillin-streptomycin were purchased from Life Technologies Corporation (Grand Island, NY, USA). Fucoidan standard, dextran sulfate, and chondroitin 6-sulfate molecular weight standards and 3-(4,5-dimethylthiazol-2-yl)-2,5-diphenyltetrazolium bromide (MTT), acridine orange, 2′ 7′-dichlorodihydrofluorescein diacetate (DCFH2-DA), propidium iodide (PI), trifluoroacetic acid, ethidium bromide, o-Toluidine blue, Hoechst 33342, agarose, low melting agarose, and sodium dodecyl sulfate were purchased from Sigma-Aldrich (St Louis, MO, USA). Polyvinylidin-fluorid (PVDF) membranes were obtained from Millipore (Schwallbach, Germany). All organic solvents used in this study were of the HPLC grade and purchased from Daejung Chemicals & Metals (Gyeonggi-do, S. Korea).

4.2. Collection and Extraction of Fucoidan Rich Fraction

Following up on the preliminary screening [25], *Sargassum polycystum* samples for the mass extraction were collected from the south-west coast of Sri Lanka. After washing with tap water, the samples were lyophilized and ground into a powder. The algae powder (350 g) was suspended in a solution of 95% ethanol for depigmentation (repeated three times). Depigmented powder was suspended in a solution of 10% formaldehyde in ethanol for 8 h at 37 °C. After filtration, the powder was washed twice with 95% ethanol and dried at 45 °C in a drying oven and lyophilized to remove any remaining moisture and ethanol. The powder (300 g) was then suspended in sterilized distilled water, and the pH was adjusted to 4.5 using 1 M HCl. Celluclast was added to the suspension, reaching a concentration of 0.5% of the substrate concentration. The mixture was incubated with continuous agitation at 50 °C for 24 h while regulating the pH at 4.5. After the digestion, the mixture was filtered through cheesecloth, and the filtrate was centrifuged to remove any particles. Celluclast was heat deactivated by incubating the supernatant at 100 °C for 10 min. The supernatant pH was adjusted to 8.0. Alcalase (0.1%, for 8 h at 50 °C) was used to hydrolyze the proteins. Alcalase was heat-inactivated by the same method above. Then the mixture was acidified to a pH of 4.0 using HCl and gradually mixed with a solution of saturated $CaCl_2$, facilitating the precipitation of alginate as calcium alginate. The mixture was then centrifuged, obtaining the supernatant. The supernatant was neutralized by using NaOH and lyophilized to reduce the water content to $1/4^{th}$ of the initial extraction volume and mixed with four volumes of 95% ethanol to precipitate the polysaccharides.

4.3. Fucoidan Purification

The precipitated polysaccharides were purified using an anion exchange chromatography on an ÄKTA chromatographic system (Uppsala, Sweden). The column (DEAE-sepharose) was equilibrated with 50.0 mM sodium acetate buffer (pH 5.3) and eluted with gradient elution using a solvent of 50.0 mM sodium acetate buffer with increasing amounts of 2.0 M NaCl in the same buffer. The eluates were collected into a hundred 15 mL conical tubes. The polysaccharide content in each tube was measured by the phenol-sulfuric assay [26].

4.4. Chemical Analysis

The proximate composition of the chemical constituents in the samples was determined according to the methods described in AOAC 2002 [27]. The adopted AOAC methods for the evaluation of ash, protein, lipid, and carbohydrates were dry ashing in a furnace at 600 °C for 5 h, Kjeldahl digestion, Soxhlet extraction, and phenol-sulfuric assay. The polysaccharide and sulfate content of the purified fractions were respectively analyzed using the standard phenol-sulfuric assay and $BaSO_4$ precipitation methods with some minor modifications [28]. Additionally, the protein and polyphenol content were estimated using the commercial BCA protein assay kit and by Folin–Ciocalteu method, respectively [29]. Monosaccharide composition was analyzed by a CarboPac PA1 cartridge column connected to an ED50Dionex electrochemical detector after hydrolysis by trifluoroacetic acid [1].

4.5. FTIR and NMR Analysis

FTIR is extensively used for the structural characterization of polymers as it allows identification of the functional groups. 10 mg of the purified polysaccharide powder were mixed with KBr and cast into pellets. The FTIR readings were taken using a Thermo Scientific NicoletTM 6700 FTIR spectrometer, MA USA. For the NMR analysis, the dialyzed polysaccharide was lyophilized, and deuterium exchanged with D_2O. The samples were then dissolved in D_2O, and a minute amount of deuterated dimethyl sulfoxide was added as an internal standard. NMR spectra were obtained using a JEOL JNMECX400, NMR spectrometer, Japan at 33 k.

4.6. Evaluation of Molecular Weight Distribution

The molecular weights of the purified fractions were analyzed using agarose gel electrophoresis following our previous method [1]. Briefly, the polysaccharide samples were electrophoresed in 1% agarose gels using a running buffer composed of Tris-Borate-EDTA (pH 8.3). The electrophoresis was carried out for 20 min at 100 V. The gel was stained with 0.02% o-Toluidine in 3% acetic acid with 0.5% Triton X-100 and destained with 3% acetic acid. Molecular weight markers used were, dextran sulfate (MW 50–500 kDa), chondroitin 6-sulfate (MW 60 kDa), Dextran sulfate (MW ≈ 50 kDa) and Dextran sulfate (MW ≈ 8 kDa).

4.7. Cell Culture

The MCF-7 cells were cultured in DMEM media and HL-60, and Vero cells were cultured in RPMI media, both of which were supplemented with 10% FBS and 1% penicillin/streptomycin mixture. Cell cultures were maintained under 37 °C in a humidified atmosphere supplemented with 5% CO_2. The cells under exponential growth were seeded for the experiments. The cancer cells were seeded in a concentration of 1×10^5 cells mL^{-1} in 96 well culture plates for 24 h and treated with different concentrations of the samples. After incubating for 24 h, the MTT assay was carried out for the determination of cell viability [30].

4.8. Evaluation of Nuclear Morphology

Nuclear fragmentation and chromatin condensation of the cancer cells were evaluated by using the nuclear staining dye Hoechst 33342 (10 μg mL^{-1}) and via the double staining method using acridine orange/ethidium bromide (100 µg mL^{-1}). Experiments were carried out, according to Fernando et al. (2018) [21]. Briefly, 24 h pre-seeded cells were treated with different concentrations of the samples and incubated for 24 h. The fluorescence dyes were then applied to the wells and incubated for 10 min. The images were visualized using a fluorescence microscope with a CoolSNAP-Pro color digital camera.

4.9. Cell Cycle Analysis

The proportion of cells in the Sub-G_1 phase of the cell cycle, which indicate apoptotic hypodiploid cells were measured using flow cytometry. The experiments were carried out according to the method described by Fernando et al. (2018) [21]. Briefly, cells (2 × 10^5 cells mL^{-1}) were incubated with different concentrations of F5 for 24 h. The cells were then harvested, washed with PBS, and fixed in 70% ethanol followed by washing with EDTA (2 mM) in PBS. Then the cells were suspended in a PI solution containing RNase, and the cell cycle analysis was carried out using a FACSCalibur flow cytometer, USA.

4.10. Analysis of DNA Damage

The DNA damage caused by F5 was analyzed by evaluating the single-cell DNA damage (comet assay) and DNA laddering analysis. The alkaline comet assay was performed by using cells incubated with different concentrations of F5 for 24 h. Experiments were carried out according to the method described by Fernando et al. (2018) [21]. For the DNA laddering analysis, the cells were incubated with samples for 24 h and harvested after PBS washing. The experiments were performed following the method described by Jayasooriya et al. (2012) [31].

4.11. Western Blot Analysis

The cells were pre-seeded in 6 well culture plates at 2 × 10^5 cells mL^{-1} for 24 h and treated with different sample concentrations. After 24 h, the cells were harvested, lysed, and centrifuged at 12,000× *g* for 20 min to remove the cellular debris. The proteins were resolved by SDS-polyacrylamide jell electrophoresis. Protein bands were blotted onto nitrocellulose membranes and incubated for 2 h with skim milk in TBST. The membranes were consequently incubated with primary (8 h under 4 °C) and secondary antibodies (2 h at room temperature). Protein bands were visualized by adding chemiluminescent substrate (Cyanagen Srl, Italy) using a FUSION SOLO Vilber Lourmat system, France [21].

4.12. Statistical Analysis

All data values are expressed as means ± SD based on at least three independent determinations. Significant differences among the data values were determined using IBM SPSS Statistics 20 software using one-way ANOVA by Duncan's multiple range test. ** P-values less than 0.05 ($p < 0.05$) were considered significant.

Author Contributions: Conceptualization, I.P.S.F. and Y.-J.J.; methodology, I.P.S.F., K.K.A.S., and A.P.J.P.V.; software, I.P.S.F.; validation, I.P.S.F., K.K.A.S., and H.-S.K.; formal analysis, I.P.S.F. and K.K.A.S.; investigation, I.P.S.F. and K.K.A.S.; resources, Y.-J.J., D.T.U.A., and J.-S.L.; data curation, I.P.S.F., K.K.A.S., and A.P.J.P.V.; writing—original draft preparation, I.P.S.F.; writing—review and editing, Y.-J.J., H.I.C.D.S., C.M.N., and D.T.U.A.; supervision, Y.-J.J., D.T.U.A., and J.-S.L.; project administration, H.G.L., D.-S.L., Y.-J.J., and D.T.U.A.; funding acquisition, D.-S.L. and Y.-J.J. All authors have read and agreed to the published version of the manuscript.

Funding: This research was supported by a grant from the Marine Biotechnology Program (20170488) funded by the Ministry of Oceans and Fisheries, Korea.

Acknowledgments: Authors wish to thank Colombo Science and Technology Cell, University of Colombo for their administrative support.

Conflicts of Interest: The authors declare no conflict of interest.

References

1. Fernando, I.P.S.; Sanjeewa, K.K.A.; Samarakoon, K.W.; Lee, W.W.; Kim, H.-S.; Kang, N.; Ranasinghe, P.; Lee, H.-S.; Jeon, Y.-J. A fucoidan fraction purified from *Chnoospora minima*; a potential inhibitor of LPS-induced inflammatory responses. *Int. J. Biol. Macromol.* **2017**, *104*, 1185–1193. [CrossRef] [PubMed]
2. Immanuel, G.; Sivagnanavelmurugan, M.; Marudhupandi, T.; Radhakrishnan, S.; Palavesam, A. The effect of fucoidan from brown seaweed *Sargassum wightii* on WSSV resistance and immune activity in shrimp Penaeus monodon (Fab). *Fish Shellfish Immunol.* **2012**, *32*, 551–564. [CrossRef] [PubMed]
3. Patankar, M.S.; Oehninger, S.; Barnett, T.; Williams, R.L.; Clark, G.F. A revised structure for fucoidan may explain some of its biological activities. *J. Biol. Chem.* **1993**, *268*, 21770–21776. [PubMed]
4. Bilan, M.I.; Grachev, A.A.; Shashkov, A.S.; Thuy, T.T.T.; Van, T.T.T.; Ly, B.M.; Nifantiev, N.E.; Usov, A.I. Preliminary investigation of a highly sulfated galactofucan fraction isolated from the brown alga *Sargassum polycystum*. *Carbohydr. Res.* **2013**, *377*, 48–57. [CrossRef] [PubMed]
5. Li, B.; Lu, F.; Wei, X.; Zhao, R. Fucoidan: Structure and Bioactivity. *Molecules* **2008**, *13*, 1671–1695. [CrossRef]
6. Ferlay, J.; Soerjomataram, I.; Ervik, M.; Dikshit, R.; Eser, S.; Mathers, C.; Rebelo, M.; Parkin, D.; Forman, D.; Bray, F. *Cancer Incidence and Mortality Worldwide: IARC CancerBase No. 11*; International Agency for Research on Cancer: Lyon, France, 2016.
7. Madigan, M.P.; Ziegler, R.G.; Benichou, J.; Byrne, C.; Hoover, R.N. Proportion of Breast Cancer Cases in the United States Explained by Well-Established Risk Factors. *Jnci: J. Natl. Cancer Inst.* **1995**, *87*, 1681–1685. [CrossRef]
8. Atashrazm, F.; Lowenthal, R.M.; Woods, G.M.; Holloway, A.F.; Dickinson, J.L. Fucoidan and cancer: A multifunctional molecule with anti-tumor potential. *Mar. Drugs* **2015**, *13*, 2327–2346. [CrossRef]
9. Chen, Q.-F.; Liu, Z.-P.; Wang, F.-P. Natural sesquiterpenoids as cytotoxic anticancer agents. *Mini Rev. Med. Chem.* **2011**, *11*, 1153–1164. [CrossRef]
10. Silchenko, A.S.; Rasin, A.B.; Kusaykin, M.I.; Kalinovsky, A.I.; Miansong, Z.; Changheng, L.; Malyarenko, O.; Zueva, A.O.; Zvyagintseva, T.N.; Ermakova, S.P. Structure, enzymatic transformation, anticancer activity of fucoidan and sulphated fucooligosaccharides from *Sargassum horneri*. *Carbohydr. Polym.* **2017**, *175* (Suppl. C), 654–660. [CrossRef]
11. Choi, E.-M.; Kim, A.-J.; Kim, Y.-O.; Hwang, J.-K. Immunomodulating activity of arabinogalactan and fucoidan in vitro. *J. Med. Food* **2005**, *8*, 446–453. [CrossRef]
12. Lee, W.; Kang, N.; Kim, E.-A.; Yang, H.-W.; Oh, J.-Y.; Fernando, I.P.S.; Kim, K.-N.; Ahn, G.; Jeon, Y.-J. Radioprotective effects of a polysaccharide purified from *Lactobacillus plantarum*-fermented *Ishige okamurae* against oxidative stress caused by gamma ray-irradiation in zebrafish in vivo model. *J. Funct. Foods* **2017**, *28*, 83–89. [CrossRef]
13. Palanisamy, S.; Vinosha, M.; Marudhupandi, T.; Rajasekar, P.; Prabhu, N.M. Isolation of fucoidan from *Sargassum polycystum* brown algae: Structural characterization, in vitro antioxidant and anticancer activity. *Int. J. Biol. Macromol.* **2017**, *102*, 405–412. [CrossRef] [PubMed]
14. Krishan, A. Rapid flow cytofluorometric analysis of mammalian cell cycle by propidium iodide staining. *J. Cell Biol.* **1975**, *66*, 188–193. [CrossRef] [PubMed]
15. Sanjeewa, K.A.; Lee, J.S.; Kim, W.-S.; Jeon, Y.-J. The potential of brown-algae polysaccharides for the development of anticancer agents: An update on anticancer effects reported for fucoidan and laminaran. *Carbohydr. Polym.* **2017**, *177*, 451–459. [CrossRef] [PubMed]
16. Tsai, H.-L.; Tai, C.-J.; Huang, C.-W.; Chang, F.-R.; Wang, J.-Y. Efficacy of Low-Molecular-Weight Fucoidan as a Supplemental Therapy in Metastatic Colorectal Cancer Patients: A Double-Blind Randomized Controlled Trial. *Mar. Drugs* **2017**, *15*, 122. [CrossRef] [PubMed]
17. Wijesinghe, W.A.J.P.; Jeon, Y.J. Enzyme-assistant extraction (EAE) of bioactive components: A useful approach for recovery of industrially important metabolites from seaweeds: A review. *Fitoterapia* **2012**, *83*, 6–12. [CrossRef]
18. Sheng, P.X.; Ting, Y.-P.; Chen, J.P.; Hong, L. Sorption of lead, copper, cadmium, zinc, and nickel by marine algal biomass: Characterization of biosorptive capacity and investigation of mechanisms. *J. Colloid Interface Sci.* **2004**, *275*, 131–141. [CrossRef]
19. Isnansetyo, A.; Lutfia, F.N.L.; Nursid, M.; Susidarti, R.A. Cytotoxicity of Fucoidan from Three Tropical Brown Algae Against Breast and Colon Cancer Cell Lines. *Pharmacogn. J.* **2017**, *9*, 14–20. [CrossRef]

20. Shi, Y. A structural view of mitochondria-mediated apoptosis. *Nat. Struct. Mol. Biol.* **2001**, *8*, 394–401. [CrossRef]
21. Fernando, I.P.S.; Sanjeewa, K.K.A.; Kim, H.-S.; Wang, L.; Lee, W.W.; Jeon, Y.-J. Apoptotic and antiproliferative properties of 3β-hydroxy-Δ5-steroidal congeners from a partially purified column fraction of *Dendronephthya gigantea* against HL-60 and MCF-7 cancer cells. *J. Appl. Toxicol.* **2018**, *38*, 527–536. [CrossRef]
22. Jänicke, R.U.; Sprengart, M.L.; Wati, M.R.; Porter, A.G. Caspase-3 is required for DNA fragmentation and morphological changes associated with apoptosis. *J. Biol. Chem.* **1998**, *273*, 9357–9360. [CrossRef] [PubMed]
23. Zhang, Z.; Teruya, K.; Eto, H.; Shirahata, S. Fucoidan extract induces apoptosis in MCF-7 cells via a mechanism involving the ROS-dependent JNK activation and mitochondria-mediated pathways. *PLoS ONE* **2011**, *6*, e27441. [CrossRef] [PubMed]
24. Zhurishkina, E.V.; Stepanov, S.I.; Shvetsova, S.V.; Kulminskaya, A.A.; Lapina, I.M. A comparison of the effect of fucoidan from alga *Fucus vesiculosus* and its fractions obtained by anion-exchange chromatography on HeLa G-63, Hep G2, and Chang liver cells. *Cell Tissue Biol.* **2017**, *11*, 242–249. [CrossRef]
25. Fernando, I.P.S.; Sanjeewa, K.K.A.; Samarakoon, K.W.; Lee, W.W.; Kim, H.-S.; Ranasinghe, P.; Gunasekara, U.K.D.S.S.; Jeon, Y.-J. Antioxidant and anti-inflammatory functionality of ten Sri Lankan seaweed extracts obtained by carbohydrase assisted extraction. *Food Sci. Biotechnol.* **2018**, *27*, 1761–1769. [CrossRef] [PubMed]
26. DuBois, M.; Gilles, K.A.; Hamilton, J.K.; Rebers, P.A.; Smith, F. Colorimetric method for determination of sugars and related substances. *Anal. Chem.* **1956**, *28*, 350–356. [CrossRef]
27. Horwitz, W. *Instructions for Inserting: Official Methods of Analysis of AOAC International*; AOAC International: Rockville, MD, USA, 2002.
28. Khan, B.M.; Qiu, H.-M.; Xu, S.-Y.; Liu, Y.; Cheong, K.-L. Physicochemical characterization and antioxidant activity of sulphated polysaccharides derived from *Porphyra haitanensis*. *Int. J. Biol. Macromol.* **2020**, *145*, 1155–1161. [CrossRef] [PubMed]
29. Draganescu, D.; Ibanescu, C.; Tamba, B.I.; Andritoiu, C.V.; Dodi, G.; Popa, M.I. Flaxseed lignan wound healing formulation: Characterization and in vivo therapeutic evaluation. *Int. J. Biol. Macromol.* **2015**, *72*, 614–623. [CrossRef]
30. Eom, S.-H.; Moon, S.-Y.; Lee, D.-S.; Kim, H.-J.; Park, K.; Lee, E.-W.; Kim, T.H.; Chung, Y.-H.; Lee, M.-S.; Kim, Y.-M. In vitro antiviral activity of dieckol and phlorofucofuroeckol-A isolated from edible brown alga *Eisenia bicyclis* against murine norovirus. *Algae* **2015**, *30*, 241. [CrossRef]
31. Jayasooriya, R.G.P.T.; Kang, S.-H.; Kang, C.-H.; Choi, Y.H.; Moon, D.-O.; Hyun, J.-W.; Chang, W.-Y.; Kim, G.-Y. Apigenin decreases cell viability and telomerase activity in human leukemia cell lines. *Food Chem. Toxicol.* **2012**, *50*, 2605–2611. [CrossRef]

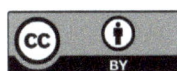

© 2020 by the authors. Licensee MDPI, Basel, Switzerland. This article is an open access article distributed under the terms and conditions of the Creative Commons Attribution (CC BY) license (http://creativecommons.org/licenses/by/4.0/).

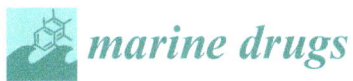

Article

Antioxidant Potential of Sulfated Polysaccharides from *Padina boryana*; Protective Effect against Oxidative Stress in In Vitro and In Vivo Zebrafish Model

Thilina U. Jayawardena [1,†], Lei Wang [1,2,†], K. K. Asanka Sanjeewa [1], Sang In Kang [3], Jung-Suck Lee [4,*] and You-Jin Jeon [1,2,*]

1. Department of Marine Life Sciences, Jeju National University, Jeju 690-756, Korea; tuduwaka@gmail.com (T.U.J.); comeonleiwang@163.com (L.W.); asanka.sanjeewa001@gmail.com (K.K.A.S.)
2. Marine Science Institute, Jeju National University, Jeju Self-Governing Province 63333, Korea
3. Department of Seafood and Aquaculture Science, Gyeongsang National University, Tongyeong 53064, Korea; sikang@gnu.ac.kr
4. Research Center for Industrial Development of Seafood, Gyeongsang National University, Tongyeong 53064, Korea
* Correspondence: jungsucklee@hanmail.net (J.-S.L.); youjin2014@gmail.com (Y.-J.J.); Tel.: +82-064-754-3475 (Y.-J.J.)
† These authors contributed equally to this work.

Received: 25 March 2020; Accepted: 13 April 2020; Published: 14 April 2020

Abstract: Elevated levels of reactive oxygen species (ROS) damage the internal cell components. *Padina boryana*, a brown alga from the Maldives, was subjected to polysaccharide extraction. The Celluclast enzyme assisted extract (PBE) and ethanol precipitation (PBP) of *P. boryana* were assessed against hydrogen peroxide (H_2O_2) induced cell damage and zebra fish models. PBP which contains the majority of sulfated polysaccharides based on fucoidan, showed outstanding extracellular ROS scavenging potential against H_2O_2. PBP significantly declined the intracellular ROS levels, and exhibited protection against apoptosis. The study revealed PBPs' ability to activate the Nrf2/Keap1 signaling pathway, consequently initiating downstream elements such that catalase (CAT) and superoxide dismutase (SOD). Further, ROS levels, lipid peroxidation values in zebrafish studies were declined with the pre-treatment of PBP. Collectively, the results obtained in the study suggest the polysaccharides from *P. boryana* might be a potent source of water soluble natural antioxidants that could be sustainably utilized in the industrial applications.

Keywords: antioxidant; Maldives; *Padina boryana*; sulfated polysaccharide; zebrafish

1. Introduction

Aerobic metabolism results reactive oxygen species (ROS) as its by-product. ROS is comprised of both radical and non-radical species. Distinctively, superoxide anion ($O_2^{-\bullet}$), hydroxyl radical ($^\bullet OH$), and hydrogen peroxide (H_2O_2) exhibit properties which discuss its involvement in biological targets. ROS possesses two faces; physiological levels support redox biology and pathological levels are explained via oxidative stress. At normal physiological amounts, ROS contributes to the activation of signaling pathways hence initiate biological processes, though oxidative stress damage cellular components including macromolecules such as DNA, lipids, and proteins [1,2]. The effect of ROS elevated levels is counterbalanced with a variety of antioxidants which are divided into two categories namely enzymatic and non-enzymatic. Superoxide dismutase (SOD), catalase (CAT), glutathione peroxidase (GTPx), and glutathione transferase (GST) are foremost components of enzymatic antioxidants. Non-enzymatic antioxidants include compounds with a low molecular weight—such as ascorbic acid (vitamin C), α-tocopherol (vitamin E), glutathione, and β-carotene [3]. However, excessive ROS accumulation makes way to countless pathologies such as inflammation, cancer, and abnormal aging. With regard, supplementary antioxidants are beneficial. Such synthetic antioxidants are butylated hydroxytoluene (BHT), and butylated hydroxyanisole (BHA) [4]. However, given its synthetic nature, the human body is vulnerable to side effects. Thus, research endeavors complying with natural antioxidants from sustainable sources have received much attention.

Seaweeds are a source of bioactive components, capable of producing a myriad of secondary metabolites. Previous literature covers antioxidant, anti-fungal, anti-inflammatory, and anti-tumor potential of compounds from vivid algal species. Though seaweeds undergo harsh environmental conditions, such as high intense light and oxygen concentrations, which support the formation of oxidizing components, they manage to prevail without any serious damage. This fact suggests possession of protective compounds and mechanisms among seaweeds [5,6].

Different species of the genus *Padina* have been subjected to experiments. A range of phytochemicals and their bioactivities were analyzed in *Padina tetrastromatica* [7]. *Padina pavonica* was extensively studied for its sulfated hetero-polysaccharides [8,9]. Inhibition of hyaluronidase activity of the *Padina pavonica* was assessed in its water extract [10].

Polysaccharides are one of the major components of the natural sources available in marine algae. These were reported as effective and non-toxic components with comparatively higher in yield and rather easy to extract, having pharmacological importance [11]. Sulfated polysaccharides inherit distinct attention among other types of polysaccharides due to its numerous bioactivities. Anti-inflammatory [11,12], anti-coagulant [13], anti-proliferative, and antioxidant [14] properties of polysaccharides purified from seaweed species have been studied previously.

This study focuses on the extraction of polysaccharides from brown algae *Padina boryana* collected from the Maldives. Antioxidant potential of the polysaccharides from *P. boryana* has not been reported yet, to the best of our knowledge. Hence, the above properties of the polysaccharides are evaluated in vitro (Vero cells) and in vivo (zebrafish) scale.

2. Results

2.1. Chemical Composition

The celluclast enzyme assisted extract of *P. boryana* (PBE) and ethanol precipitated component PBP were subjected to chemical composition analysis. The results are given in Table 1. The total phenol content of PBE was 1.32 ± 0.17% while PBP exhibited 1.14 ± 0.26%. Sulfated polysaccharide content was higher in the PBP (56.34%). Monosaccharide analysis revealed, high contents of fucose and galactose in PBP compared to PBE.

Table 1. Chemical composition of PBE and PBP obtained from *P. boryana*.

Sample		PBE	PBP
Polysaccharides content %		42.14 ± 0.86	49.36 ± 0.79
Sulfates content %		4.57 ± 0.64	6.98 ± 0.35
Phenolic content %		1.32 ± 0.17	1.14 ± 0.26
Mono sugars %	Fucose	39.84	57.51
	Galactose	15.11	21.35
	Mannose	18.24	13.21
	other	24.81	5.63

The analyzed Fourier transform infrared (FTIR) data are illustrated in Figure 1. Glycosidic bonds are formed among multiple monomer units to form polysaccharides and are represented via the

1025 cm^{-1} (C-O-C stretching vibrations) fingerprint peak. An intense peak at the 1200 cm^{-1} is observed due to the sulfate stretching vibrations (S=O). While the bending sulfate vibrations are represented via the absorptions at 845 cm^{-1} (C-O-S). The moisture content available in the sample was observed via the H-O-H bending vibrations in the 1625 cm^{-1} region [12,15,16]. Results suggest the PBP possesses a close correlation with commercial fucoidan.

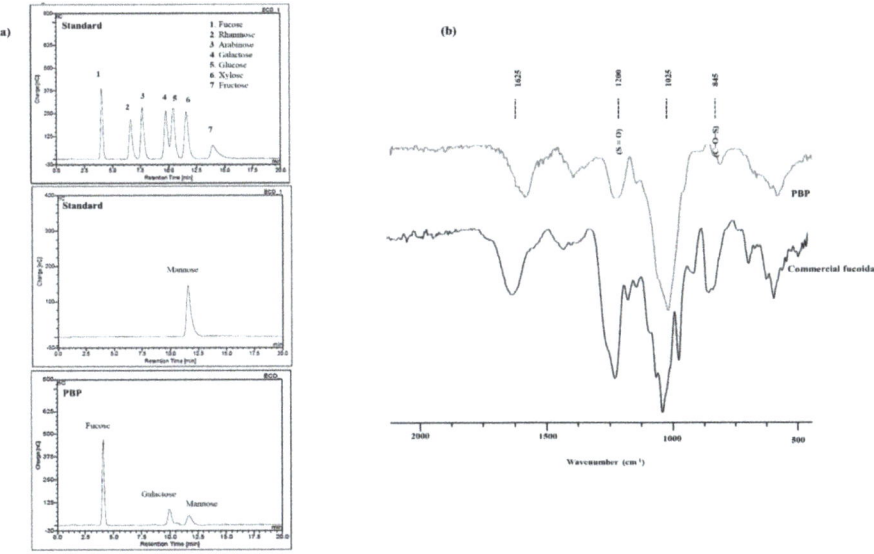

Figure 1. Chemical characterization of PBP. (**a**) Standard monosaccharide and PBP analyzed by HPAE-PAD spectrum. (**b**) ATR-FTIR spectra of PBP and commercial fucoidan.

2.2. Free Radical and Hydrogen Peroxided Scavenging Activity

The individual radical scavenging activities corresponding to each sample is expressed in Table 2. Both samples exhibited potent scavenging activities where PBP was more active compared to PBE. Interestingly, H_2O_2 chemical assay analysis for scavenging also exhibited PBP as the potent, significant scavenger of radicals. Hence, further experiments were planned with the PBP sample.

Table 2. Free radical/ROS scavenging activities of PBE and PBP.

	Free Radical/ROS Scavenging Activity (IC$_{50}$, mg/mL)			
	DPPH	Alkyl	Hydroxyl	H_2O_2
PBE	4.26 ± 0.14	3.88 ± 0.13	1.96 ± 0.17	1.17 ± 0.11
PBP	3.66 ± 0.44	2.87 ± 0.07	1.06 ± 0.21	0.58 ± 0.04

All results expressed as means ± SE, based on triplicated trials.

2.3. Protective Effect of PBP in H_2O_2 Stimulated Cells

The PBP exhibited protective effects against the H_2O_2 induced cells. The cell viability which was declined with the H_2O_2 treatment was reinstated with the PBP treatment. Similarly, the intracellular ROS level which was increased against the H_2O_2 stimulation was effectively downregulated with the treatment of PBP. Furthermore, the results exhibited a dose dependent recovery of each indicator (Figure 2).

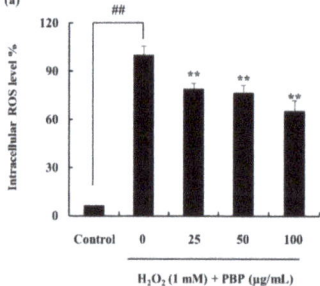 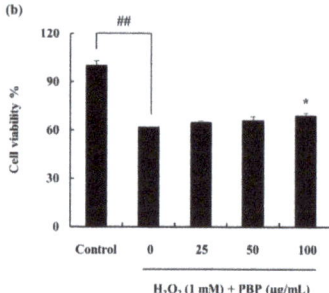

Figure 2. Hydrogen peroxide stimulated Vero cells exhibit oxidative stress. (**a**) Intracellular reactive oxygen species (ROS) scavenging ability of PBP. (**b**) PBPs' potential to protect cells against hydrogen peroxide. Experiments were triplicated and data shown as mean ± SE; * $p < 0.05$, ** $p < 0.01$. (# denotes significance compared to control while * represents significance compared to H_2O_2 treated group).

2.4. PBP Protects Cells from H_2O_2 Induced Apoptosis

Earlier studies have revealed the effect of H_2O_2 on DNA damage leading to apoptosis [17]. Hence, the effect was evaluated through nuclear staining methods. This particular study followed the Hoechst 33342 staining method. Viable cells are indicated via homogeneously stained nuclei while fragmented and chromatin condensed nuclei are an indication of apoptotic cells [18]. As indicated in Figure 3, cells that were exposed to H_2O_2 were associated with increased cell death, indicating higher intensity in the nuclei region. The number of apoptotic bodies was significantly decreased with the PBP treatment, which was indicative of its potential to act as a protective substance against ROS.

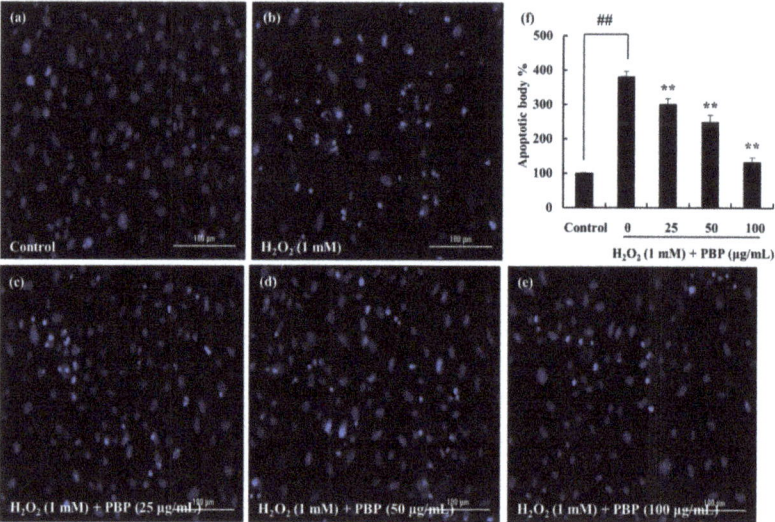

Figure 3. PBP protects Vero cells against H_2O_2-induced apoptosis. The apoptotic body formation was observed using Hoechst 33342 staining method under a fluorescence microscope. (**a**) non-treated group, (**b**) H_2O_2 treated (1 mM) cells, H_2O_2 stimulated cells treated with PBP (**c**) 25 µg/mL, (**d**) 50 µg/mL, (**e**) 100 µg/mL, (**f**) quantitative representation. The intensity levels were analyzed using ImageJ software. Triplicated experiments were conducted and results are represented as mean ± SE; * $p < 0.05$, ** $p < 0.01$. (# denotes significance compared to control while * represents significance compared to H_2O_2 treated group).

2.5. Effect of PBP on Antioxidant Enzymes and Pathway Proteins

CAT and SOD are important enzymes in the process of degrading hydrogen peroxide to protect the cells against oxidative damage. It was observed that the particular enzyme protein levels were significantly declined with the H_2O_2 treatment. The co-treatment of the PBP recovered the enzyme levels dose dependently overcoming the effect of H_2O_2 (Figure 4a,b). Further, the effect was examined in the Nrf2-Keap1 pathway proteins. The cytoplasm nuclear factor E2-related factor 2 (Nrf2) level was increased while Kelch-like ECH-associated protein 1 (Keap1) exhibited declining intensities. It was observed that PBP encouraged the Nrf2 protein expression and stabilized the Keap1 protein allowing successful translocation of Nrf2 to the nucleus (Figure 4c,d). Collectively, the results obtained suggested the potential of PBP to promote Nrf2 expression and nuclear translocation to induce transcription of antioxidant enzymes such as CAT and SOD.

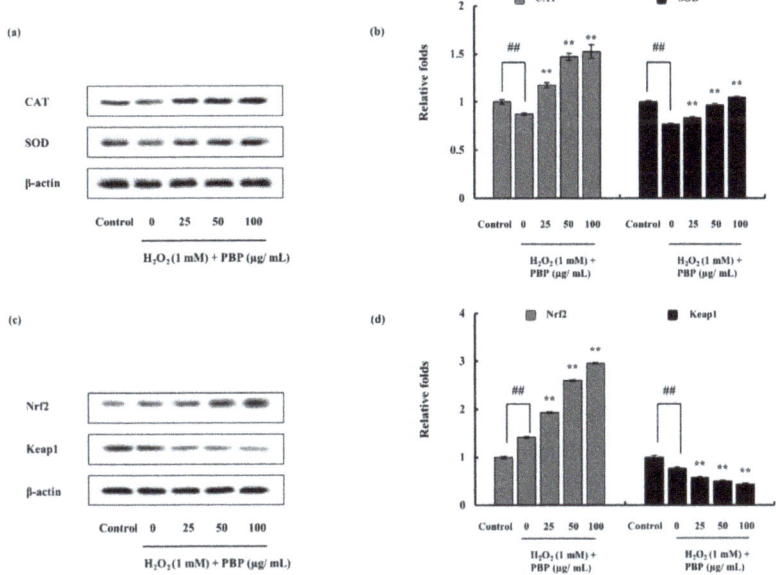

Figure 4. Effect of PBP on the H_2O_2 induced antioxidant related protein in Vero cells. (**a**) CAT and SOD, (**b**) relevant quantitative data, (**c**) Nrf2 and Keap1 in cytosol western blot, and (**d**) relevant quantitative data. β-actin was used as internal control. Quantification was assisted with the ImageJ software. Results are represented as mean ± SE; * $p < 0.05$, ** $p < 0.01$. (# denotes significance compared to control while * represents significance compared to H_2O_2 treated group).

2.6. Potential of PBP to Protect H_2O_2 Induced Zebrafish in Lipid Peroxidation, ROS Accumulation, and Cell Death

The survival rate and the heartbeat rate were recorded against the PBP treatment in H_2O_2 stimulated zebrafish (Figure 5). The ROS production in the zebrafish embryos treated with H_2O_2 was investigated by 2,7-dichlorofluorescein diacetate (DCF-DA). The results are interpreted as an indication of the fluorescence intensity. The H_2O_2 treated embryos expressed significantly high fluorescence intensity compared to the non-treated group. PBP pre-treated embryos exhibited a downregulation of fluorescence intensities dose dependently, subduing the effect generated via H_2O_2. This reflects the gradual decrement of ROS production, which implies PBPs' ability to work as a protective agent (Figure 6a,b). The amount of lipid peroxidation was measured using the diphenyl-1-pyrenylphosphine (DPPP) staining. Similarly, the results indicated a decline in the amount of lipid peroxidation with the PBP treatment, (Figure 6c,d). The cell death which was evaluated through the acridine orange staining exhibited the fluorescent intensities to be declined significantly in H_2O_2 induced zebrafish embryos with the PBP treatment (Figure 6e,f). The cell death percentage which was 290 in the H_2O_2 treated group was declined up to 170 with the PBP (100 μg/mL) treatment. These results reveal the prospective of PBP to act as a potent protector against H_2O_2 stimulated oxidative stress.

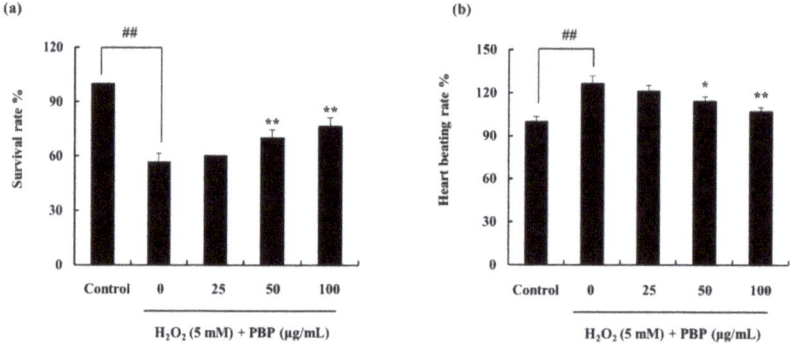

Figure 5. Embryos pre-treated with H_2O_2 (5 mM) and followed by PBP treatment (25, 50, 100 μg/mL). (**a**) survival rate, and (**b**) heart beating rate. Experimental procedure followed triplication and data indicated as mean ± SE; * $p < 0.05$, ** $p < 0.01$. (# denotes significance compared to control while * represents significance compared to H_2O_2 treated group).

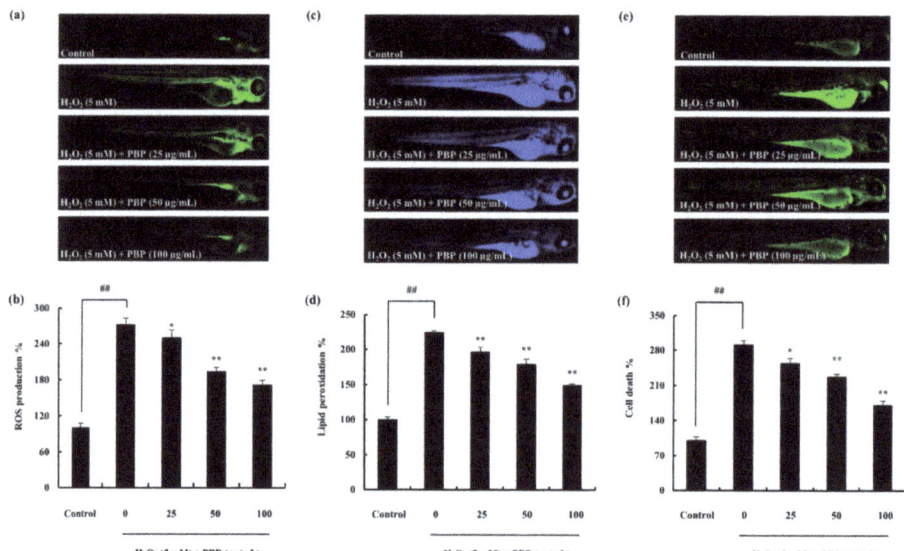

Figure 6. in vivo evaluation of antioxidant potential of PBP. (**a**) Hydrogen peroxide induced ROS production with DCF-DA staining, (**c**) Hydrogen peroxide-induced lipid peroxidation production stained with DPPP, (**e**) PBP protects zebrafish embryos against H_2O_2-induced death, stained with acridine orange and captured under fluorescence microscope. Quantitative results of each analysis are represented in (**b**), (**d**), and (**f**) respectively, measured via ImageJ software. Triplicated experiments were conducted and results are represented as mean ± SE; * $p < 0.05$, ** $p < 0.01$. (# denotes significance compared to control while * represents significance compared to H_2O_2 treated group).

3. Discussion

Marine organisms are reported to be immense sources of secondary metabolites that possess novel biological activities. These sources have proven to be useful in the treatment of diseases and hence be utilized prospectively in pharmacology and medicinal sectors [19]. The antioxidant activity of Hawaiian marine algae has been studied by Kelman et al. (2012), providing an extensive report on different marine algal species including red, brown, and green algae [20]. The sulfated polysaccharides from marine algae as a source of antioxidant secondary metabolite were reviewed by Wijesekara et al. (2011) [21]. Brown algae *Ecklonia cava* was reported as a source of antioxidant components further conducting its abilities in vitro scale. The secondary metabolite of interest; phlorotannin derivatives were reported to be exhibiting noteworthy antioxidant potential [22].

Padina is a genus of brown algae in which the thallus is calcified. The seaweed is fan shaped, widely distributed in warm tropical waters from lower intertidal to deep subtidal zones [23]. *Padina boryana*, in particular, has previously been studied by Sanjeewa et al. (2019), purifying fucoidan and evaluating its anti-inflammatory properties [24]. The structure of fucoidan was widely evaluated by Usoltseva et al. (2017) [25]. The species form the Maldives has not been deeply studied for its secondary metabolites specifically against antioxidant potentials. Hence, this study aimed to extract water soluble sulfated polysaccharide from the above under-explored brown algae and to investigate its antioxidant properties, specifically on the ethanol precipitation (PBP) which is rich in fucose.

Polysaccharides among other metabolites receive much attention due to their high availability, and diversified structure with vivid functional groups attached to its backbone [26]. Polysaccharides lack structural homogeneity. Fucoidan is one such polysaccharide containing fucose as its main component. Sulfate groups are substituted in the structure of fucose forming ester bonds. Fucoidan is unique due to its higher content of L-fucose and sulfate groups [27]. Different insertions into the backbone of the structure are also possible (mannose, glucose, and galactose). The point of sulfation and the degree of sulfation could be altered form one species to another. The bioactive properties of fucoidans prevail and increase due to the substitution of sulfate groups. One such report emphasized the action of the anionic sulfate group is that it enhances the nonspecific binding of proteins [28]. Hence, the potential of PBP is attributed to the higher degree of polysaccharide content and its sulfate substitution percentage. Another important component of crude polysaccharide is alginate. The chemical composition indicates higher polysaccharide yield in the PBP and sulfate content exhibits a similar trend. The yield of the polysaccharide is justifiable via the activity of celluclast enzyme to breakdown the cell wall. Furthermore, the dielectric constant of the solution is lowered by the addition of ethanol and polysaccharides are precipitated. The structural characterization of the PBP was supported by the FTIR analysis. The FTIR spectral data collectively revealed the correspondence of PBP to commercial fucoidan.

Previous literature reveals the potential of crude polysaccharides to act as antioxidants. The composition including its functional groups and monosaccharides are reported to synergistically induce the free radical scavenging activity [29,30]. Therefore, monosaccharide composition of the samples was analyzed and results indicate an increment in fucose and galactose contents. Higher values of fucose and galactose composition were available in PBP compared to PBE accrediting PBPs' elevated potential to act as an antioxidant.

DCF-DA assay was used in the evaluation of intracellular ROS scavenging activities. The stain is absorbed into the cells through the membrane and converted to DCFH, a non-fluorescent component, via the cellular esterases. Thus, intracellular ROS converts DCFH to fluorescent active DCF and detectable with a fluorimeter. Intracellular ROS levels were observed to be upregulated with H_2O_2 pre-treatment while treatment with PBP dose-dependently downregulated it. Furthermore, the protective effects of PBP against H_2O_2 were observed by cell viability analysis.

Oxidative stress is caused due to the presence of reactive oxygen species (ROS). Cellular metabolism and environmental factors contribute to the production of ROS. At moderate concentrations, ROS plays an important role in the function of physiological cell processes while high concentrations lead to adverse effects [31]. The highly reactive molecules damage cell structures including macromolecules thus alter the physiological functions. Moreover, the imbalance between the ROS and its counterpart antioxidants creates oxidative stress. Cell viability, proliferation rate, and further functions are affected by oxidative stress. Even though aerobic organisms possess integrated antioxidant systems, under pathological conditions these systems can be overwhelmed [3]. H_2O_2 is a distinct ROS species with physiological significance among others such as superoxide anion ($O_2^{-\bullet}$) and hydroxyl radical ($^\bullet OH$). H_2O_2 is produced in the cells upon phagocytosis due to the superoxide burst and converted. Xanthine oxidase, NAD(P)H oxidase, and amino acid oxidase contribute in the production of hydrogen peroxide [32]. In the presence of transition metal ions, H_2O_2 break down and result in OH^- and $^\bullet OH$ via the Fenton reaction [33]. Therefore, this study focuses on the stimulation via H_2O_2 under both in vivo and in vitro conditions.

The genetic material is modified by the ROS via different mechanisms involving DNA strand breakage, sugar moiety modifications, base unit degradation, deletions, and translocations [34]. Possible DNA modifications lead to carcinogenesis, aging, and numerous diseases. The effect was evaluated in the study via nuclear staining methods. It was evident the effect of H_2O_2 on the condensation and fragmentation of the nuclear material which was dose dependent and down regulated via the treatment of PBP.

Superoxide anion radicals are scavenged via SOD, while CAT plays an important role in the detoxification of the H_2O_2. Hence, these could eliminate free radicals and help the conversion of reactive toxic components to non-toxic elements and protect the live organelles from oxidative damage. The antioxidant enzymes were initially hampered by the excess ROS created via the effect of H_2O_2, though the potential of PBP recovered the enzyme expression hence reducing ROS production. Keap1 is an inhibitor protein, a cysteine-rich protein that is anchored to the actin cytoskeleton. It is responsible for the cytosolic sequestration of Nrf2 under physiological conditions. Keap1 promotes ubiquitination and degradation of Nrf2 under normal physiological conditions. Under stressful conditions in which the Nrf2-dependent cellular mechanism is active (electrophiles and oxidants are rich in this stage), the Nrf2 is rapidly released from Keap1. Dissociated Nrf2 is translocated to the nucleus and binds to antioxidant response element (ARE). Keap1 also receives redox information or environmental cues via its highly reactive cysteine residues and referred to as the sensor of the Nrf2-Keap1 system [35]. The dissociation of the system is a relatively rapid event. The breakdown of the system leads to Keap1 stabilization. Nrf2 also increases its half-life [36]. This allows successful nuclear translocation and cytoprotective gene transcription. A similar effect of antioxidant polysaccharides was reported by Zhou et al. (2019) [37].

The membrane lipid bilayer is disrupted via ROS stimulated lipid peroxidation thus membrane bound receptor activities are altered leading to increased tissue permeability [38]. Lipid peroxidation results in unsaturated aldehydes which are potent inactivators of cellular proteins through the formation of cross linkages [3]. The effect of ROS was evaluated in vivo scale using zebrafish. The ROS production levels examined via DCFDA fluorescent staining initially indicated the decline of intensities revealing the protective effect of PBP. Furthermore, DPPP staining exhibited the lipid peroxidation intensities to be upregulated under H_2O_2 stimulation and significant decline under PBP pre-treatment. The results confirmed the antioxidant potential of PBP against H_2O_2 induced oxidative stress. Thus, zebrafish cell death was successfully downregulated dose-dependently as indicated. The results obtained in the study well aligns with an earlier report on polysaccharide extracts from *Hizikia fusiforme* [39]. Furthermore, fucoidan purified from brown algae has incorporated zebrafish studies as an in vivo model [12,40].

Zebrafish involvement in developmental biology and drug discovery has been recognized and the implementation was advanced throughout the years. The size, husbandry, and early morphology is a distinct advantage of the usage of zebrafish over other vertebrate species. This provides researchers to minimize the costs in maintenance as well as in quantities of dosing samples, further in histological assessments [41]. High fertility including transparent embryos makes the species a valuable source [42]. Fluorescent staining methods implemented in the present study also support the above fact.

4. Material and Methods

4.1. Materials

African monkey kidney cell line (Vero) was purchased from the Korean cell line bank (KCLB, Seoul, Korea). Media for the cell line maintenance (Roswell Park Memorial Institute-1640; RPMI-1640) and serum (fetal bovine serum; FBS) including antibiotics (penicillin, streptomycin) were purchased from Gibco-BRL (Grand Island, NY, USA). 3-(4,5-dimethylthiazol-2-yl)-2,5-diphenyltetrazolium bromide (MTT), 1-diphenyl-2-picrylhydrazyl (DPPH), 2,2-azobis(2-amidinopropane) hydrochloride (AAPH), 5,5-dimethyl-1-pyrolin N-oxide (DMPO), and α-(4-Pyridyl-1-oxide)-N-tert-butylnitrone (POBN) were purchased from Sigma (St. Louis, MO, USA). H_2O_2 and $FeSO_4 \cdot 7H_2O$ used were purchased from Fluka Co. (Buchs, Switzerland). Furthermore, dimethyl sulfoxide (DMSO), 2,7-dichlorofluorescein diacetate (DCF-DA), and 2,2′-azino-bis(3-ethylbenzthiazoline)-6-sulfonic acid (ABTS) were obtained from Sigma-Aldrich (St. Louis, MO, USA).

4.2. Collection of Seaweed and Extraction

P. boryana samples were collected from the shores of Fulhadhoo Island (4.8849 °N, 72.9350 °E), the Maldives in January of 2018. Samples were immediately washed with running water to remove epiphytes and sand. Samples were then lyophilized and ground into powder. A sample portion (50 g) was added to 500 mL of distilled water. Optimal pH value was obtained via the addition of 1M of HCL. Celluclast assisted extraction was carried out in a period of 24 h under shaking kinetics with optimal conditions (pH 4.5, 50 °C). Following the extraction, the enzyme was inactivated via heating the mixture in 100 °C for 10 min. The filtrate was obtained and pH was brought back to neutral value. The sample was identified as enzymatic extract of *P. boryana* (PBE).

4.3. Crude Polysaccharide Preparation

The above enzymatic extract was mixed with 95% ethanol (1:3) and was maintained in 4 °C for >8 h period. The precipitate was polysaccharide from *P. boryana* and was designated as PBP.

4.4. Chemical Analysis

The chemical composition of both the PBE and PBP was analyzed using several methods. Official methods of analysis of the Association of Official Analytical Chemists (AOAC) was used to obtain the total polysaccharide content [43]. The polyphenol content was measured accordingly with the method described by Chandler and Dodds (1983) with minor modifications [44]. The sulfate content was evaluated by $BaCl_2$ gelation method [45].

Samples were hydrolyzed in 4M triflouroacetic acid (4 h, 100 °C). This was subjected to CarboPac PA1 cartridge column (4.5 × 50 mm) for separation and detected with an ED50 Dionex electrochemical detector (Dionex) concerning monosugar analysis [46].

The attenuated total reflectance Fourier transform infra-red (ATR-FTIR) spectrum was obtained with a Bruker FTIR, Alpha II (Bruker, Karlsruhe, Germany) instrument in the 400–4000 cm^{-1} wavenumber range. Commercial grade fucoidan was analyzed at the same time.

4.5. Radical Scavenging Activity Evaluation via Electron Spin Resonance (ESR) Spectrometer

Both PBE and PBP were analyzed for its radical scavenging activities. DPPH, alkyl, and hydroxyl radical scavenging activities were evaluated using electron spin resonance spectroscopy (ESR, JES-FA200; JEOL, Tokyo, Japan). The DPPH radical scavenging was assessed via the method defined by Nanjo et al. (1996) [47]. The method, in brief, equal volumes of sample and DPPH was mixed vigorously, transferred to a capillary tube and inserted to the ESR spectrometer for measurement.

Alkyl radical scavenging followed the method described by Hiramoto et al. (1993) [48]. The radical was generated via a reaction mixture of AAPH and 4-POBN with tested sample which was incubated in water bath (37 °C, 30 min) and subjected to analysis. The method explained by Finkelstein et al. (1980) was used in the evaluation of the hydroxyl radical scavenging potential [49]. This used the Fenton reaction as the basis and mixed sample in phosphate buffer solution (pH 7.4) with equal volumes of 0.3 M DMPO, 10 mM $FeSO_4$, and 10 mM H_2O_2 (200 µL) for analysis.

4.6. Chemical Assay for Hydrogen Peroxide

A colorimetric assay described by Kim et al. (2014) was implemented in the evaluation of the hydrogen peroxide scavenging [50]. The method in brief; each sample was mixed with 0.1 M phosphate buffer (pH 5.0, 100 µL) in a micro well plate. Hydrogen peroxide (20 µL) was added and was incubated (37 °C, 5 min). ABTS (1.25 mM, 30 µL) and peroxidase (1 unit/mL, 30 µL) was added to the above and further incubated at 37 °C for 10 min. The absorbance measurements were collected using an ELISA reader at 405 nm.

4.7. Protective Effects of PBP via In Vitro Methods

4.7.1. Cell Culture

RPMI-1640 medium supplemented with heat-inactivated FBS and antibiotics (penicillin and streptomycin) was used to culture the Vero cells. The cells were maintained in controlled environment (humidified, 5% CO_2). Periodic subculture was continued and cells were subjected to experiments at its exponential growth phase.

4.7.2. Cell Viability and Intracellular ROS Scavenging Activity in H_2O_2 Stimulated Vero Cells

Cells were seeded (1×10^5 cells/mL) and were incubated for 16 h, samples were treated and incubated for 1 h. Following the cells were stimulated with H_2O_2 (1 mM). The cell viability was measured given 24 h incubation time using the MTT assay [51]. The intracellular ROS scavenging potential of the samples was measured using the dichloro- fluorescein diacetate (DCF-DA) assay [52]. Initially, the cells were seeded (1×10^5 cells/mL), incubated and treated with different sample concentrations. Cells were stimulated with H_2O_2 given 1 h incubation time and DCF-DA (500 µg/mL, stock) was treated to each well. The results were detected as a fluorescence measurement (Ex-485 nm, Em-530 nm) with a microplate reader (BioTech, Winooski, VT, USA).

4.7.3. H_2O_2 Induced Cell Apoptosis through Nuclear Staining

The cells were seeded as explained above, treated with samples and was induced with H_2O_2. Following a 24 h incubation period, the cells were stained with cell permeable DNA dye Hoechst 33342 (10 µg/mL). Given 10 min incubation period, the cells were observed by a fluorescence microscope equipped with a CoolSNAP-Pro color digital camera (Olympus, Tokyo, Japan) [53,54].

4.7.4. Western Blot Analysis

Protein expression levels of catalase (CAT), superoxide dismutase (SOD), nuclear factor E2-related factor 2 (Nrf2), and Kelch-like ECH-associated protein 1 (Keap1) were analyzed via western blotting. Cells were seeded in 6 well culture plates and samples were treated given 24 h period, following 1 h incubation cells were stimulated with H_2O_2. Cells were harvested after complete incubation and lysed. Protein content was measured and standardized. Following electrophoresis, it was transferred on to nitrocellulose membranes. Blocked membranes (5% skim milk) were incubated with primary and secondary antibodies step wisely (Santa Cruz Biotechnology, Paso Robles, CA, USA). The bands were developed and photographed via a FUSION SOLO Vilber Lourmat system. ImageJ program was assisted in the quantification of the band intensities [55,56].

4.8. In Vivo Antioxidant Effects of PBP Using Zebrafish Model

4.8.1. Zebrafish Maintenance

Zebrafish in their adult stage were purchased from Seoul Aquarium, Korea. The fish were maintained in acrylic tanks under controlled conditions (28.5 °C, with a 14/10 h light/dark cycle). Fish were fed with tetramin flake, including live brine shrimp, three times per day in equal intervals for 6 days of the week. Natural spawning was stimulated with lights on conditions to obtain the embryos and completed collection within 30 min.

4.8.2. Polysaccharide Application to Zebrafish Embryos

The embryos were transferred to 12 well plates after 7–9 h post-fertilization (hpf). The embryos were maintained in an embryo medium. Samples were treated and incubated for 1 h and stimulated with H_2O_2 (5 mM) and continued incubation for 24 hpf. The live embryos were counted after 3 days of post-fertilization (dpf) to obtain the survival rate.

4.8.3. Intracellular ROS, Lipid Peroxidation, and Viability Analysis

At 2 days of post fertilization (dpf), the heartbeat rate was evaluated. Both the atrium and ventricle heartbeat rate was assessed under microscope for 1 min. The zebrafish were initially treated with sample and was induced with H_2O_2 [57].

DCF-DA was used to detect the intracellular ROS levels in the zebrafish embryos while lipid peroxidation was assessed via DPPP. Moreover, cell death was evaluated with acridine orange staining. Following each staining method, the embryos, zebrafish larvae were rinsed with embryo media and anaesthetized with 2-phenox ethanol. A microscope equipped with CoolSNAP-Pro color digital camera (Olympus, Tokyo, Japan) was assisted in observation and photography. The intensity quantification was completed with the ImageJ program [58].

4.9. Statistical Analysis

The experiments were triplicated and expressed data as the mean ± standard error (SE). One-way ANOVA was implemented in the comparison of mean values. Significance among the treatments were evaluated by Student's t-test ($p < 0.05$, $p < 0.01$).

5. Conclusions

This study evaluated sulfated polysaccharide from marine brown alga *P. boryana* ethanol precipitation (PBP) as a source of natural antioxidants. Preliminary chemical characterization revealed its composition and the contribution of sulfate content, fucose, and galactose towards the bioactive properties. Results suggest the ability of PBP to protect ROS mediated cell damage and to inhibit oxidative stress in zebrafish. The increased antioxidant pathway protein expression of Nrf2 and its resulting CAT, SOD protein levels accompanied the effect of PBP. Hence, PBP is a potential source of antioxidants that could be successfully utilized in healthy functional and cosmeceutical sectors.

Author Contributions: Conceived and designed the experiments: Y.-J.J.; Performed the experiments: L.W., T.U.J.; Analyzed data: L.W., T.U.J.; Contributed reagents/materials/analysis tools: K.K.A.S., S.I.K., J.-S.L.; Wrote the paper: T.U.J. All authors have read and agreed to the published version of the manuscript.

Funding: This research was financially supported by a grant from the "Marine Biotechnology program—20170488", funded by the Ministry of Oceans and Fisheries, Korea.

Acknowledgments: This research was financially supported by a grant from the "Marine Biotechnology program—20170488", funded by the Ministry of Oceans and Fisheries, Korea.

Conflicts of Interest: The authors declare to possess no competing interests.

References

1. Schieber, M.; Chandel, N.S. ROS function in redox signaling and oxidative stress. *Curr. Biol.* **2014**, *24*, R453–R462. [CrossRef]
2. Finkel, T. Signal transduction by reactive oxygen species. *J. Cell Biol.* **2011**, *194*, 7–15. [CrossRef] [PubMed]
3. Birben, E.; Sahiner, U.M.; Sackesen, C.; Erzurum, S.; Kalayci, O. Oxidative stress and antioxidant defense. *World Allergy Organ. J.* **2012**, *5*, 9–19. [CrossRef] [PubMed]
4. Kang, M.C.; Kim, S.Y.; Kim, Y.T.; Kim, E.A.; Lee, S.H.; Ko, S.C.; Wijesinghe, W.A.; Samarakoon, K.W.; Kim, Y.S.; Cho, J.H.; et al. In vitro and in vivo antioxidant activities of polysaccharide purified from aloe vera (*Aloe barbadensis*) gel. *Carbohydr. Polym.* **2014**, *99*, 365–371. [CrossRef] [PubMed]
5. Chew, Y.L.; Lim, Y.Y.; Omar, M.; Khoo, K.S. Antioxidant activity of three edible seaweeds from two areas in South East Asia. *LWT - Food Sci. Technol.* **2008**, *41*, 1067–1072. [CrossRef]
6. Chanda, S.; Dave, R.; Kaneria, M.; Nagani, K. Seaweeds: A novel, untapped source of drugs from sea to combat infectious diseases. *Curr. Res. Technol. Educ. Top. Appl. Microbiol. Microb. Biotech.* **2010**, *1*, 473–480.
7. Ponnanikajamideen, M.; Malini, M.; Malarkodi, C.; Rajeshkumar, S. Bioactivity and phytochemical constituents of marine brown seaweed (*Padina tetrastromatica*) extract from various organic solvents. *Int. J. Pharm. Ther.* **2014**, *5*, 108–112.
8. Magdel-Din Hussein, M.; Abdel-Aziz, A.; Mohamed Salem, H. Some structural features of a new sulphated heteropolysaccharide from Padina pavonia. *Phytochemistry* **1980**, *19*, 2133–2135. [CrossRef]
9. Magdel-Din Hussein, M.; Abdel-Aziz, A.; Mohamed Salem, H. Sulphated heteropolysaccharides from Padina pavonia. *Phytochemistry* **1980**, *19*, 2131–2132. [CrossRef]
10. Fayad, S.; Nehme, R.; Tannoury, M.; Lesellier, E.; Pichon, C.; Morin, P. Macroalga Padina pavonica water extracts obtained by pressurized liquid extraction and microwave-assisted extraction inhibit hyaluronidase activity as shown by capillary electrophoresis. *J. Chromatogr. A* **2017**, *1497*, 19–27. [CrossRef]
11. Ananthi, S.; Raghavendran, H.R.; Sunil, A.G.; Gayathri, V.; Ramakrishnan, G.; Vasanthi, H.R. In vitro antioxidant and in vivo anti-inflammatory potential of crude polysaccharide from *Turbinaria ornata* (Marine Brown Alga). *Food Chem. Toxicol.* **2010**, *48*, 187–192. [CrossRef] [PubMed]
12. Jayawardena, T.U.; Fernando, I.P.S.; Lee, W.W.; Sanjeewa, K.K.A.; Kim, H.S.; Lee, D.S.; Jeon, Y.J. Isolation and purification of fucoidan fraction in *Turbinaria ornata* from the Maldives; Inflammation inhibitory potential under LPS stimulated conditions in in-vitro and in-vivo models. *Int. J. Biol. Macromol.* **2019**, *131*, 614–623. [CrossRef] [PubMed]
13. Athukorala, Y.; Lee, K.W.; Kim, S.K.; Jeon, Y.J. Anticoagulant activity of marine green and brown algae collected from Jeju Island in Korea. *Bioresour. Technol.* **2007**, *98*, 1711–1716. [CrossRef] [PubMed]
14. Athukorala, Y.; Kim, K.N.; Jeon, Y.J. Antiproliferative and antioxidant properties of an enzymatic hydrolysate from brown alga, Ecklonia cava. *Food Chem. Toxicol.* **2006**, *44*, 1065–1074. [CrossRef]
15. Marais, M.F.; Joseleau, J.P. A fucoidan fraction from Ascophyllum nodosum. *Carbohydr. Res.* **2001**, *336*, 155–159. [CrossRef]
16. Lim, S.J.; Wan Aida, W.M.; Maskat, M.Y.; Mamot, S.; Ropien, J.; Mazita Mohd, D. Isolation and antioxidant capacity of fucoidan from selected Malaysian seaweeds. *Food Hydrocoll.* **2014**, *42*, 280–288. [CrossRef]
17. Hemnani, T.; Parihar, M.S. Reactive oxygen species and oxidative DNA damage. *Indian J. Physiol. Pharmacol.* **1998**, *42*, 440–452.
18. Ahn, G.; Lee, W.; Kim, K.N.; Lee, J.H.; Heo, S.J.; Kang, N.; Lee, S.H.; Ahn, C.B.; Jeon, Y.J. A sulfated polysaccharide of Ecklonia cava inhibits the growth of colon cancer cells by inducing apoptosis. *EXCLI J.* **2015**, *14*, 294–306.
19. Takamatsu, S.; Hodges, T.W.; Rajbhandari, I.; Gerwick, W.H.; Hamann, M.T.; Nagle, D.G. Marine natural products as novel antioxidant prototypes. *J. Nat. Prod.* **2003**, *66*, 605–608. [CrossRef]
20. Kelman, D.; Posner, E.K.; McDermid, K.J.; Tabandera, N.K.; Wright, P.R.; Wright, A.D. Antioxidant activity of Hawaiian marine algae. *Mar. Drugs* **2012**, *10*, 403–416. [CrossRef]
21. Wijesekara, I.; Pangestuti, R.; Kim, S.-K. Biological activities and potential health benefits of sulfated polysaccharides derived from marine algae. *Carbohydr. Polym.* **2011**, *84*, 14–21. [CrossRef]
22. Li, Y.; Qian, Z.J.; Ryu, B.; Lee, S.H.; Kim, M.M.; Kim, S.K. Chemical components and its antioxidant properties in vitro: An edible marine brown alga, Ecklonia cava. *Bioorg. Med. Chem.* **2009**, *17*, 1963–1973. [CrossRef] [PubMed]

23. Win, N.N.; Hanyuda, T.; Arai, S.; Uchimura, M.; Prathep, A.; Draisma, S.G.; Phang, S.M.; Abbott, I.A.; Millar, A.J.; Kawai, H. A Taxonomic Study of the Genus Padina (Dictyotales, Phaeophyceae) Including the Descriptions of Four New Species from Japan, Hawaii, and the Andaman Sea(1). *J. Phycol.* **2011**, *47*, 1193–1209. [CrossRef] [PubMed]
24. Asanka Sanjeewa, K.K.; Jayawardena, T.U.; Kim, H.S.; Kim, S.Y.; Shanura Fernando, I.P.; Wang, L.; Abetunga, D.T.U.; Kim, W.S.; Lee, D.S.; Jeon, Y.J. Fucoidan isolated from Padina commersonii inhibit LPS-induced inflammation in macrophages blocking TLR/NF-kappaB signal pathway. *Carbohydr. Polym.* **2019**, *224*, 115195. [CrossRef]
25. Usoltseva, R.V.; Anastyuk, S.D.; Ishina, I.A.; Isakov, V.V.; Zvyagintseva, T.N.; Thinh, P.D.; Zadorozhny, P.A.; Dmitrenok, P.S.; Ermakova, S.P. Structural characteristics and anticancer activity in vitro of fucoidan from brown alga Padina boryana. *Carbohydr. Polym.* **2018**, *184*, 260–268. [CrossRef]
26. Fernando, I.P.S.; Sanjeewa, K.K.A.; Samarakoon, K.W.; Lee, W.W.; Kim, H.-S.; Kim, E.-A.; Gunasekara, U.K.D.S.S.; Abeytunga, D.T.U.; Nanayakkara, C.; De Silva, E.D.; et al. FTIR characterization and antioxidant activity of water soluble crude polysaccharides of Sri Lankan marine algae. *Algae* **2017**, *32*, 75–86. [CrossRef]
27. Li, B.; Lu, F.; Wei, X.; Zhao, R. Fucoidan: Structure and bioactivity. *Molecules* **2008**, *13*, 1671–1695. [CrossRef]
28. Mulloy, B. The specificity of interactions between proteins and sulfated polysaccharides. *An. Acad. Bras. Cienc.* **2005**, *77*, 651–664. [CrossRef]
29. Chen, Y.; Xie, M.-Y.; Nie, S.-P.; Li, C.; Wang, Y.-X. Purification, composition analysis and antioxidant activity of a polysaccharide from the fruiting bodies of Ganoderma atrum. *Food Chem.* **2008**, *107*, 231–241. [CrossRef]
30. Lo, T.C.-T.; Chang, C.A.; Chiu, K.-H.; Tsay, P.-K.; Jen, J.-F. Correlation evaluation of antioxidant properties on the monosaccharide components and glycosyl linkages of polysaccharide with different measuring methods. *Carbohydr. Polym.* **2011**, *86*, 320–327. [CrossRef]
31. Valko, M.; Rhodes, C.J.; Moncol, J.; Izakovic, M.; Mazur, M. Free radicals, metals and antioxidants in oxidative stress-induced cancer. *Chem. Biol. Interact.* **2006**, *160*, 1–40. [CrossRef] [PubMed]
32. Dupuy, C.; Virion, A.; Ohayon, R.; Kaniewski, J.; Deme, D.; Pommier, J. Mechanism of hydrogen peroxide formation catalyzed by NADPH oxidase in thyroid plasma membrane. *J. Biol. Chem.* **1991**, *266*, 3739–3743. [PubMed]
33. Winterbourn, C.C. Toxicity of iron and hydrogen peroxide: The Fenton reaction. *Toxicol. Lett.* **1995**, *82–83*, 969–974. [CrossRef]
34. Sallmyr, A.; Fan, J.; Rassool, F.V. Genomic instability in myeloid malignancies: Increased reactive oxygen species (ROS), DNA double strand breaks (DSBs) and error-prone repair. *Cancer Lett.* **2008**, *270*, 1–9. [CrossRef] [PubMed]
35. Loboda, A.; Damulewicz, M.; Pyza, E.; Jozkowicz, A.; Dulak, J. Role of Nrf2/HO-1 system in development, oxidative stress response and diseases: An evolutionarily conserved mechanism. *Cell Mol. Life Sci.* **2016**, *73*, 3221–3247. [CrossRef] [PubMed]
36. Canning, P.; Sorrell, F.J.; Bullock, A.N. Structural basis of Keap1 interactions with Nrf2. *Free Radic. Biol. Med.* **2015**, *88*, 101–107. [CrossRef]
37. Zhou, T.Y.; Xiang, X.W.; Du, M.; Zhang, L.F.; Cheng, N.X.; Liu, X.L.; Zheng, B.; Wen, Z.S. Protective effect of polysaccharides of sea cucumber Acaudina leucoprocta on hydrogen peroxide-induced oxidative injury in RAW264.7 cells. *Int. J. Biol. Macromol.* **2019**, *139*, 1133–1140. [CrossRef]
38. Dhindsa, R.S.; Plumb-Dhindsa, P.; Thorpe, T.A. Leaf Senescence: Correlated with Increased Levels of Membrane Permeability and Lipid Peroxidation, and Decreased Levels of Superoxide Dismutase and Catalase. *J. Exp. Bot.* **1981**, *32*, 93–101. [CrossRef]
39. Wang, L.; Oh, J.Y.; Kim, H.S.; Lee, W.; Cui, Y.; Lee, H.G.; Kim, Y.-T.; Ko, J.Y.; Jeon, Y.-J. Protective effect of polysaccharides from Celluclast-assisted extract of Hizikia fusiforme against hydrogen peroxide-induced oxidative stress in vitro in Vero cells and in vivo in zebrafish. *Int. J. Biol. Macromol.* **2018**, *112*, 483–489. [CrossRef]
40. Fernando, I.P.S.; Sanjeewa, K.K.A.; Samarakoon, K.W.; Lee, W.W.; Kim, H.-S.; Kang, N.; Ranasinghe, P.; Lee, H.-S.; Jeon, Y.-J. A fucoidan fraction purified from Chnoospora minima: A potential inhibitor of LPS-induced inflammatory responses. *Int. J. Biol. Macromol.* **2017**, *104*, 1185–1193. [CrossRef]
41. Hill, A.J.; Howard, C.V.; Cossins, A.R. Efficient embedding technique for preparing small specimens for stereological volume estimation: Zebrafish larvae. *J. Microsc.* **2002**, *206*, 179–181. [CrossRef] [PubMed]

42. Hill, A.J.; Teraoka, H.; Heideman, W.; Peterson, R.E. Zebrafish as a model vertebrate for investigating chemical toxicity. *Toxicol. Sci.* **2005**, *86*, 6–19. [CrossRef] [PubMed]
43. Cunniff, P. Official methods of analysis of the Association of Official Analytical Chemists International. *Arlingt. AOAC Int.* **1995**, *11*, 6–7.
44. Chandler, S.F.; Dodds, J.H. The effect of phosphate, nitrogen and sucrose on the production of phenolics and solasodine in callus cultures of solanum laciniatum. *Plant. Cell. Rep.* **1983**, *2*, 205–208. [CrossRef]
45. Dodgson, K.S.; Price, R.G. A note on the determination of the ester sulphate content of sulphated polysaccharides. *Biochem. J.* **1962**, *84*, 106–110. [CrossRef]
46. Sanjeewa, K.K.A.; Fernando, I.P.S.; Kim, S.Y.; Kim, H.S.; Ahn, G.; Jee, Y.; Jeon, Y.J. In vitro and in vivo anti-inflammatory activities of high molecular weight sulfated polysaccharide; containing fucose separated from Sargassum horneri: Short communication. *Int. J. Biol. Macromol.* **2018**, *107*, 803–807. [CrossRef]
47. Nanjo, F.; Goto, K.; Seto, R.; Suzuki, M.; Sakai, M.; Hara, Y. Scavenging effects of tea catechins and their derivatives on 1,1-diphenyl-2-picrylhydrazyl radical. *Free Radic. Res. Commun.* **1996**, *21*, 895–902. [CrossRef]
48. Hiramoto, K.; Johkoh, H.; Sako, K.; Kikugawa, K. DNA breaking activity of the carbon-centered radical generated from 2,2′-azobis(2-amidinopropane) hydrochloride (AAPH). *Free Radic. Res. Commun.* **1993**, *19*, 323–332. [CrossRef]
49. Finkelstein, E.; Rosen, G.M.; Rauckman, E.J. Spin trapping of superoxide and hydroxyl radical: Practical aspects. *Arch. Biochem. Biophys.* **1980**, *200*, 1–16. [CrossRef]
50. Kim, H.-S.; Zhang, C.; Lee, J.-H.; Ko, J.-Y.; Kim, E.-A.; Kang, N.; Jeon, Y.-J. Evaluation of the Biological Activities of Marine Bacteria Collected from Jeju Island, Korea, and Isolation of Active Compounds from their Secondary Metabolites. *Fish. Aquat. Sci.* **2014**, *17*, 215–222. [CrossRef]
51. Samarakoon, K.W.; Ko, J.-Y.; Shah, M.M.R.; Lee, J.-H.; Kang, M.-C.; Kwon, O.N.; Lee, J.-B.; Jeon, Y.-J. In vitro studies of anti-inflammatory and anticancer activities of organic solvent extracts from cultured marine microalgae. *Algae* **2013**, *28*, 111–119. [CrossRef]
52. Yang, X.; Kang, M.-C.; Lee, K.-W.; Kang, S.-M.; Lee, W.-W.; Jeon, Y.-J. Antioxidant activity and cell protective effect of loliolide isolated from *Sargassum ringgoldianum* subsp. coreanum. *Algae* **2011**, *26*, 201–208. [CrossRef]
53. Fernando, I.P.S.; Sanjeewa, K.K.A.; Kim, H.S.; Wang, L.; Lee, W.W.; Jeon, Y.J. Apoptotic and antiproliferative properties of 3beta-hydroxy-Delta5-steroidal congeners from a partially purified column fraction of Dendronephthya gigantea against HL-60 and MCF-7 cancer cells. *J. Appl. Toxicol.* **2018**, *38*, 527–536. [CrossRef] [PubMed]
54. Jayawardena, T.U.; Lee, W.W.; Fernando, I.P.S.; Sanjeewa, K.K.A.; Wang, L.; Lee, T.G.; Park, Y.J.; Ko, C.-I.; Jeon, Y.-J. Antiproliferative and apoptosis-inducing potential of 3β-hydroxy-Δ5-steroidal congeners purified from the soft coral Dendronephthya putteri. *J. Ocean. Limnol.* **2018**, *37*, 1382–1392. [CrossRef]
55. Jayawardena, T.U.; Kim, H.-S.; Sanjeewa, K.K.A.; Kim, S.-Y.; Rho, J.-R.; Jee, Y.; Ahn, G.; Jeon, Y.-J. Sargassum horneri and isolated 6-hydroxy-4,4,7a-trimethyl-5,6,7,7a-tetrahydrobenzofuran-2(4H)-one (HTT); LPS-induced inflammation attenuation via suppressing NF-κB, MAPK and oxidative stress through Nrf2/HO-1 pathways in RAW 264.7 macrophages. *Algal Res.* **2019**, *40*, 101513. [CrossRef]
56. Fernando, I.P.S.; Lee, W.W.; Jayawardena, T.U.; Kang, M.-C.; Ann, Y.-S.; Ko, C.-I.; Park, Y.J.; Jeon, Y.-J. 3β-Hydroxy-Δ5-steroidal congeners from a column fraction of Dendronephthya puetteri attenuate LPS-induced inflammatory responses in RAW 264.7 macrophages and zebrafish embryo model. *RSC Adv.* **2018**, *8*, 18626–18634. [CrossRef]
57. Ko, J.Y.; Kim, E.A.; Lee, J.H.; Kang, M.C.; Lee, J.S.; Kim, J.S.; Jung, W.K.; Jeon, Y.J. Protective effect of aquacultured flounder fish-derived peptide against oxidative stress in zebrafish. *Fish Shellfish Immunol.* **2014**, *36*, 320–323. [CrossRef]
58. Kim, E.A.; Lee, S.H.; Ko, C.I.; Cha, S.H.; Kang, M.C.; Kang, S.M.; Ko, S.C.; Lee, W.W.; Ko, J.Y.; Lee, J.H.; et al. Protective effect of fucoidan against AAPH-induced oxidative stress in zebrafish model. *Carbohydr. Polym.* **2014**, *102*, 185–191. [CrossRef]

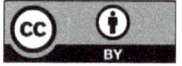

© 2020 by the authors. Licensee MDPI, Basel, Switzerland. This article is an open access article distributed under the terms and conditions of the Creative Commons Attribution (CC BY) license (http://creativecommons.org/licenses/by/4.0/).

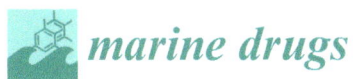

Article

Fucoidan Induces Apoptosis of HT-29 Cells via the Activation of DR4 and Mitochondrial Pathway

Xu Bai [1], Yu Wang [1], Bo Hu [1], Qi Cao [1], Maochen Xing [1], Shuliang Song [1,*] and Aiguo Ji [1,2,*]

[1] Marine College, Shandong University, Weihai 264209, China; 15634407267@163.com (X.B.); wy392191187@163.com (Y.W.); hobophar@163.com (B.H.); sddxcqq@163.com (Q.C.); sddxxmc@163.com (M.X.)
[2] School of Pharmaceutical Sciences, Shandong University, Jinan 250012, China
* Correspondence: songshuliang@sdu.edu.cn (S.S.); jiaiguo@sdu.edu.cn (A.J.)

Received: 23 March 2020; Accepted: 15 April 2020; Published: 20 April 2020

Abstract: Fucoidan has a variety of pharmacological activities, but the understanding of the mechanism of fucoidan-induced apoptosis of colorectal cancer cells remains limited. The results of the present study demonstrated that the JNK signaling pathway is involved in the activation of apoptosis in colorectal cancer-derived HT-29 cells, and fucoidan induces apoptosis by activation of the DR4 at the transcriptional and protein levels. The survival rate of HT-29 cells was approximately 40% in the presence of 800 µg/mL of fucoidan, but was increased to 70% after DR4 was silenced by siRNA. Additionally, fucoidan has been shown to reduce the mitochondrial membrane potential and destroy the integrity of mitochondrial membrane. In the presence of an inhibitor of cytochrome C inhibitor and DR4 siRNA or the presence of cytochrome C inhibitor only, the cell survival rate was significantly higher than when cells were treated with DR4 siRNA only. These data indicate that both the DR4 and the mitochondrial pathways contribute to fucoidan-induced apoptosis of HT-29 cells, and the extrinsic pathway is upstream of the intrinsic pathway. In conclusion, the current work identified the mechanism of fucoidan-induced apoptosis and provided a novel theoretical basis for the future development of clinical applications of fucoidan as a drug.

Keywords: fucoidan; apoptosis; DR4; mitochondrial pathway

1. Introduction

Fucoidan is a water-soluble heteropolysaccharide, derived mostly from brown algae, such as *Fucus vesiculosus* (Figure 1) [1–5]. Recent studies have shown that the research on fucoidan mainly focuses on two aspects—one is to explore ways to increase the yield of fucoidan [6–9], while the other is to explore the various pharmacological activities of fucoidan [10–12], including anti-inflammatory [13,14], anti-tumor, anti-virus, hypolipidemic, antithrombotic, and so on [15], but less research exists on its mechanism. Owing to the characteristics of high incidence and high mortality of tumor, the prevention and treatment of tumor has become a global research trend. Fucoidan can exert anti-tumor effects mainly by inducing apoptosis [16,17], arresting cell cycle [18], inhibiting cell migration [18–20], and so on.

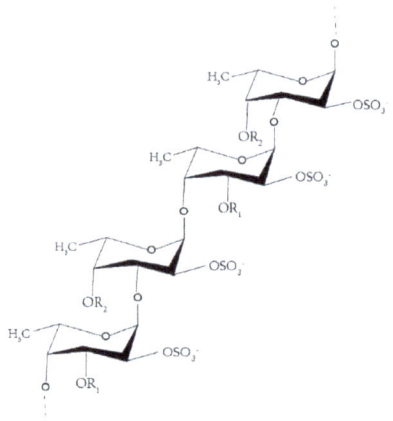

Figure 1. Fucoidan structure from *Fucus vesiculosus*.

Studies have shown that fucoidan can induce apoptosis [16]. There are two main apoptotic pathways currently studied. One is the extrinsic pathway, the death receptor pathway, which activates apopain in cells through extrinsic signal transduction [21]; the TRAIL receptor directly recruits procaspase-8, which is activated to form caspase-8, and then activates downstream effector molecules. The other is the intrinsic pathway [21,22], the mitochondrial pathway, where external stimulation leads to the enhancement of mitochondrial outer membrane permeability and apoptosis-related proteins in the mitochondrial inner. Moreover, outer membrane spaces, such as cytochrome C, form apoptosome with apaf-1; activate cascades; and further activate caspase -3, -6, and -7. Both ways can activate the downstream effector molecule caspase, which may lead to the activation of nuclease and the degradation of important proteins [23]. If the activated caspase-8 is sufficient, caspase-3 will be activated directly to induce cell apoptosis through the receptor; if the activated caspase-8 is insufficient, caspase-8 will activate the mitochondrial pathway [24,25]. In this study, the receptor of fucoidan in the process of inducing HT-29 cell apoptosis was determined at the level of gene and protein, determining that the extrinsic pathway was involved in the process of cell apoptosis; at the same time, it was found that fucoidan could affect the mitochondrial membrane potential and induce cell apoptosis through the mitochondrial pathway.

Apoptosis is usually mediated by a variety of signaling pathways, including NF-kB, PI3K, JNK, and so on [26–29]. The activation of JNK is stress-induced and plays an important role in the process including cell proliferation, differentiation, and tumor transformation.

In this study, we found that fucoidan can affect the migration, cycle, and apoptosis of HT-29 cells, and the effect of inducing apoptosis of HT-29 cells was the most significant. Thus, the purpose of this study was to explore the receptor and mechanism of fucoidan-induced apoptosis in HT-29 cells preliminarily. On one hand, it can lay a theoretical foundation for the application of fucoidan in dietary supplements and drugs; on the other hand, it can provide research support for the high-value development of kelp resources.

2. Results

2.1. Cytotoxicity of Fucoidan

Fucoidan administered at concentrations up to 800 µg/mL was not cytotoxic to human normal cell 293T cells (Figure 2A). However, fucoidan induced death of HeLa, MCF-7, and HT-29 cells in a dose-dependent manner (Figure 2B–D). The cytotoxic effect of fucoidan was most pronounced in HT-29 cells, with the cell survival rate of only approximately 40% at 800 µg/mL of the compound. Therefore, HT-29 cells and fucoidan concentrations of up to 800 µg/mL were selected for further experiments.

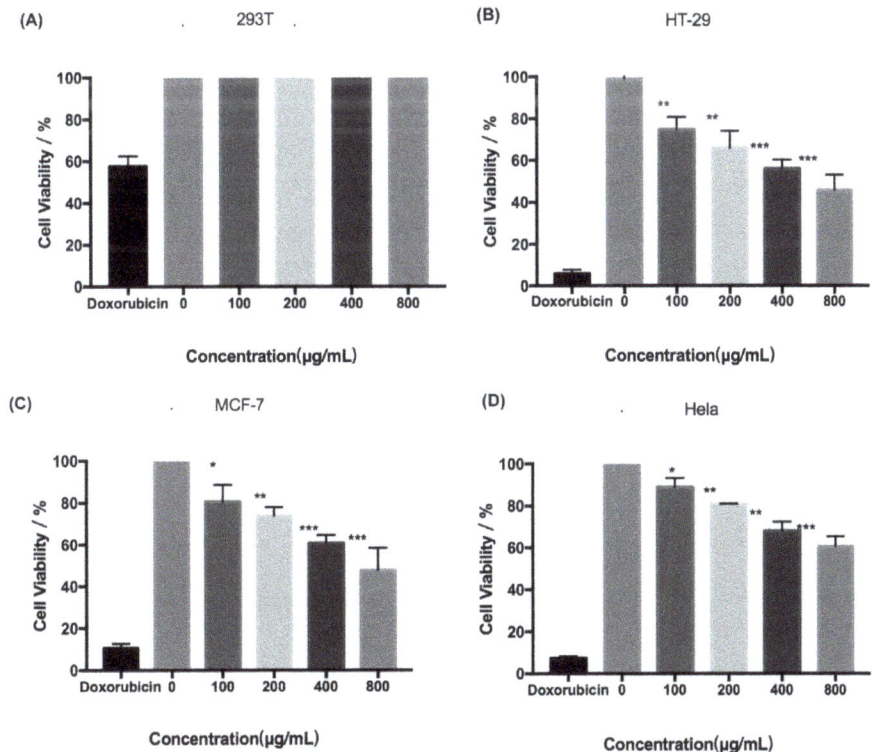

Figure 2. Cytotoxicity of fucoidan. (**A**) Toxicity of fucoidan to 293T cell is expressed as the means ± SD (n = 3). (**B**) Toxicity of fucoidan to HT-29 cells is expressed as the means ± SD (n = 3). (**C**) Toxicity of fucoidan to MCF-7 cell is expressed as the means ± SD (n = 3). (**D**) Toxicity of fucoidan to HeLa cell is expressed as the means ± SD (n = 3). *, $p < 0.05$; **, $p < 0.01$; ***, $p < 0.001$.

2.2. Pharmacological Activity of Fucoidan on HT-29 Cells

To explore the pharmacological effects of fucoidan on HT-29 cells, apoptosis, migration, and cell cycle were analyzed. We can find that the treatment increased the rate of apoptosis of HT-29 cells in a dose-dependent fashion, with 80% of the cells in the late stage of apoptosis at 800 µg/mL of fucoidan (Figure 3A,D). However, fucoidan blocked the cells in the G0/G1 phase of the cell cycle, with 50% of the cells in the G0/G1 phase of the cell cycle at 800 µg/mL of fucoidan, and the fraction of arrested cells increased with higher fucoidan concentrations (Figure 3B,E). Additionally, the migration of HT-29 cells tended to decrease with increasing fucoidan concentration and incubation time, but the reduction in migratory activity did not reach statistical significance, remaining at approximately 30% at 800 µg/mL (Figure 3C,F). These findings indicated that fucoidan affected apoptosis more significantly than migration and cell cycle.

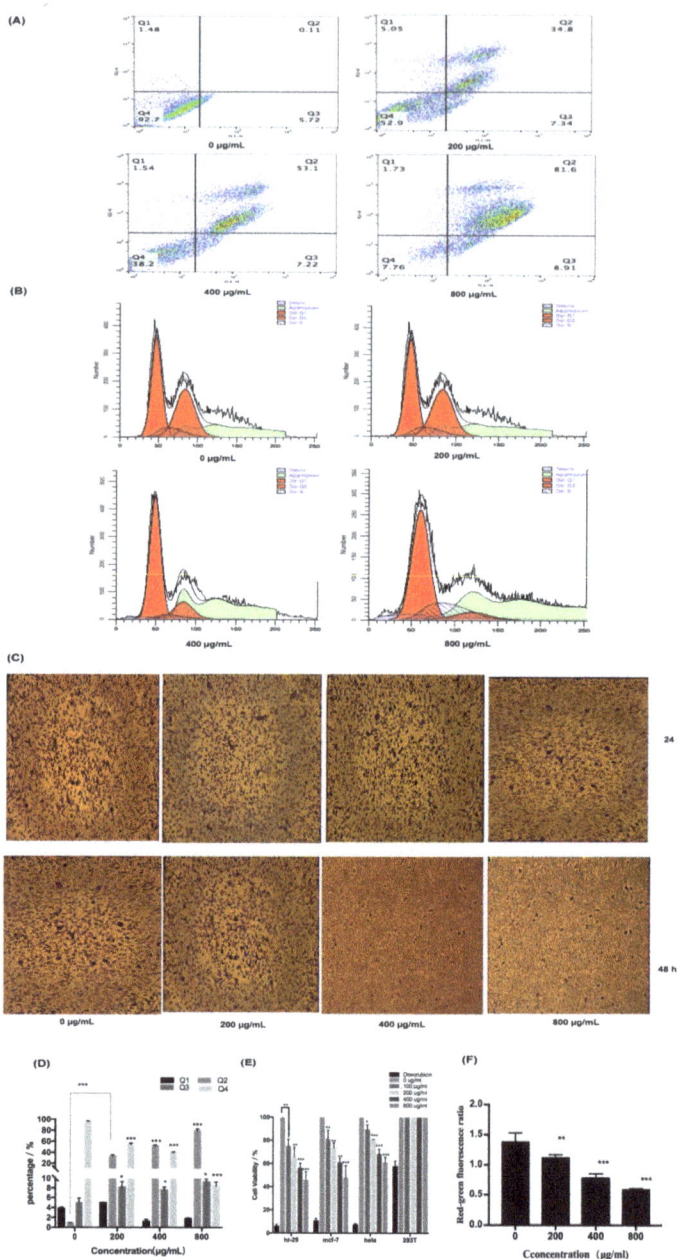

Figure 3. Pharmacological activity of fucoidan on cells. (**A**) Detection of apoptosis by flow cytometry. (**B**) Detection of cell cycle by flow cytometry. (**C**) Detection of cell migration. (**D**) Statistical results of apoptosis are expressed as the means ± SD (n = 3). (**E**) Statistical results of cell cycle are expressed as the means ± SD (n = 3). (**F**) Statistical results of cell migration are expressed as the means ± SD (n = 3). *, $p < 0.05$; **, $p < 0.01$; ***, $p < 0.001$.

2.3. Analysis of Fucoidan-Induced Apoptosis of HT-29 Cells

2.3.1. Fucoidan Can Induce Apoptosis Through the Extrinsic Pathway

To explore the involvement of receptors in the activation of apoptosis by fucoidan, the expression of DR4 and related proteins at the transcriptional and translational level was determined. All examined proteins, including DR4 and caspase-3, -6, and -9, were upregulated by fucoidan in a concentration-dependent manner (Figure 4A). The expression level of DR4 increased with the increase of fucoidan concentration at the gene level and the result demonstrated that DR4 was required for the induction of apoptosis by fucoidan (Figure 4B). To determine whether DR4 was required for the induction of apoptosis by fucoidan, siRNA was used to silence its expression, whose silence rate was about 65% (Figure 4C). However, although the expression of all examined proteins was suppressed in the presence of siRNA targeting DR4 (Figure 4D), these proteins did not decrease significantly with the increasing concentration in comparison, which may be because of DR4's low silence rate. However, DR4 silencing decreased the cytotoxicity of fucoidan (800 μg/mL) on HT-29 cells, resulting in an increase in the survival rate from 40% to 75% (Figure 4E). These results demonstrated that fucoidan can induce apoptosis of HT-29 cells by upregulating DR4.

2.3.2. Fucoidan Can Induce Apoptosis Through the Intrinsic Pathway

To determine whether the mitochondrial pathway can contribute to fucoidan-induced apoptosis of HT-29 cells, the changes in mitochondrial membrane potential were determined by the JC-1 probe, and the expression of cytochrome C protein was assessed by Western blotting. It can be seen that, with an increase in fucoidan concentration, the red-to-green ratio of JC-1 fluorescence decreased from 1.3 to 0.6, indicating a reduction in the inner mitochondrial membrane potential and an increase in its permeability (Figure 5A,B). Concurrently, cytochrome C was released from the mitochondria into the cytoplasm; this effect was also dependent on fucoidan concentration, and the ratio of cytochrome C expression in the experimental group to the control group was 1.56 at 800 μg/mL (Figure 5C). The release of cytochrome C initiated the caspase cascade, leading to apoptosis. These results showed that fucoidan activated not only the extrinsic pathway through surface death receptors, but also the intrinsic mitochondrial pathway-mediated apoptosis of HT-29 cells.

2.3.3. Relationship Between the Extrinsic and Intrinsic Pathways

Cells in this experiment were divided into three groups: the first group, cells treated with siRNA for DR4; the second group, cells treated with cytochrome C inhibitor; and the third group, cells treated simultaneously with cytochrome C inhibitor and DR4 siRNA. We can find that in cells treated only with DR4 siRNA at 800 μg/mL, the ratio of cytochrome C expression in the experimental group to the control group decreased from 1.56 to 1.32 (Figures 5C and 6A,B), and the cell survival rate was increased from 40% to about 75%(Figures 2B and 6C). When cells were treated only with the inhibitor of cytochrome C or treated simultaneously with cytochrome C inhibitor and DR4 siRNA, there was no significant difference in the ratio and cell survival rate between the second and third group. In the second and third group, it can be seen that the ratio decreased from 1.56 to 1.15 and 1.13 at 800 μg/mL, respectively (Figures 5C and 6D–H), both lower than the ratio after inhibiting the death receptor pathway; besides, at 800 μg/mL, the cell survival rate was increased from 40% to about 80% (Figures 2B and 6F,I), both higher than 75%.Therefore, the difference of cell survival rate and cytochrome C expression indicated that the mitochondrial pathway was downstream of the DR4 pathway.

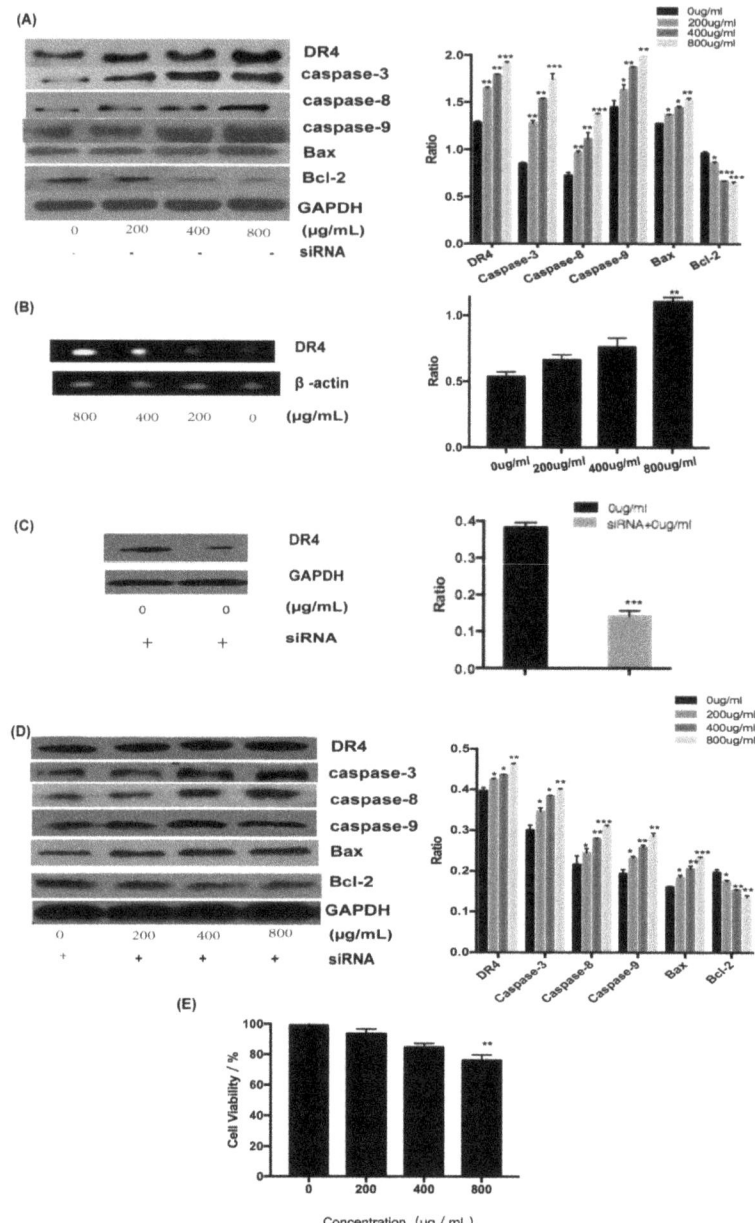

Figure 4. Fucoidan induced apoptosis through DR4. (**A**) Results of Western blotting of proteins. (**B**) Results of Reverse Transcription-Polymerase Chain Reaction (RT-PCR) with DR4. (**C**) Results of Western blotting of proteins with the silent DR4. (**D**) Expression of proteins after DR4 was silenced. (**E**) The toxicity of fucoidan to HT-29 cells with silent DR4 is expressed as the means ± SD (n = 3). *, $p < 0.05$; **, $p < 0.01$; ***, $p < 0.001$.

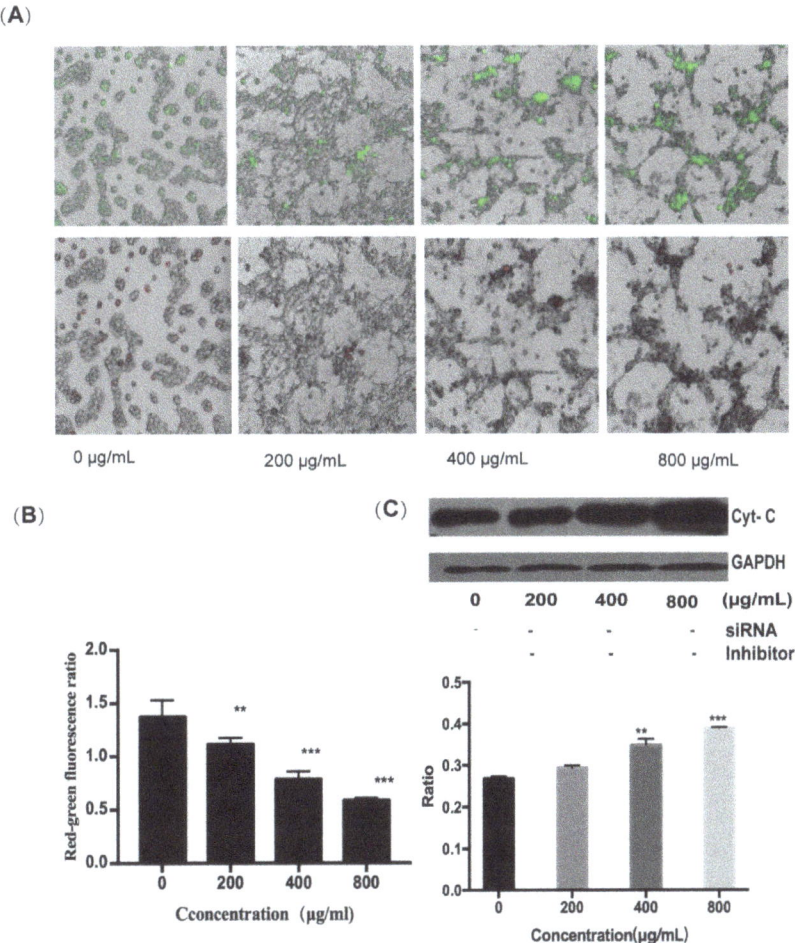

Figure 5. Changes of membrane potential induced by fucoidan in HT-29 cells. (**A**) Results of JC-1 staining. (**B**) Results of red-green fluorescence ratio. (**C**) Results of Western blotting of cytochrome C. **, $p < 0.01$; ***, $p < 0.001$.

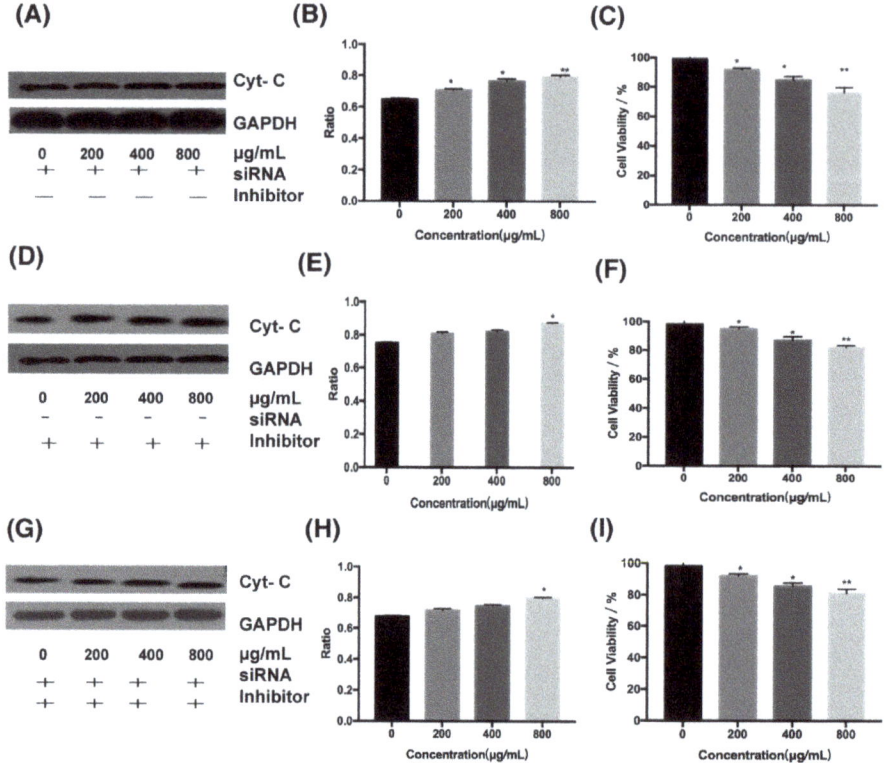

Figure 6. Effects of cytochrome C inhibitor on HT-29 cells. (**A**) Results of Western blotting of cytochrome C with the silent DR4. (**B**) Results of Western blotting of cytochrome C with cytochrome C inhibitor. (**C**) Results of Western blotting of cytochrome C with cytochrome C inhibitor and silent DR4. (**D**) Results of protein expression ratio at different concentrations with the silent DR4. (**E**) Results of protein expression ratio at different concentrations with cytochrome C inhibitor. (**F**) Results of protein expression ratio at different concentrations with cytochrome C inhibitor and silent DR4. (**G**) The toxicity of fucoidan to HT-29 cells with the silent DR4 is expressed as the means ± SD (n = 3). (**H**) The toxicity of fucoidan to HT-29 cells with cytochrome C inhibitor is expressed as the means ± SD (n = 3). (**I**) The toxicity of fucoidan to HT-29 cells with cytochrome C inhibitor and silent DR4 is expressed as the means ± SD (n = 3). *, $p < 0.05$; **, $p < 0.01$.

2.4. Effect of Fucoidan on the JNK Signaling Pathway in HT-29 Cells

The role of the JNK signal pathway in the induction of apoptosis in HT-29 cells was determined by RT-PCR and Western blotting. At the mRNA level, the expression of ras, raf, MEK1, MEK2, and JNK were upregulated with increasing concentrations of fucoidan (Figure 7A,B). Moreover, fucoidan increased the level of JNK protein and its phosphorylated form, P-JNK, in a dose-dependent fashion, as assessed by Western blot analysis (Figure 7C); the ratio of p-JNK/JNK increased from 2.9 to about 5.2 at 800 µg/mL (Figure 7D). Therefore, the JNK signaling pathway was essential for the activation of apoptosis of HT-29 cells by fucoidan.

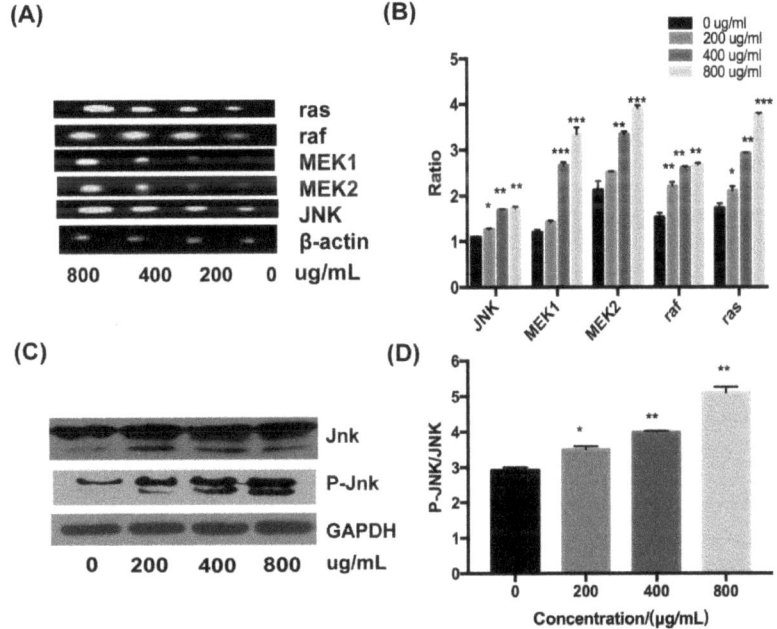

Figure 7. Effects of fucoidan on JNK signaling pathway in HT-29 cells. (**A**) Results of RT-PCR. (**B**) Ratio of related expression factors at mRNA level. (**C**) Results of Western blotting of related proteins. (**D**) Ratio of JNK to p-JNK. *, $p < 0.05$; **, $p < 0.01$; ***, $p < 0.001$.

3. Discussion

Cancer is the leading cause of death worldwide, and colorectal cancer has become a common type of cancer. Given the high incidence, morbidity, and mortality of colorectal cancer, significant research effort is focused on its prevention and treatment. The current work documented that fucoidan affects the migration, apoptosis, and cell cycle progression of colorectal cancer-derived HT-29 cells. Among these effects, the induction of apoptosis was the most potent one. Further analysis of the mechanisms implicated in triggering apoptosis indicated that fucoidan induced this process in HT-29 cells through simultaneous activation of the intrinsic and extrinsic pathways by the JNK signaling pathway.

In the presence of 800 µg/mL of fucoidan, the cell survival rate was approximately 40%, and the induction of apoptosis in HT-29 cells was accompanied by the increase in expression of DR4 at the mRNA and protein levels. After silencing DR4 with siRNA, the difference in the expression of DR4 gradually decreased after inhibiting the extrinsic pathway. Although the expression of the protein was not significantly different from that when DR4 is not silenced, the fraction of surviving cells increased from 40% to 75% at 800 µg/mL of fucoidan, further documenting the critical role DR4 played in the apoptosis of HT-29 cells. In addition, the red-to-green ratio of JC-1 fluorescence decreased from 1.3 to 0.6, suggesting that fucoidan can destroy mitochondrial membrane integrity. These changes triggered the intrinsic apoptotic pathway by the release of cytochrome C into the cytoplasm.

To explore the relationship between the intrinsic and extrinsic pathways, inhibitor of cytochrome C inhibitors and siRNA targeting DR4 siRNA were added. In this experiment, at 800 µg/mL, the cell survival rate was increased from 40% to about 75% when cells were treated only with DR4 siRNA. When the intrinsic pathway or both pathways were inhibited simultaneously, the cell survival rates were improved without significant differences, both from 40% to about 80%, which were higher than the cell survival rates after inhibiting the extrinsic pathway. In addition, the difference in the expression of cytochrome C gradually decreased after inhibiting the extrinsic pathway; the ratio of the expression of cytochrome C in the experimental group to that of the control group decreased from 1.56 to 1.32 at the concentration of 800 μg/mL. When the intrinsic pathway or both pathways were inhibited simultaneously, the difference in cytochrome C expression was significantly reduced without significant differences, and the ratio decreased from 1.56 to 1.15 and 1.13, respectively, at 800 μg/mL, both lower than the ratio after inhibiting the extrinsic pathway. Therefore, the ratios of cytochrome C expression and cell survival after inhibiting the intrinsic pathway were similar to those after inhibiting both pathways, which were different from those after inhibiting the extrinsic pathway, indicating that the intrinsic pathway was in the downstream of the extrinsic pathway.

It was established that fucoidan inhibited the proliferation activity of HT-29 cells through simultaneous activation of the intrinsic and extrinsic pathways by the JNK signaling pathway, and the intrinsic pathway was downstream of the extrinsic pathway. However, there was still much controversy about whether the intrinsic and extrinsic pathways played an important role in inducing apoptosis in HT-29 cells owing to the lack of untransfected control within the same experiment, which must be improved in order to get more convincing results. In addition, a study showed that the cell survival rate was only approximately 80% with cells treated with cytochrome C inhibitor or with cytochrome C inhibitor and DR4 siRNA simultaneously; not all cells survived. On one hand, the silencing of DR4 or inhibition of the expression of cytochrome C could not be completed; on the other hand, fucoidan can play other roles besides inducing apoptosis, such as fucoidan significantly blocking the cell cycle, while inducing apoptosis with the increase in concentration. Therefore, future studies should address the impact of fucoidan on both apoptosis and cycle of HT-29 cells. These studies may reveal the inevitable connection between cell cycle and apoptosis and further clarify the mechanism of the induction of HT-29 cell death by fucoidan.

4. Materials and Methods

4.1. Materials

HT-29, MCF-7, Hela, and 293T cells were purchased from Kunming Institute of Zoology, Chinese Academy of Sciences Kunming Cell Bank; Dulbecco's minimum essential medium (DMEM) was purchased from GE Healthcare HyClone, USA; trypsin was purchased from Invitrogen, US; penicillin and streptomycin were purchased from Invitrogn, USA; Methylthiazolyldiphenyl-tetrazolium bromide (MTT) was purchased from Beyotime Biotechnology, China; Ddimethylsulphoxide (DMSO) was purchased from Sigma-Aldrich, USA; fucoidan from *F. vesiculosus* was provided by Shandong University, where the average molecular weight of fucoidan is about 1300 kDa, as analyzed by size exclusion chromatography (fucose content is about 80%, galactose is about 9%, glucuronic acid is about 7%, glucose is about 2%, xylose is about 1%, and rhamnose is about 1%, which were detected by high performance liquid chromatography (HPLC) after acid hydrolysis) [30,31]; Cytochrome C inhibitor was purchased from abcam, UK; cell cycle and apoptosis analysis kit was purchased from Beyotime, China; mitochondrial membrane potential assay kit with JC-1 was purchased from Beyotime, China; Transwell chamber (8.0 μm) was purchased from corning, USA; primary antibodies against Bcl-2 (product number: AB112), BAX (product number: AB026), P-JNK/SAPK (product number: AJ516), JNK/SAPK (product number: AJ518), caspase-8 (product number: AC056), caspase-9 (product number: AC062), GAPDH (product number: AG019), and cytochrome C (product number: AC909) were purchased from Beyotime, China; primary antibodies against DR4 (product number: 24063-1-AP) and caspase-3 (product number: 66470-2-Ig) were purchased from Proteintech, USA; horseradish peroxidase-conjugated anti-rabbit (product number: A0208) and anti-mouse (product number: A0216) secondary antibodies were purchased from Beyotime, China; diluent was purchased from Beyotime, China; siRNA (DR4) was purchased from Sangon Biotech, China; Lipo8000 transfection reagent was purchased from Beyotime, China; PCR primer was purchased from Sangon Biotech, China; revert aid first strand cDNA synthesis kit was purchased from ThermoFisher, USA; and dream taq green PCR master mix (2X) was purchased from ThermoFisher, USA.

4.2. Cell Culture

Colon cancer cell line (HT-29), breast cancer cell line (MCF-7), cervical cancer cell line (HeLa), and renal epithelial cell line (293T) were cultured in DMEM medium supplemented with 20% (v/v) fetal bovine serum (FBS) and 1% (v/v) antibiotics. The cells were incubated in a 5% CO_2 incubator at 37 °C.

4.3. MTT Assay for Cell Viability

The cytotoxicity of fucoidan toward HT-29, Hela, MCF-7, and 293T cells was determined using the MTT assay. The cells were seeded in a 96-well plate (6×10^3 cells/well), and fucoidan (0, 100, 200, 400, and 800 μg/mL) was added after 24 h, Doxorubicin, 5 μg/mL, was used as a positive control. After incubation for 48 h, a 10 μL aliquot of MTT solution (5 mg/mL) was added to each well, and the cells were incubated for an additional 4 h. The medium was then aspirated, 100 μL of DMSO was added to each well, and the plates were vortexed for 3 min until thoroughly mixed. The absorbance of each well was measured at a wavelength of 490 nm using a microplate reader (Sunrise, Tecan, Austria).

4.4. Cell Cycle Analysis

After treatment with fucoidan, the cells were harvested with trypsin and washed twice with cold phosphate buffer saline (PBS). Subsequently, the cell nuclei were stained using the cell cycle and apoptosis analysis kit following the manufacturer's instructions. The cells were analyzed by flow cytometry and the relative DNA content was determined using the Modfit software (5.0.9., Verity, Topsham, VT, USA).

4.5. Cell Migration Assay

For cell migration assay, HT-29 cells were grown to 80% confluence, harvested, and seeded in 24-well Transwell plates with 8 μm pores at the density of 5×10^4 cells/well. DMEM containing 10% FBS was added to the lower chamber. After 24 h, 0, 200, 400, and 800 μg/mL of fucoidan was added to the upper chamber, and the cells were cultured for 24 h and 48 h, respectively. At the end of incubation, cells were stained with crystal violet, photographed, and counted under an inverted microscope (DM100FL, Leica, Germany).

4.6. Quantification of Apoptosis with the Annexin V/Propidium Iodide Assay

Cells in log-phase growth were seeded in six-well plates at a density of 1×10^5 cells/well. After 24 h, 0, 200, 400, and 800 μg/mL of fucoidan was added and the cultures were incubated for 48 h. The cells were then harvested, washed, and resuspended in the binding buffer containing Annexin V and propidium iodide (PI). After incubation for 15 min at room temperature, the stained cells were analyzed by flow cytometry. Data were analyzed using FlowJo software (10.0.7., BD, Franklin, NJ, USA).

4.7. Total RNA Extraction and Reverse Transcription-Polymerase Chain Reaction

RNA was isolated and reverse-transcribed into cDNA using the revert aid first strand cDNA synthesis kit, according to the manufacturer's protocol. For PCR, the cDNA was mixed with forward and reverse primers (for the list of primers, see Table 1) and dream taq green PCR master mix (2x). The amplification included 30 cycles of denaturation for 30 s at 95 °C, annealing for 30 s at 57 °C, and elongation for 30 s at 72 °C. The PCR products were subjected to electrophoresis on 1% agarose gel. The gel was analyzed using the Image J software, and the amount of cDNA was determined and normalized to the amount of β-actin cDNA.

Table 1. Primer sequence table.

	Primers	Sequences	Product Size
Ras	Forward	5′-CGACACAGCAGGTCAAGAGG-3′	20
	Reverse	5′-GGCATCATCAACACCCTGTCT-3′	21
Raf	Forward	5′-CAGCGAATCAGCCTCACCTTCAG-3′	23
	Reverse	5′-CGCAGAACAGCCACCTCATTCC-3′	22
β-actin	Forward	5′-CGTGGACATCCGCAAAGAC-3′	19
	Reverse	5′-GCATTTGCGGTGGACGAT-3′	18
DR4	Forward	5′-CTGATCACCCAACAAGACCTAG-3′	22
	Reverse	5′-GATGCAATCTCTACCGCTTCT-3′	22
JNK	Forward	5′-GGAATGGCCTGCCTTACGATGAC-3′	23
	Reverse	5′-GGCTCTGTTGCTGCCACTGC-3′	20
MEK1	Forward	5′-CAGCTCTGCGGAGACCAACTTG-3′	22
	Reverse	5′-CTGATCTCGCCATCGCTGTAGAAC-3′	24
MEK2	Forward	5′-ACTTGACGAGCAGCAGAAGAAGC-3′	23
	Reverse	5′-GAGCCGCCGTCCATGTGTTC-3′	20

4.8. Silencing the Expression of DR4 by siRNA

The cells in the logarithmic phase of growth were seeded in a six-well plate at a density of 2×10^5 cells/well. After 24 h, a mixture of 6 µL Lipo 8000 and 150 µL siRNA (sense: 5′-GCU GUUCUUUGACAAGUUUTT3′, antisense: 5′ AAACUUGUCAAAGAACAGCTT-3′) was added, and the medium was replenished to 2 mL. The mixture was aspirated after 6 h, and the cells were incubated with 0, 200, 400, and 800 µg/mL of fucoidan for an additional 48 h.

4.9. Detection of Mitochondrial Membrane Potential by JC-1 Staining

The cells in the logarithmic phase of growth were seeded in a six-well plate at a density of 6×10^3 cells/well. After 24 h, 0, 200, 400, and 800 µg/mL of fucoidan were added. The cells were stained 48 h later using the mitochondrial membrane potential detecting kit (JC-1); the manufacturer's protocol was employed. Stained cells were photographed and counted using a multi-function microplate reader.

4.10. Inhibition of Cytochrome C Expression

The cells in the logarithmic phase of growth were seeded in a six-well plate at a density of 6×10^3 cells/well. Then, 3 µM cytochrome C inhibitor was added after 24 h. One hour later, the inhibitor was washed out, and the cells were incubated for an additional 48 h in the presence of 0, 200, 400, and 800 µg/mL of fucoidan.

4.11. Western Blot Analysis

Cells were lysed with RIPA lysis buffer containing a phosphatase inhibitor and PMSF. Extracted proteins were subjected to electrophoresis on 10% SDS-polyacrylamide gel and transferred to a PVDF membrane. The membrane was blocked with 5% (w/v) skim milk powder in TBST for 1 h, and incubated with primary antibodies at 4 °C overnight, according to the manufacturer's protocol (dilution ratio of all proteins was 1:1000, except for cytochrome c, which was 1:200). After washing, membranes were incubated with peroxidase-conjugated secondary antibodies (dilution ratio was 1:1000), and protein bands were visualized using the hypersensitive enhanced chemiluminescence (ECL) chemiluminescence kit. Densitometric analysis was performed using the Image J software (1.8.0, NIH, US), and the intensity of specific bands was normalized to the GAPDH band.

4.12. Statistical Analysis

All data in graphs were presented as the mean value ± standard deviation from three independent measurements. The statistical analysis was used in statistical software (SPSS, Chicago, IL, USA) and GraphPad Prism 7.00 (GraphPad Software, CA, USA). $p < 0.05$ was considered significant.

Author Contributions: X.B. designed the project, performed data analysis, and wrote the paper. Y.W. performed data analysis, and B.H. contributed to the paper writing. Q.C. and M.X. contributed to data processing. S.S. and A.J. guided the experiment. All authors have read and agreed to the published version of the manuscript.

Funding: This research received no external funding.

Acknowledgments: In this section you can acknowledge any support given which is not covered by the author contribution or funding sections. This may include administrative and technical support, or donations in kind (e.g., materials used for experiments).

Conflicts of Interest: The authors declare no conflicts of interest.

References

1. Bai, X.; Zhang, E.; Hu, B.; Liang, H.; Song, S.; Ji, A. Study on Absorption Mechanism and Tissue Distribution of Fucoidan. *Molecules* **2020**, *25*, 1087. [CrossRef]
2. Gabbia, D.; Saponaro, M.; Sarcognato, S.; Guido, M.; Ferri, N.; Carrara, M.; de Martin, S. Fucus vesiculosus and Ascophyllum nodosum Ameliorate Liver Function by Reducing Diet-Induced Steatosis in Rats. *Mar. Drugs* **2020**, *18*, 62. [CrossRef] [PubMed]
3. Bae, H.; Lee, J.Y.; Yang, C.; Song, G.; Lim, W. Fucoidan Derived from Fucus vesiculosus Inhibits the Development of Human Ovarian Cancer via the Disturbance of Calcium Homeostasis, Endoplasmic Reticulum Stress, and Angiogenesis. *Mar. Drugs* **2020**, *18*, 45. [CrossRef] [PubMed]
4. Pozharitskaya, O.N.; Shikov, A.N.; Faustova, N.M.; Obluchinskaya, E.D.; Kosman, V.M.; Vuorela, H.; Makarov, V.G. Pharmacokinetic and Tissue Distribution of Fucoidan from Fucus vesiculosus after Oral Administration to Rats. *Mar. Drugs* **2018**, *16*, 132. [CrossRef] [PubMed]
5. Luthuli, S.; Wu, S.; Cheng, Y.; Zheng, X.; Wu, M.; Tong, H. Therapeutic Effects of Fucoidan: A Review on Recent Studies. *Mar. Drugs* **2019**, *17*, 487. [CrossRef]
6. Usoltseva, R.V.; Shevchenko, N.M.; Malyarenko, O.S.; Ishina, I.A.; Ivannikova, S.I.; Ermakova, S.P. Structure and anticancer activity of native and modified polysaccharides from brown alga Dictyota dichotoma. *Carbohydr. Polym.* **2018**, *180*, 21–28. [CrossRef]
7. Dobrincic, A.; Balbino, S.; Zoric, Z.; Pedisic, S.; Kovacevic, D.B.; Garofulic, I.E.; Dragovic-Uzelac, V. Advanced Technologies for the Extraction of Marine Brown Algal Polysaccharides. *Mar. Drugs* **2020**, *18*, 168. [CrossRef]
8. Garcia-Vaquero, M.; Rajauria, G.; Tiwari, B.; Sweeney, T.; O'Doherty, J. Extraction and Yield Optimisation of Fucose, Glucans and Associated Antioxidant Activities from Laminaria digitata by Applying Response Surface Methodology to High Intensity Ultrasound-Assisted Extraction. *Mar. Drugs* **2018**, *16*, 257. [CrossRef]
9. Obluchinskaya, E.D.; Makarova, M.N.; Pozharitskaya, O.N.; Shikov, A.N. Effects of Ultrasound Treatment on the Chemical Composition and Anticoagulant Properties of Dry Fucus Extract. *Pharm. Chem. J.* **2015**, *49*, 183–186. [CrossRef]
10. Blaszczak, W.; Lach, M.S.; Barczak, W.; Suchorska, W.M. Fucoidan Exerts Anticancer Effects against Head and Neck Squamous Cell Carcinoma In Vitro. *Molecules* **2018**, *23*, 3302. [CrossRef]
11. Wei, H.; Gao, Z.; Zheng, L.; Zhang, C.; Liu, Z.; Yang, Y.; Teng, H.; Hou, L.; Yin, Y.; Zou, X. Protective Effects of Fucoidan on Abeta25-35 and d-Gal-Induced Neurotoxicity in PC12 Cells and d-Gal-Induced Cognitive Dysfunction in Mice. *Mar. Drugs* **2017**, *15*, 77. [CrossRef] [PubMed]
12. Niu, Q.; Li, G.; Li, C.; Li, Q.; Li, J.; Liu, C.; Pan, L.; Li, S.; Cai, C.; Hao, J.; et al. Two different fucosylated chondroitin sulfates: Structural elucidation, stimulating hematopoiesis and immune-enhancing effects. *Carbohydr. Polym.* **2020**, *230*, 115698. [CrossRef] [PubMed]
13. Liu, J.; Wu, S.Y.; Chen, L.; Li, Q.J.; Shen, Y.Z.; Jin, L.; Zhang, X.; Chen, P.C.; Wu, M.J.; Choi, J.I.; et al. Different extraction methods bring about distinct physicochemical properties and antioxidant activities of Sargassum fusiforme fucoidans. *Int. J. Biol. Macromol.* **2019**. [CrossRef]
14. Amin, M.L.; Mawad, D.; Dokos, S.; Koshy, P.; Martens, P.J.; Sorrell, C.C. Immunomodulatory properties of photopolymerizable fucoidan and carrageenans. *Carbohydr. Polym.* **2020**, *230*, 115691. [CrossRef] [PubMed]
15. Liu, M.; Liu, Y.; Cao, M.J.; Liu, G.M.; Chen, Q.; Sun, L.; Chen, H. Antibacterial activity and mechanisms of depolymerized fucoidans isolated from Laminaria japonica. *Carbohydr. Polym.* **2017**, *172*, 294–305. [CrossRef]
16. Ji, X.; Peng, Q.; Wang, M. Anti-colon-cancer effects of polysaccharides: A mini-review of the mechanisms. *Int. J. Biol. Macromol.* **2018**, *114*, 1127–1133. [CrossRef]

17. Bovet, L.; Samer, C.; Daali, Y. Preclinical Evaluation of Safety of Fucoidan Extracts from Undaria pinnatifida and Fucus vesiculosus for Use in Cancer Treatment. *Integr. Cancer* **2019**, *18*, 1534735419876325. [CrossRef]
18. Paternot, S.; Bockstaele, L.; Bisteau, X.; Kooken, H.; Coulonval, K.; Roger, P.P. Rb inactivation in cell cycle and cancer: The puzzle of highly regulated activating phosphorylation of CDK4 versus constitutively active CDK-activating kinase. *Cell Cycle* **2010**, *9*, 689–699. [CrossRef]
19. Ishikawa, C.; Senba, M.; Mori, N. Mitotic kinase PBK/TOPK as a therapeutic target for adult Tcell leukemia/lymphoma. *Int. J. Oncol.* **2018**, *53*, 801–814.
20. Zayed, A.; Ulber, R. Fucoidan production: Approval key challenges and opportunities. *Carbohydr. Polym.* **2019**, *211*, 289–297. [CrossRef]
21. Chen, M.C.; Hsu, W.L.; Hwang, P.A.; Chou, T.C. Low Molecular Weight Fucoidan Inhibits Tumor Angiogenesis through Downregulation of HIF-1/VEGF Signaling under Hypoxia. *Mar. Drugs* **2015**, *13*, 4436–4451. [CrossRef]
22. Wang, F.; Ye, X.; Zhai, D.; Dai, W.; Wu, Y.; Chen, J.; Chen, W. Curcumin-loaded nanostructured lipid carrier induced apoptosis in human HepG2 cells through activation of the DR5/caspase-mediated extrinsic apoptosis pathway. *Acta Pharm.* **2020**, *70*, 227–237. [CrossRef] [PubMed]
23. Xue, M.; Ji, X.; Xue, C.; Liang, H.; Ge, Y.; He, X.; Zhang, L.; Bian, K.; Zhang, L. Caspase-dependent and caspase-independent induction of apoptosis in breast cancer by fucoidan via the PI3K/AKT/GSK3beta pathway in vivo and in vitro. *Biomed. Pharm.* **2017**, *94*, 898–908. [CrossRef] [PubMed]
24. Liu, D.; Liu, M.; Wang, W.; Pang, L.; Wang, Z.; Yuan, C.; Liu, K. Overexpression of apoptosis-inducing factor mitochondrion-associated 1 (AIFM1) induces apoptosis by promoting the transcription of caspase3 and DRAM in hepatoma cells. *Biochem. Biophys. Res. Commun.* **2018**, *498*, 453–457. [CrossRef]
25. Wu, Q.; Deng, J.; Fan, D.; Duan, Z.; Zhu, C.; Fu, R.; Wang, S. Ginsenoside Rh4 induces apoptosis and autophagic cell death through activation of the ROS/JNK/p53 pathway in colorectal cancer cells. *Biochem. Pharm.* **2018**, *148*, 64–74. [CrossRef] [PubMed]
26. Amarante-Mendes, G.P.; Griffith, T.S. Therapeutic applications of TRAIL receptor agonists in cancer and beyond. *Pharmacol. Ther.* **2015**, *155*, 117–131. [CrossRef] [PubMed]
27. Bittner, S.; Knoll, G.; Ehrenschwender, M. Death receptor 3 mediates necroptotic cell death. *Cell Mol. Life Sci.* **2017**, *74*, 543–554. [CrossRef]
28. Flusberg, D.A.; Sorger, P.K. Surviving apoptosis: Life-death signaling in single cells. *Trends Cell Biol.* **2015**, *25*, 446–458. [CrossRef]
29. Jin, J.O.; Song, M.G.; Kim, Y.N.; Park, J.I.; Kwak, J.Y. The mechanism of fucoidan-induced apoptosis in leukemic cells: Involvement of ERK1/2, JNK, glutathione, and nitric oxide. *Mol. Carcinog.* **2010**, *49*, 771–782. [CrossRef]
30. Vishchuk, O.S.; Ermakova, S.P.; Zvyagintseva, T.N. Sulfated polysaccharides from brown seaweeds Saccharina japonica and Undaria pinnatifida: Isolation, structural characteristics, and antitumor activity. *Carbohydr. Res.* **2011**, *346*, 2769–2776. [CrossRef]
31. Lim, S.J.; Aida, W.M.W.; Maskat, M.Y.; Latip, J.; Badri, K.H.; Hassan, O.; Yamin, B.M. Characterisation of fucoidan extracted from Malaysian Sargassum binderi. *Food Chem.* **2016**, *209*, 267–273. [CrossRef] [PubMed]

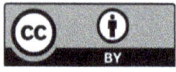 © 2020 by the authors. Licensee MDPI, Basel, Switzerland. This article is an open access article distributed under the terms and conditions of the Creative Commons Attribution (CC BY) license (http://creativecommons.org/licenses/by/4.0/).

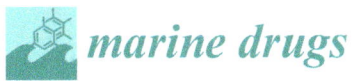

Review

Brown Seaweed Fucoidan in Cancer: Implications in Metastasis and Drug Resistance

María Elena Reyes [1,†], Ismael Riquelme [2,†], Tomás Salvo [1], Louise Zanella [1], Pablo Letelier [3] and Priscilla Brebi [1,*]

1. Laboratory of Integrative Biology (LIBi), Center of Excellence in Translational Medicine- Scientific and Technological Bioresource Nucleus (CEMT-BIOREN), Universidad de La Frontera, Temuco 4710296, Chile; m.reyes14@ufromail.cl (M.E.R.); tomas.salvo.e@gmail.com (T.S.); zanella.bio@gmail.com (L.Z.)
2. Instituto de Ciencias Biomédicas, Facultad de Ciencias de la Salud, Universidad Autónoma de Chile, Temuco 4810101, Chile; ismael.riquelme.contreras@gmail.com
3. Precision Health Research Laboratory, Departamento de Procesos Diagnósticos y Evaluación, Facultad Ciencias de la Salud, Universidad Católica de Temuco, Temuco 4813302, Chile; pletelier@uct.cl
* Correspondence: priscilla.brebi@ufrontera.cl; Tel.: +56-9-92659362
† María Elena Reyes & Ismael Riquelme contributed equally to this work.

Received: 16 March 2020; Accepted: 19 April 2020; Published: 28 April 2020

Abstract: Fucoidans are sulphated polysaccharides that can be obtained from brown seaweed and marine invertebrates. They have anti-cancer properties, through their targeting of several signaling pathways and molecular mechanisms within malignant cells. This review describes the chemical structure diversity of fucoidans and their similarity with other molecules such as glycosaminoglycan, which enable them to participation in diverse biological processes. Furthermore, this review summarizes their influence on the development of metastasis and drug resistance, which are the main obstacles to cure cancer. Finally, this article discusses how fucoidans have been used in clinical trials to evaluate their potential synergy with other anti-cancer therapies.

Keywords: fucoidan; cancer; metastasis; epithelial mesenchymal transition; nanoparticles

1. Introduction

Fucans are a family of polymeric molecules composed by a simple and long structure based on fucose and sulphate. Fucoidans are a subgroup within the fucan family, consisting of polysaccharides that are composed of sulphated L-fucose (6-deoxy-L-galactose) produced mainly by brown algae and, to a lesser extent, by marine invertebrates [1].

Due to the structural similarity between fucoidans and certain sulphated polysaccharides from animal cells, there has been increasing interest to study the biological properties of these algae polysaccharides within animal cells. An example for this are proteoglycans, which are found on the surface of animal cells and the extracellular matrix (ECM) and participate in structural and support functions. They have been shown to regulate a series of intercellular signaling pathways and interactions with cytokines and growth factors [2]. The structure of proteoglycans is similar to fucoidans, being composed of a protein (central chain) with glycosaminoglycans (GAGs) ramifications (e.g., chondroitin, dermatan, keratan, heparan sulphates, and heparin). This finding has sparked a renewed interest for studying the numerous potential biological properties including the anticoagulant [3], antioxidant [4], antiviral, immunomodulatory, anticomplement, and antitumor [5] characteristics of fucoidans isolated from different brown algae species.

The chemical variety of fucans in algae and invertebrate, their abundant bioavailability in nature as a renewable natural resource available from our coasts [5] and their potential use for biomedicine, make these polysaccharides an interesting material to study. This review will reveal not only structural characteristics but also the cellular/molecular aspects of fucoidans and their potential applications for cancer due to their properties to reduce metastasis and drug resistance in the different in vivo and in vitro cancer models.

2. General Structure of Fucoidans

Fucoidans from algae have been extensively studied since 1913 when Prof. Kylin discovered and described fucoidans [6]. Then, in 1957 these molecules were also shown to have anticoagulant functions and subsequently their anticancer activities were demonstrated (1970) [7].

As described above, fucoidans are polysaccharide composed by sulphated L-fucose (6-deoxy-L-galactose) [8]. Although many fucoidans consist of fucose and sulphate groups as is typical for fucans in general, fucoidans—in contrast to other fucans—consist of up to 10% of other monosaccharides (mannose, galactose, glucose, xylose, etc.), uronic acids, or branches of one or more monosaccharides [5]. In addition, there are fucoidans with different monosaccharide residues alternating with α (1→3) and α (1→4) bonds. Therefore, fucoidans constitute a highly variable and versatile subgroup of fucans [9] (Figure 1).

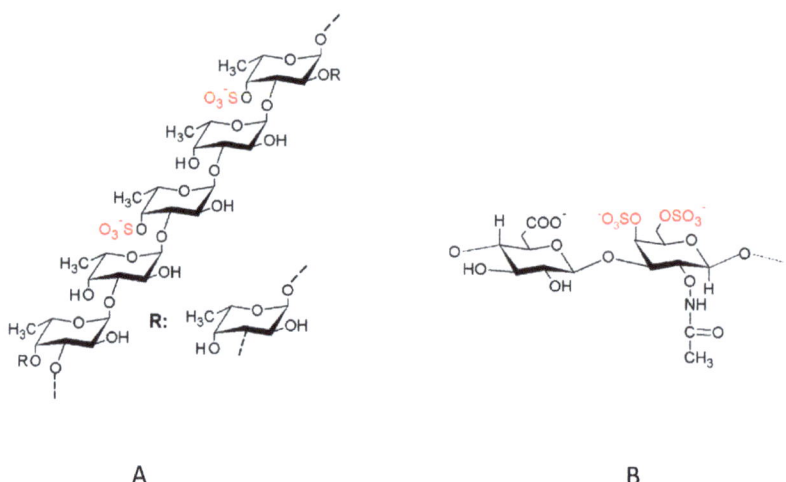

Figure 1. Comparison between fucoidan and glycosaminoglycan structures. (**A**) Structure of fucoidan from the brown alga *Fucus vesiculosus* and (**B**) structure of chondroitin sulphate. It is important to remark the similarity in the sugar skeleton and the presence of sulphate groups (red) in both structures. "R" represents a fucose subunit without sulphate.

For instance, fucoidans from *Fucus vesiculosus* are composed of L-fucopyranosil residues linked through α (1→2) bonds with 4-position sulphate groups [10]. In addition, next generation techniques have shown that the scaffold is also composed by fucose residues linked through α (1→3) bonds with 4-position sulphate groups from some of the fucose residues disposed every two or three units of the main chain [11]. In contrast, other algae species contain the typical fucan complexes. *Sargassum stenophyllum* contains two types of fucans: (1) fucans containing predominantly α-L-fucose with high percentage of glucuronic acid and low amounts of sulphate located in different positions in the sugar [12] (2) fucans containing high amounts of sulphate but lower content of uronic acids distributed along the fucose chains or the only other sugar, galactose [12].

A wide range of L-fucose polymers has been found by fractionating the extracts from different algae species within the brown seaweed genus [3,13–20]. These fucoidans range from fractions of typical sulphated fucoidans to heteropolymer fractions of low-sulphate fucose and others containing glucosamine. The fucoidan structures vary from species to species, by season, location and maturity [21]. This structural variations are important for industrial applications to identify the optimum harvesting times and to ensure a consistent product composition. For instance, Fletcher et al., 2017 found that the highest quantity of fucoidans can be extracted from three algae *F. serratus*, *F. vesiculosus*, and *Ascophyllum nodosum* in autumn, whereas in spring the amount that can be obtained is at a minimum [21].

In addition to brown seaweed species, also marine invertebrates contain this type of sulphated polysaccharides. The viscous liquid containing sea urchin eggs, such as that of the *Strongylocentrotus franciscanus* species, contains a compound composed by sulphate acids residues only in position 2 bonds through α (1→3) bonds [22]. Other fucoidans have been found in the skin of the sea cucumber species *Stichopus japonicas* [23] and the recently commercially important *Holothuria tubulosa* [24].

The great diversity of fucoidans and their capability to be chemically modified make them molecules with great potential to be used as adjuvant agents in the treatment of cancer.

3. Fucoidans and Metastasis

In cancer, many cells develop the ability to invade adjacent tissue components of its primary organ and spread to other organs [25]. This process is called metastasis and involves several steps including altered cellular adhesions, cell motility, resistance to extracellular death signals, and disruption of the basement membrane and ECM [26]. Metastasis is responsible for more than 90% of cancer deaths [27] due to its systemic nature and higher drug resistance. Therefore, new molecular or clinical strategies are needed to counteract this aggressive feature [28]. In general, the metastasis process can be divided into 4 steps: (1) Certain tumor cells obtain characteristics of epithelial–mesenchymal transition (EMT), dissociating and detaching from the primary tumor to escapes from this area. (2) The dissociated tumor cells infiltrate into the surrounding stroma and invade and migrate through the basement membrane supporting the endothelium of local blood and/or lymphatic vessels. (3) The dissociated tumor cells cross the ECM resulting in intravasation. This involves dissemination of tumor cells to distant organs through blood or lymph vessels. These tumor cells can then forma new tumor in other organs or tissues (secondary tumor) through mesenchymal to epithelial transition (MET), which is another mechanism that enables metastatic colonization (neoplasm) and that is the contrary to EMT (e.g., re-expression of E-cadherin). (4) The final dormancy step is characterized by invading tumor cells that can remain silent for many years in the distant organ [29]. Both step 1 (EMT) and 2 (infiltration and invasion into stroma) are characterized by morphological changes from the epithelial cell monolayer with an apical-basal polarity, to dispersed, spindle-shaped mesenchymal cells with migratory protrusions [30]. In particular, EMT involves changes in the expression of cell–cell junction proteins, cytokeratin intermediate filaments, increase vimentin filaments and fibronectin [31]. In this case, sulphated fucoidans have been shown to maintain the endothelium adhesion by binding to endothelial cell receptors, especially when the polysaccharides that normally bind to these receptors decrease, confirming that fucoidans have antimetastatic effects and can prevent EMT [32]. A recent study demonstrated this using fucoidan from *F. vesiculosus*, which was able to inhibit the EMT and, therefore, an important step in the metastasis development [33]. In addition, fucoidan has been shown to decrease the activity or expression of transforming growth factor receptors (TGFRs) in vitro and in vivo. This blocks the EMT process and its morphological changes by upregulating epithelial markers, downregulating mesenchymal markers and decreasing the expression of transcriptional repressors such as SNAIL, SLUG, and TWIST, which subsequently induce migration and invasion inhibition [34]. Moreover, fucoidans are also able to reduce TGFR downstream signaling events, including SMAD2/3 and non-SMAD pathways: AKT, ERK1/2, and Focal Adhesion Kinase (FAK) phosphorylation. Fucoidans decrease TGFR proteins by ubiquitination proteasome pathway (UPP)-mediated degradation of TGFRs and by the promotion of SMURF2 and SMAD7 that conjugate to TGFRs, resulting in TGFR degradation [35].

Post-transcriptional mechanisms have also been implicated in the control of EMT and their relationship to TGF-β signaling through microRNAs (miRs). In this context, fucoidan of *S. hemiphyllum*, increases the miR-29 family expression that suppresses *DNMT3B* expression, which results in the upregulation of the tumor suppressor gene *MTSS1*. This fucoidan also downregulates TGF-β signaling, increases E-cadherin expression, decreases N-cadherin, *ADAM12*, and *PTEN* expression, and finally prevents ECM degradation by overexpressing *TIMP-1* and reducing the expression of matrix metalloproteinase enzymes MMP2 and MMP9, secreted by cancer cells to degrade ECM and induce cell migration [36,37]. Furthermore, an oligo-fucoidan extracted from *S. hemiphyllum* has been shown to inhibit the signaling of chemokine CCL2, which has a chemoattractant activity for monocytes, T cells, mast cells and basophils, and promotes invasion and metastasis via JAK-STAT and MAPK signaling pathways. Therefore, this CCL2 inhibition induces an inflammatory response, anti-tumor immunity and tissue conservation to avoid metastasis and angiogenesis [18]. Another example is the fucoidan of *S. fusiforme* which has an antimetastatic effect on liver cancer cells by inactivating the integrin αVβ3 and prevent the invadopodia formation [38].

Another characteristic of metastasis is the involvement of cell migration and invasion properties through ECM [30]. As fucoidans have structural similarities with heparin, these polysaccharides not only have anticoagulant features but also are able to decrease the expression and activity of matrix metalloproteinases, resulting in an incapability of tumor cells to cross the capillary wall [39]. For example, fucoidan derived from *Undaria pinnatifida sporophylls* inhibits in vitro cell growth, migration, invasion, and adhesion capabilities probably by downregulating the VEGFC/VEGFR3 axis, inactivating the NF-kB pathway and increasing the protein levels of TIMPs [40]. Other fucoidans decrease the expression levels of MMP2 in a dose dependent manner and downregulate the PI3K/Akt/mTOR signaling pathway [41].

Fucoidan of *Laminaria japonica* reduce the migratory and invasive features of triple-negative breast cancer (TNBC) cell models by suppressing the activation of MAPK and PI3K pathways and subsequently inhibiting AP-1 and NF-κB signaling. Additionally, this fucoidan was shown to inhibit micrometastasis in an in vivo transgenic zebrafish model [42].

Hypoxia in tumoral microenvironment is another phenomenon that can lead to metastasis. Fucoidan derived from *U. pinnatifida sporophylls* inhibit hypoxia in cancer cells through nuclear translocation, activity of HIF-1α and reduction in the levels of phosphorylated-PI3K (p-PI3K), p-Akt, p-mTOR, p-ERK, NF-κB, MMP-2, and MMP-9, but increased TIMP-1 levels. In addition, this fucoidan can decrease the levels of VEGF-C and HGF [43]. The most complete studies about inhibition of metastasis and drug resistance by fucoidans are shown in Table 1 and the main signaling pathways involved in these processes are shown in Figure 2.

Given the biological activities and implications of fucoidans in cancer, particularly in metastasis, the sulphated polysaccharides are candidates to generate functional foods and drugs as well as for their applications in prevention, synergism with chemotherapy, and nanotechnology. For instance, one nanotechnology application is the utilization of polysaccharides by eco-friendly synthesis of fucoidan-stabilized gold nanoparticles for charge interaction [44]. This demonstrates the potential of fucoidan to be used as a therapeutic agent and as technological material.

Table 1. Sources, characteristics and effects of fucoidans on the metastatic and drug-resistant phenotype of cancer models.

Source	Fucoidan Structure	Cancer Type/Model	Effects/Pathways	Refs
		Hepatocellular carcinoma (HCC)		
		In vitro Huh-7 and SNU-761 cell lines	Effects on metastasis by avoiding invasion ↑p42/44MAPK-dependent NDRG-1/CAP43 ↑p42/44 MAPK-dependent VMP-1	[45]
		In vivo Distant metastasis model in C3H mice	Effects on metastasis by avoiding invasion ↓MMPs (MMP-2) ↓NF-κB ↓VEGF	
		In vitro MHCC-97H cell line	Nanoparticle drug resistance fucoidan downregulate chemokines and cytokines involved in chemoresistance	[46]
		Lung cancer		
		In vitro NSCLC CL1-5 human cells A549 human cells LLC1 mouse cells	Effects on metastasis by avoiding migration and proliferation ↓TGFRI and TGFRII ↓p-SMAD2/3 ↓AKT ↓ERK1/2 ↓p-FAK	[35]
Fucus vesiculosus	This fucoidan has a central core formed by α-L-fucose (1,3)-linked, sulphated at C4. In addition, several branching points (every two or three fucose residues) were present in α-(1,2) or α-(1,4)-linked, on the main chain.	In vivo Xenograft	Drug resistance and Combined therapy ↑ Cisplatin cytotoxicity ↑Caspase 3, PARP and apoptosis	[47]
		Lung cancer cell line In vitro	Synergize with gefitinib and ↑apoptosis	[48]
		Breast cancer		
		In vitro MDA-MB-231 and MCF-7 human breast cancer cells In vivo 4T1 mouse breast adenocarcinoma	Effects on metastasis by avoiding EMT ↑E-Cadherin, ↑γ-Catenin ↓N-Cadherin ↓SNAIL, SLUG and TWIST ↓p-SMAD2/3 ↓SMAD4 ↓TGFRI and TGFRII ↓MMP-9	[34]
		In vitro MDA-MB-231 cells	Effects on metastasis by avoiding EMT ↓N-Cadherin and ↓vimentin ↑ZO-1, ↑E-Cadherin ↓Nuclear translocation of HIF-1α ↓TWIST-1, SNAIL, CAIX and GLUT-1	[49]
		In vitro MCF-7 and ZR-75 In vivo Orthotopic Mouse model	Combined therapy increase effect Tamoxifen	[50]
		In vitro MDA-MB-231 human breast cancer cells, 4T1 mouse breast cells and J774.1A mouse macrophage cells. In vivo BALB/c mice	Nanoparticle combined therapy ↑ immunostimulatory activity and increase doxorubicin effect	[51]

Table 1. Cont.

Source	Fucoidan Structure	Cancer Type/Model	Effects/Pathways	Refs
		Proliferative vitreoretinopathy (PVR)		
		In vitro Human primary RPE cells In vivo PVR model in rabbits	Effects on metastasis by avoiding EMT ↓TGF-β1-induced SMAD2/3 phosphorylation ↓α-SMA and fibronectin ↓E-cadherin	[52]
		Colorectal cancer (CRC)		
		In vitro HT29 human cells	Effects on proliferation ↓Cyclin D1/E and ↓CDK2/4 Effects on apoptosis ↓BCL2 ↑BAX, ↑Caspase-3, ↑PARP1	[41,53]
		In vitro HT29 human colon cancer cells	Effects on metastasis by avoiding migration ↓MMP-2 ↓PI3K-AKT-mTOR drug resistance by effect in P38 and JNK pathways	[41]
			Drug resistance related decrease prion protein and decrease cell survival and could	[54]
		HCT-8 human ileocecal In vitro	Combined therapy ↑cytotoxicity than those treated with cisplatin alone	[55]
		Pancreatic cancer		
		In vitro AsPC-3 and BxPC-3 human pancreatic cancer cell lines	Effects on metastasis by avoiding hypoxia and angiogenesis ↓Hypoxia induced radioresistance ↓HIF-1α ↓Tumor growth and angiogenesis	[56]
		In vivo Xenograft	Combined therapy	
		Prostate cancer		
		In vitro DU-145 human cells In vivo Xenograft	Effects on metastasis by avoiding angiogenesis ↓CD31 and CD105 ↓p-JAK and p-STAT3 ↓VEGF, Bcl-xL, Cyclin D1	[57]
		Breast cancer		
Cladosiphon navae-caledoniae	Low molecular weight fraction (72%, MW < 500 Da) and non-digested fractions (less than 28%, peak MW: 800 kDa). Fucose (73%), xylose (12%) and mannose (7%). The ratio of sulphation was 14.5%.	In vitro ER-positive MCF-7 cells ER-negative MDA-MB-231 cells	Effects on metastasis and apoptosis ↓p-ERK and ↓AKT in MDA-MB-231 cells ↑p-ERK in MCF-7 cells ↑IC-ROS and ↓GSH in both cell lines	[58]
			Effects on drug resistance ↑cisplatin, tamoxifen and paclitaxel efficacy ↓Cell growth, ↑apoptosis ↓Bcl-xL, ↓Mcl-1 ↑ROS Combined therapy	

Table 1. Cont.

Source	Fucoidan Structure	Cancer Type/Model	Effects/Pathways	Refs
		Hepatocellular carcinoma (HCC)		
Undaria pinnatifida	This sulphated galactofucan is composed of: Galactose 44.6% and Fucose 50.9%. Xylose (4.2%) Mannose (0.3%), uronic acids were not detected. A significant number of O-acetyl groups	In vitro Hca-F cell line	Effects on metastasis ↓VEGF C/VEGFR 3 ↓HGF/c-MET, cyclin D1. ↓PI3K, p-AKT, p-ERK 1/2, and NF-κB Effects on metastasis by avoiding hypoxia ↓HIF-1α ↓p-PI3K, ↓p-AKT, ↓p-mTOR ↓p-ERK ↓NF-κB ↓MMP-2, ↓MMP-9 ↑TIMP-1	[20,40,43]
		In vivo Hca-F cells were inoculated subcutaneously into the footpads of the mice	Effects on metastasis by deregulating adhesion/invasion ↓ L-Selectin ↑TIMPs Effects on metastasis by avoiding lymph angiogenesis and lymphatic infiltration ↓VEGF-C, ↓HGF	
		Melanoma cancer		
		In vitro WM266-4, WM115 (mutated BRAF), SKMEL2 (RAS mutated), MeWo and FEMX (wild type)	Effects on drug resistance and combined therapy Fucoidan increase Lapatinib (ERBB inhibitor) effect in drug resistance cell	[59]
		Breast cancer		
		In vitro MCF-7 and ZR-75 In vivo Orthotopic Mouse model	Combined therapy Increase effect in Tamoxifen treatment	[50]
Sargassum hemiphyllum		**Colorectal cancer (CRC)**		
		Double-Blind Randomized Controlled Trial	Fucoidan as a supplemental therapy to chemotarget agents in patients with metastatic CRC	[60]
		Hepatocellular carcinoma (HCC)		
		In vitro Huh6, Huh7, SK-Hep1 and HepG2 human cells.	Effects on metastasis by avoiding EMT ↑miR-29b, ↓DNMT3B, ↑MTSS1 ↑E-Cadherin, ↓N-Cadherin ↑TIMP-1, ↓MMP-2/9	[36]
		Breast Cancer		
		In vitro MCF-10A, MCF-7	Effects on metastasis by avoiding migration and invasion ↑miR-29c, ↓ADAM12 ↓miR-17-5p, ↑PTEN	[37]
		MDA-MB-231 human cells.	Effects on metastasis by avoiding EMT ↑E-Cadherin, ↓N-Cadherin	
Ascophyllum nodosum	This fucoidan is composed of fucose (52.1%), galactose (6.1%), glucose (21.3%), and xylose (16.5%). Sulphate content is 19%. Two main size fractions (47 and 420 kDa).	**NSCLC (Lung cancer)**		
		In vitro NSCLC-N6	Effects on cell cycle arrest	[61,62]
		In vivo Xenograft		

Table 1. Cont.

Source	Fucoidan Structure	Cancer Type/Model	Effects/Pathways	Refs
Turbinaria ornate	The results showed that the fucoidan has a sulphate content of 25.6% and is mainly composed of fucose and galactose residues (Fuc:Gal ≈ 3:1). The fucoidan has a backbone of 3-linked α-L-Fucose residues with branches, →4)-Galp(1→ at C-4 of the fucan chain. Sulphate groups are attached mostly at C-2 and sometimes at C-4 of both fucose and galactose residues.	NSCLC (Lung cancer)		[63,64]
		In vitro NSCLC-N6	Effects on cell cycle arrest	
Cladosiphon okamuranus	The fucoidan is composed of 70.13 ± 0.22 wt% fucose and 15.16 ± 1.17 wt% sulphate. Other minor monosaccharides are D-xylose, D-galactose, D-mannose, D-glucose, D-arabinose, D-rhamnose and D-glucuronic acid. Linkage analysis revealed that fucopyranoside units along the backbone are linked, through α-1,3-glycosidic bonds, with fucose branching at C-2, and one sulphate group at C-4 per every three fucose units, i.e. the structure of fucoidan from Japanese Cladosiphon okamuranus is [→3)-α-fuc(1→]0.52[→3)-α-fuc-4-OSO3-(1→]0.33[→2)-α-fuc]0.14.	Breast cancer		[65,66]
		In vitro MCF-7 ADR (drug resistant human breast cancer cell line)	Combination therapy (Synergistic effect doxorubicin and photothermal nanocarrier) ↑doxorubicin delivery ↑morphology-control in Pt-nanoparticles	
		In vivo Xenograft		
Sargassum fusiforme	The fucoidan is composed of fucose, xylose, galactose, mannose, glucuronic acid, and 20.8% sulphate. The 17 sulphate groups are attached to diverse positions of fucose, xylose, mannose, and galactose residues. The backbone consists of alternate 1, 2-linked α-D-Mannose and 1, 4-linked β-D-GlcpA	Hepatocellular carcinoma (HCC)		[38]
		In vitro SMMC-7721, Huh7 and HCCLM3 cells	Effects on metastasis by avoiding migration and invasion	
		In vivo Xenograft	↓Invadopodia-related proteins (Src, Cortactin, N-WASP, ARP3, CDC42, MMP2, MT1-MMP) ↓Integrin αVβ3	

α-SMA: α-smooth muscle actin. CDK: Cyclin dependent kinase. CRC: Colorectal cancer. CTGF: Connective tissue growth factor. EMT. Epithelial-mesenchymal transition. ER: Estrogen receptor. FAK: Focal adhesion kinase. FE: Fucoidan extract. GSH: Glutathione. HCC: Hepatocellular carcinoma. HGF: hepatocyte growth factor. CRC: colorectal cancer. NSCLC: Non-small-cells human bronchopulmonary carcinoma. IC-ROS: Intra cellular reactive oxygen species. LMWF: Low molecular weight fucoidan. MMP: Matrix metalloproteinase. NDRG: N-myc downstream-regulated gene. PTEN: phosphatase and tensin homolog. PVR: Proliferative vitreoretinopathy. ROS: Oxygen reactive species. RPE: Retinal pigment epithelial. TGFR: Transforming growth factor-b receptor. TIMP: Tissue inhibitor of metalloproteinase. VEGF: Vascular endothelial growth factor. VMP: vacuole membrane protein.

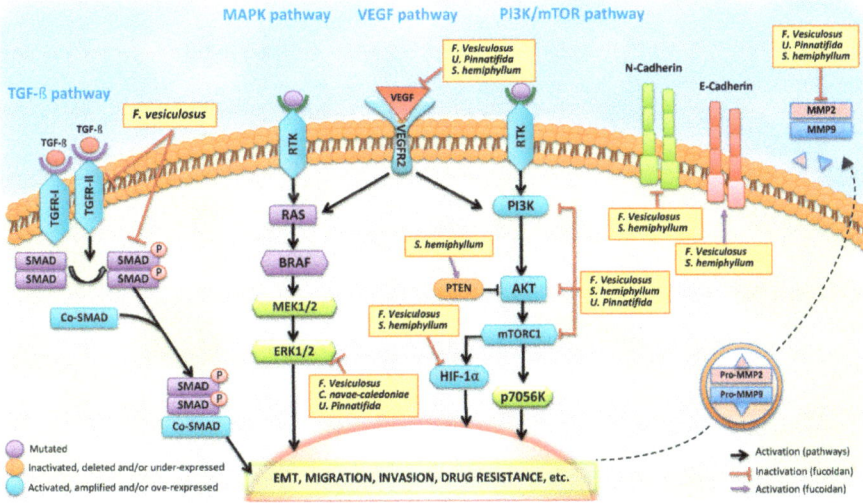

Figure 2. Summary of the main signaling pathways involved in the fucoidan function during the processes of metastasis and drug resistance.

4. Fucoidans and Drug Resistance in Cancer

There are many types of cancer treatments, including surgery, radiation, chemotherapy, hormone therapy and, more recently, target therapy (e.g., chemokine receptors), stem cells transplantation, and immunotherapy [67]. One of the major complications in cancer treatment is the appearance of chemotherapy resistance, which is defined as the development of innate and/or acquired ability by cancer cells to evade the effects of chemotherapeutics [68]. Some cancer cells are intrinsically resistant to chemotherapy and others are able to develop a resistance phenotype, either by their own characteristics as tumor cells or by external conditions such as the tumor microenvironment [69]. For instance, repeated chemotherapeutic stimulation can induce pro-survival biological changes in tumor cells, allowing them to evade cell death under drug pressure by using host or tumor-related factors [70]. Most chemotherapeutic agents in cancer therapy (e.g., platinum drugs, taxanes) induce cell stress on "sensitive cells" resulting in cell death mediated predominantly by the apoptosis pathway [71]. Despite the effectiveness of programmed cell death induced by drugs, because tumors are heterogeneous in nature, certain cancer cells can display a drug-resistant behavior. This constitutes the main obstacle for anticancer therapeutic success [72]. There are four major mechanisms that contribute to drug resistance in cancer cells: (1) Decreased uptake of water soluble drugs [73]; (2) changes in intracellular pathways that affect the potential of cytotoxic drugs to kill cells, including alterations in the cell cycle, DNA repair, apoptosis pathways, metabolism/elimination of drugs, or others [73–75]; (3) increased energy-dependent efflux of hydrophobic drugs mediated via overexpression of a family of energy-dependent transporters (known as ATP-binding cassette transporters) such as P-glycoprotein 1 (P-gp, ABCB1) or breast cancer resistance protein (ABCG2) amongst others [73]; and (4) intracellular detoxifiers such as antioxidants (e.g., glutathione) [76,77]. Multiple signaling pathways have been implicated in resistance to chemotherapy, and innovative therapeutic strategies to overcome these are urgently needed [78].

Some fucoidans have been implicated in the decrease of the cancer drug resistant phenotype (Table 1). For example, fucoidans from *A. nodosum* showed an arrest in G1 phase of the cell cycle and a reduction in the chemoresistance to cisplatin of non-small-cell human bronchopulmonary carcinoma (NSCLC-N6) cells, a type of chemoresistant cell line [62]. The same study also showed an antitumor effect at sub-toxic doses of fucoidan in vivo in NSCLC-bearing nude mice [62]. Similarly, a sulphated fucan-like polysaccharide with aminosugar obtained from *Turbinaria ornate* was shown to arrest cell cycle in G1 phase in NSCLC-N6 cells [63]. A fucoidan obtained from *F. veciculosus* was able to decrease the expression of cellular prion protein (PrPC) HT29 colon cancer cell lines. PrPC is a protein whose overexpression is involved in increasing cell survival and proliferation, and inhibition of stress-response proteins p38, JNK, and p53, which could induce drug resistance [54,79].

More recently, cytokines have been shown not only to directly influence cancer progression by inducing cancer cell proliferation, migration, metastasis, reprogramming of tumor microenvironment (TME), immune evasion and the formation of new blood vessel within tumors [80,81] but are also often associated with chemoresistance and overall poor prognosis [80,82–86]. In this context, certain oligo-fucoidan have been shown to produce pro-inflammatory cytokines and chemokines (e.g., IL-6 and CCL2/MCP-1 respectively) and decrease the side effects of chemotherapy [18]. Also, other fucoidans can downregulate some cytokines and chemokines (e.g., M2-type chemokine CCL22) to inhibit tumor cell migration and lymphocytes recruitment via NF-κB-dependent transcription, which may be a novel and promising mechanism for tumor immunotherapy [46].

Fucoidans can also function as adjuvant agents along with chemotherapy. For instance, it has been demonstrated that sulphated polysaccharides can increase the bioavailability of certain oral drugs, like doxorubicin [87]. Fucoidans from *U. pinnatifida* and *F. vesiculosus* have been studied in combination with tamoxifen and paclitaxel in orthotopic mouse models of breast cancer and ovarian cancer. The results showed that both fucoidans improved the effect of tamoxifen, but not paclitaxel, in breast cancer. In the ovarian cancer model, only fucoidan from *F. vesiculosus* was able to improve the activity of tamoxifen, but not paclitaxel [50]. Fucoidan from *F. vesiculosus* has been shown to increase cytotoxicity of cisplatin on lung cancer cell lines via upregulation of cleaved caspase-3 and poly (ADP ribose) polymerase (PARP) expression, which induces apoptosis in these cells [47]. In addition, this fucoidan can also act synergistically with gefitinib to induce apoptosis in lung cancer cells [48].

Fucoidan from *U. pinnatifida* has also been investigated in melanoma, which is an intrinsically aggressive and therapy-resistant cancer that can develop resistance to the ERBB inhibitor, lapatinib. While, lapatinib alone inhibited 60% of tumor growth, in combination with fucoidan it decreased 85% of tumor growth. In addition, the use of fucoidan can counteract the morbidity associated with prolonged lapatinib treatment. This ability to avoid side effects provides an additional advantage for the potential use of fucoidan extracts [59]. Another fucoidan extracted from *Cladosiphon navae-caledoniae* Kylin in combination with cisplatin, tamoxifen or paclitaxel can improve outcomes in breast cancer treatment. These co-treatments significantly inhibited cell growth in MDA-MB-231 and MCF-7 breast cancer cells. Furthermore, they enhanced apoptosis in these cells by downregulating anti-apoptotic proteins Bcl-xL and Mcl-1 and promoting higher intracellular ROS levels [58].

Fucoidans have particular chemical characteristics (backbone with fucose sugar and sulphate group) that confer them a negative surface and favor interaction with other chemical compounds or cellular molecules. This makes them an interesting material for the development of nanoparticles. Hwang et al. designed fucoidan-cisplatin nanoparticles with high cisplatin content and loading efficiency. These were used to treat macrophage cells (RAW264.7) to assess immune protection from the cytotoxicity of cisplatin [88]. Indeed, the cells treated with fucoidan-cisplatin conjugation were more protected in comparison to cells treated with cisplatin alone. Moreover, the fucoidan-cisplatin nanoparticles showed stronger cytotoxicity against colon cancer cell lines than those treated with cisplatin alone, which suggests that fucoidan-based nanoparticles with high drug encapsulation have a potential application in immunotherapy and chemotherapy [88]. Other nanoparticles with fucoidan-coated manganese dioxide were applied in pancreatic cancer cell models associated to hypoxia as a mechanism of resistance to radiation therapy [56]. The nanoparticles not only showed a significant decrease of HIF-1 expression under a hypoxic condition, but they were also able to reverse hypoxia-induced radioresistance. The latter was shown by a decrease of clonogenic survival and an increase of DNA damage and apoptosis in response to radiation therapy. In vivo studies showed that fucoidan-coated manganese dioxide nanoparticles along with radiotherapy also decrease tumor growth in comparison to radiation alone [56]. Therefore, fucoidan-coated manganese dioxide nanoparticles have clinical potential in the treatment of hypoxic, radioresistant pancreatic cancer [56] (Figure 2). Furthermore, a combinational synergistic effect between fucoidan (natural compound), doxorubicin (chemotherapeutic drug) and photothermal nanocarrier (Pt nanoparticle) has been observed as it was possible to reverse the drug resistance of breast cancer cells submitted to photothermal therapy [66]. In this case, the fucoidan was applied as a biocompatible surfactant and surface-coating biopolymer in the fucoidan-coated photothermal nanocarrier. As a result, the biological–chemo–thermo combination treatment showed a promising therapeutic efficiency against multidrug resistant breast cancer cell MCF-7 ADR both in in vitro and in vivo breast cancer models [66]. Fucoidan from *F. vesiculosus* assembled within nanoparticles bearing doxorubicin improved significantly the chemotherapy response in breast cancer cell lines by enhancing their immunostimulatory activity [51].

The molecular mechanisms of drug resistance have been classified into pre-target (alterations that precede the binding to DNA), on-target (alterations that are directly related to drug-DNA interaction), post-target (mechanisms downstream of DNA damage with effect in cell death signaling pathways) and off-target (influencing on molecular processes that are not directly associated with drug-elicited signals) [78]. In this context, the potential mechanisms in which fucoidans can reverse the drug resistance are versatile. Fucoidans can inhibit chemokine/chemokine receptors interaction as a pre-target mechanism [18]. The increase of cell cytotoxicity and arrest of the cell cycle demonstrates their effect on on-target mechanisms [62].They can influence post-target mechanisms, for example through the downregulation of anti-apoptotic proteins Bcl-xL and Mcl-1.and finally, the promotion of higher intracellular ROS levels, is an example for their role in an off-target mechanisms [58].

5. Fucoidan Clinical Trials

In general, clinical trials are used to assess if a new treatment is more effective and/or has less harmful side effects than the standard treatment. Currently, only few clinical trials have been performed to assess fucoidan in cancer. These studies tested fucoidan either as a new therapeutic agent or as diet supplement (Table 2).

Table 2. Fucoidans tested in clinical trials.

Source	Cancer Type (No Patients)	Fucoidan Dosage	Effects	Refs
Undaria pinnatifida	Breast cancer (20 patients)	Capsule of 500 mg twice a day for 3 weeks	Letrozole (n = 10) or Tamoxifen (n = 10) co-administration with fucoidan no decrease drugs in steady-state plasma and was well tolerated.	[89]
Sargassum hemiphyllum	Colorectal cancer (54 patients)	4 g twice a day for 6 months	Supplemental therapy, fucoidan combined with FOLFIRI chemotherapy plus Bevacizumab improved disease control rate.	[60]
Cladosiphon okamuranus	Unresectable advanced or recurrent cases of colorectal cancer (20 patients).	4.05 g for day	Decreases toxicity of chemotherapy FOLFOX or FOLFIRI.	[90]
	Survivors of diverse cancer types (11 patients).	1.5 g twice a day for 6 months	Activation of NK cells in male cancer survivors	[91]
	Advanced cases of several types of cancer (20 patients).	4 g for day for 4 weeks	Anti-inflammatory effect, decreases IL-1β, IL-6 and TNF-α	[92]
Nemacystis decipiens	Cervical cancer (1 case study)	200 mL/day	No concluded information	[93]
	Kidney cancer (1 case study)	60 mL×3L/day		
	Breast cancer (1 case study)	200 mL/day		

FOLFIRI: Combination chemotherapy with Irinotecan plus 5-Fuorouracil/leucovorin; FOLFOX: Combination chemotherapy with Oxaliplatin plus 5-Fuorouracil/leucovorin; NK: Natural Killer; IL-1β: Interleukin 1-β; IL-6: Interleukin 6; TNF-α: Tumor Necrosis Factor-α.

There are some examples of the use of fucoidan as a complementary therapy or food supplement in complementary alternative medicine in the treatment of cancer. A review, combining five case studies, showed clinical improvement in cancer patients, mainly using low molecular weight fucoidan supplements [93]. Other clinical trials in colorectal cancer [60] and breast cancer [89] in which fucoidans were used as a co-adjuvant treatment showed a better life quality cancer survivors [91] and in patients with advanced cancers [92]. The main fucoidan effects reported in cancer patients have been the improvement of negative effects of the chemotherapy and improved immune regulation. The fucoidan from *Cladosiphon okamuranus* for instance, decreases the cytotoxic effect from long-term colon cancer therapy (FOLFOX and FOLFIRI). The fucoidan in this case prevents the occurrence of fatigue during chemotherapy and increases patient survival. By ameliorating side effects, it enables the constant application of therapeutic drugs [90]. Fucoidan therefore has high potential for adjuvant therapy and may improve current clinical outcomes for cancer patients [55]. However, more clinical trials and further development of fucoidan applications are required.

6. Concluding Remarks

Fucoidans are a family of sulphated polysaccharides with great diversity in their structures due to their different sulphation patterns and the types of monosaccharides that in addition to fucose make up their backbone.

In some cancer types, fucoidans can inhibit metastasis processes including EMT, migration, invasion and MET processes. Fucoidans function by altering signaling axes such as TGFR/TGF-β, PI3K/AKT, VEGF, NF-κB, or ERK1/2 pathways and by inhibiting MMPs from cancer cells. Other mechanisms in which fucoidans may prevent EMT are TGF-β inhibition regulation of microRNAs. However, many questions regarding the functional mechanisms in which fucoidans affect EMT remain, leaving the door open for future research.

The molecular characteristics of fucoidans (e.g., molecular weight and sulphation grade) enable chemical or enzymatic modifications, which make them good candidates for therapeutic use, or to use them as adjuvants to increase the therapeutic efficiency of known chemotherapeutics. Moreover, the molecular versatility of fucoidans has made them excellent precursors for the development nanoparticles. Studies have demonstrated their potential to improve the efficiency of drug delivery into the tumor and/or to achieve a synergistic effect with other cancer drugs.

However, despite these auspicious/promising results, there is a lack of information about fucoidan structure, molecular weight, sulphate amount, etc. This will be important to better understand the possible influence of fucoidans on intracellular biological activity. In addition, the use of fucoidans in different cancer models and the interpretation of the results remains challenging. Most of the time, there are controversies related to the vague establishment of the studying variables or the scarce explanation of them, which makes it difficult to compare different studies.

Although there are still multiple challenges to overcome before fucoidans can be clinically used, it is predicted that in the near future, fucoidan-based approaches may provide important advances in overcoming the most complicated cancer drawbacks including metastasis and drug resistance and improving chemotherapy response and quality of life in cancer patients. Further studies are needed to discover more fucoidans and fucoidan-related targets to acquire a better understanding of how these molecules can arrest the mechanisms of metastasis and multidrug resistance in different cancer types.

Author Contributions: Conceptualization, M.E.R., I.R., P.B.; Validation, M.E.R., I.R., T.S., P.L., P.B.; Formal analysis, M.E.R., I.R.; Data curation, M.E.R., I.R., L.Z., T.S., P.L.; Writing—original draft preparation, M.E.R., I.R.; Writing—review and editing, M.E.R., I.R., L.Z., T.S., P.L.; Visualization, M.E.R., I.R.; Supervision, P.B. All authors have read and agreed to the published version of the manuscript.

Funding: This research was funded by National Commission for Scientific and Technological Research (CONICYT) Grant 21201835 (MER). National Funding for Scientific and Technologic Development of Chile (FONDECYT) Grant 11150802 (PB), National Funding for Scientific and Technologic Development of Chile (FONDECYT) Grant 3170826 (IR).

Acknowledgments: The authors want to thank Hannah Desmond for her help in editing the English for this article.

Conflicts of Interest: The authors declare no conflict of interest.

Abbreviations

DNMT3B	DNA methyltransferase 3B
MTSS1	metastasis suppressor 1
ADAM12	a disintegrin and metalloproteinase 12
PTEN	phosphatase and tensin homolog
TGF-β	Transforming growth factor beta (β)
TGFRs	Transforming growth factor b receptors
VEGFC	vascular endothelial growth factor C
VEGFR3	VEGF receptor 3
TIMPs	tissue inhibitor of metalloproteinases
MMP	matrix metalloproteinase
NF-κB	nuclear factor kappa-beta
ECM	extracellular matrix
GAGs	glycosaminoglycans
EMT	epithelial-mesenchymal transition
FAK	Focal adhesion kinase
UPP	ubiquitination proteasome pathway
miRs	microRNAs
P-gp	P-glycoprotein 1
ABCB1	ATP Binding Cassette Subfamily B Member 1
ABCG2	breast cancer resistance protein
PrPC	cellular prion protein
TME	tumor microenvironment
IL-6	interleukin-6
CCL2/MCP-1	chemokine (C-C motif) ligand 2/ monocyte chemoattractant protein 1
ROS	reactive oxygen species
HIF-1	Hypoxia Inducible Factor
FOLFIRI	Combination chemotherapy with Irinotecan plus 5-Fuorouracil/leucovorin
FOLFOX	Combination chemotherapy with Oxaliplatin plus 5-Fuorouracil/leucovorin

References

1. Mourão, P.A.; Pereira, M.S. Searching for alternatives to heparin: Sulfated fucans from marine invertebrates. *Trends Cardiovasc. Med.* **1999**, *9*, 225–232. [CrossRef]
2. Iwamoto, R.; Mine, N.; Kawaguchi, T.; Minami, S.; Saeki, K.; Mekada, E. HB-EGF function in cardiac valve development requires interaction with heparan sulfate proteoglycans. *Development* **2010**, *137*, 2205–2214. [CrossRef]
3. Nishino, T.; Nishioka, C.; Ura, H.; Nagumo, T. Isolation and partial characterization of a novel amino sugar-containing fucan sulfate from commercial Fucus vesiculosus fucoidan. *Carbohydr. Res.* **1994**, *255*, 213–224. [CrossRef]
4. Barahona, T.; Chandía, N.P.; Encinas, M.V.; Matsuhiro, B.; Zúñiga, E.A. Food Hydrocolloids Antioxidant capacity of sulfated polysaccharides from seaweeds. A kinetic approach. *Food Hydrocoll.* **2011**, *25*, 529–535. [CrossRef]
5. Li, B.; Lu, F.; Wei, X.; Zhao, R. Fucoidan: Structure and Bioactivity. *Molecules* **2008**, *13*, 1671–1695. [CrossRef]
6. Kylin, H. Zur Biochemie der Meeresalgen. *Z. für Physiol. Chem.* **1913**, *83*, 171–197. [CrossRef]
7. Springer, G.F.; Wurzel, H.A.; McNeal, G.M.; Ansell, N.J.; Doughty, M.F. Isolation of Anticoagulant Fractions from Crude Fucoidin. *Exp. Biol. Med.* **1957**, *94*, 404–409. [CrossRef]
8. Kadam, S.; Alvarez, C.; Tiwari, B.; O'Donnell, C.P. Extraction of biomolecules from seaweeds. *Seaweed Sustain.* **2015**, 243–269. [CrossRef]
9. Chevolot, L.; Foucault, A.; Chaubet, F.; Kervarec, N.; Sinquin, C.; Fisher, A.-M.; Boisson-Vidal, C. Further data on the structure of brown seaweed fucans: Relationships with anticoagulant activity. *Carbohydr. Res.* **1999**, *319*, 154–165. [CrossRef]

10. Percival, E.; McDowell, R.H. *Chemistry and Enzymology of Marine Algal Polysaccharides*, 1st ed.; Academic Press: Cambridge, MA, USA, 1967.
11. Patankar, M.S.; Oehninger, S.; Barnett, T.; Williams, R.L.; Clark, G.F. A revised structure for fucoidan may explain some of its biological activities. *J. Biol. Chem.* **1993**, *268*, 21770–21776.
12. Duarte, M.E.R.; A Cardoso, M.; Noseda, M.D.; Cerezo, A.S. Structural studies on fucoidans from the brown seaweed Sargassum stenophyllum. *Carbohydr. Res.* **2001**, *333*, 281–293. [CrossRef]
13. Percival, E.E.; Jara, M.F.V.; Weigel, H. Carbohydrates of the brown seaweed lessonia nigrescens. *Phytochem.* **1983**, *22*, 1429–1432. [CrossRef]
14. Chandía, N.; Matsuhiro, B. Characterization of a fucoidan from Lessonia vadosa (Phaeophyta) and its anticoagulant and elicitor properties. *Int. J. Biol. Macromol.* **2008**, *42*, 235–240. [CrossRef]
15. Lim, S.J.; Aida, W.M.W.; Maskat, M.Y.; Latip, J.; Badri, K.H.; Hassan, O.; Yamin, B.M. Characterisation of fucoidan extracted from Malaysian Sargassum binderi. *Food Chem.* **2016**, *209*, 267–273. [CrossRef]
16. Bilan, M.I.; Grachev, A.A.; Shashkov, A.S.; Nifantiev, N.E.; Usov, A.I. Structure of a fucoidan from the brown seaweed *Fucus serratus* L. *Carbohydr. Res.* **2006**, *341*, 238–245. [CrossRef]
17. Usoltseva, R.V.; Anastyuk, S.D.; Ishina, I.; Isakov, V.V.; Zvyagintseva, T.N.; Thinh, P.D.; Zadorozhny, P.A.; Dmitrenok, P.S.; Ermakova, S.P. Structural characteristics and anticancer activity in vitro of fucoidan from brown alga Padina boryana. *Carbohydr. Polym.* **2018**, *184*, 260–268. [CrossRef]
18. Chen, L.-M.; Liu, P.-Y.; Chen, Y.-A.; Tseng, H.-Y.; Shen, P.-C.; Hwang, P.-A.; Hsu, H.-L. Oligo-Fucoidan prevents IL-6 and CCL2 production and cooperates with p53 to suppress ATM signaling and tumor progression. *Sci. Rep.* **2017**, *7*, 11864. [CrossRef]
19. Chen, A.; Lan, Y.; Liu, J.; Zhang, F.; Zhang, L.; Li, B.; Zhao, X. The structure property and endothelial protective activity of fucoidan from Laminaria japonica. *Int. J. Biol. Macromol.* **2017**, *105*, 1421–1429. [CrossRef]
20. Synytsya, A.; Kim, W.-J.; Kim, S.-M.; Pohl, R.; Synytsya, A.; Kvasnicka, F.; Čopíková, J.; Park, Y.I. Structure and antitumour activity of fucoidan isolated from sporophyll of Korean brown seaweed Undaria pinnatifida. *Carbohydr. Polym.* **2010**, *81*, 41–48. [CrossRef]
21. Fletcher, H.; Biller, P.; Ross, A.; Adams, J. The seasonal variation of fucoidan within three species of brown macroalgae. *Algal Res.* **2017**, *22*, 79–86. [CrossRef]
22. Vilela-Silva, A.C.E.S.; Alves, A.-P.; Valente, A.P.; Vacquier, V.D.; Mourão, P.A. Structure of the sulfated -L-fucan from the egg jelly coat of the sea urchin Strongylocentrotus franciscanus: Patterns of preferential 2-O- and 4-O-sulfation determine sperm cell recognition. *Glycobiology* **1999**, *9*, 927–933. [CrossRef]
23. Kariya, Y.; Mulloy, B.; Imai, K.; Tominaga, A.; Kaneko, T.; Asari, A.; Suzuki, K.; Masuda, H.; Kyogashima, M.; Ishii, T. Isolation and partial characterization of fucan sulfates from the body wall of sea cucumber Stichopus japonicus and their ability to inhibit osteoclastogenesis. *Carbohydr. Res.* **2004**, *339*, 1339–1346. [CrossRef]
24. Chang, Y.; Hu, Y.; Yu, L.; McClements, D.J.; Xu, X.; Liu, G.; Xue, C. Primary structure and chain conformation of fucoidan extracted from sea cucumber Holothuria tubulosa. *Carbohydr. Polym.* **2016**, *136*, 1091–1097. [CrossRef]
25. Jiang, W.G.; Sanders, A.J.; Katoh, M.; Ungefroren, H.; Gieseler, F.; Prince, M.; Thompson, S.K.; Zollo, M.; Spano, D.; Dhawan, P.; et al. Tissue invasion and metastasis: Molecular, biological and clinical perspectives. *Semin. Cancer Biol.* **2015**, *35*, 244–275. [CrossRef]
26. Gupta, G.P.; Massagué, J. Review Cancer Metastasis: Building a Framework. *Cell* **2006**, *127*, 679–695. [CrossRef]
27. Lambert, A.W.; Pattabiraman, D.R.; Weinberg, R.A. Review Emerging Biological Principles of Metastasis. *Cell* **2016**, *168*, 670–691. [CrossRef]
28. Fontebasso, Y.; Dubinett, S.M. Drug Development for Metastasis Prevention. *Crit. Rev. Oncog.* **2015**, *20*, 449–473. [CrossRef]
29. Alizadeh, A.M.; Shiri, S.; Farsinejad, S. Metastasis review: From bench to bedside. *Tumor Biol.* **2014**, *35*, 8483–8523. [CrossRef]
30. Yang, J.; Weinberg, R.A. Review Epithelial-Mesenchymal Transition: At the Crossroads of Development and Tumor Metastasis. *Dev. Cell.* **2008**, *14*, 818–829. [CrossRef]
31. Zhang, X.; Pei, Z.; Ji, C.; Zhang, X.; Xu, J.; Wang, J. Chapter 15: Novel Insights into the Role of the Cytoskeleton in Cancer. In *Cytoskeleton-Structure, Dynamics, Function and Disease*; IntechOpen: London, UK, 2017; pp. 299–313.

32. Coombe, D.R.; Parish, C.R.; Ramshaw, I.A.; Snowden, J.M. Analysis of the inhibition of tumour metastasis by sulphated polysaccharides. *Int. J. Cancer* **1987**, *39*, 82–88. [CrossRef]
33. He, X.; Xue, M.; Jiang, S.; Li, W.; Yu, J.; Xiang, S. Fucoidan Promotes Apoptosis and Inhibits EMT of Breast Cancer Cells. *Biol. Pharm. Bull.* **2019**, *42*, 442–447. [CrossRef]
34. Hsu, H.-Y.; Lin, T.-Y.; Hwang, P.-A.; Tseng, L.-M.; Chen, R.-H.; Tsao, S.-M.; Hsu, J. Fucoidan induces changes in the epithelial to mesenchymal transition and decreases metastasis by enhancing ubiquitin-dependent TGF receptor degradation in breast cancer. *Carcinogenesis* **2012**, *34*, 874–884. [CrossRef]
35. Hsu, H.-Y.; Lin, T.-Y.; Wu, Y.-C.; Tsao, S.-M.; Hwang, P.-A.; Shih, Y.-W.; Hsu, J. Fucoidan inhibition of lung cancer in vivo and in vitro: Role of the Smurf2-dependent ubiquitin proteasome pathway in TGFβ receptor degradation. *Oncotarget* **2014**, *5*, 7870–7885. [CrossRef]
36. Yan, M.-D.; Lai, G.-M.; Chow, J.-M.; Chang, C.-L.; Hwang, P.-A.; Chuang, S.-E.; Whang-Peng, J.; Lai, G.-M. Fucoidan Elevates MicroRNA-29b to Regulate DNMT3B-MTSS1 Axis and Inhibit EMT in Human Hepatocellular Carcinoma Cells. *Mar. Drugs* **2015**, *13*, 6099–6116. [CrossRef]
37. Wu, S.; Yan, M.; Wu, A.T.H.; Yuan, K.S.; Liu, S.H. Brown Seaweed Fucoidan Inhibits Cancer Progression by Dual Regulation of mir-29c / ADAM12 and miR-17-5p/PTEN Axes in Human Breast Cancer Cells. *J. Cancer* **2016**, *7*, 2408–2419. [CrossRef]
38. Pan, T.; Li, L.; Zhang, J.; Yang, Z.; Shi, D.; Yang, Y. Antimetastatic Effect of Fucoidan-Sargassum against Liver Cancer Cell Invadopodia Formation via Targeting Integrin α V β 3 and Mediating α V β 3 / Src / E2F1 Signaling. *J. Cancer* **2019**, *10*, 4777–4792. [CrossRef]
39. Atashrazm, F.; Lowenthal, R.; Woods, G.M.; Holloway, A.; Dickinson, J. Fucoidan and Cancer: A Multifunctional Molecule with Anti-Tumor Potential. *Mar. Drugs* **2015**, *13*, 2327–2346. [CrossRef]
40. Wang, P.; Liu, Z.; Liu, X.; Teng, H.; Zhang, C.; Hou, L.; Zou, X. Anti-Metastasis Effect of Fucoidan from Undaria pinnatifida Sporophylls in Mouse Hepatocarcinoma Hca-F Cells. *PLoS ONE* **2014**, *9*, e106071. [CrossRef]
41. Han, Y.S.; Lee, J.; Lee, S. Fucoidan inhibits the migration and proliferation of HT-29 human colon cancer cells via the phosphoinositide-3 kinase / Akt / mechanistic target of rapamycin pathways. *Mol. Med. Rep.* **2015**, *12*, 3446–3452. [CrossRef]
42. Hsu, W.; Lin, M.; Kuo, T.; Chou, C. Fucoidan from luminaria japonica exerts antitumor effects on angiogenesis and micrometastasis in triple-negative breast cancer cells. *Int. J. Biol Macromol.* **2020**, *149*, 600–608. [CrossRef]
43. Teng, H.; Yang, Y.; Wei, H.; Liu, Z.; Liu, Z.; Ma, Y.; Gao, Z.; Hou, L.; Zou, X. Fucoidan Suppresses Hypoxia-Induced Lymphangiogenesis and Lymphatic Metastasis in Mouse Hepatocarcinoma. *Mar. Drugs* **2015**, *13*, 3514–3530. [CrossRef] [PubMed]
44. Soisuwan, S.; Warisnoicharoen, W. Eco-Friendly Synthesis of Fucoidan-Stabilized Gold Nanoparticles Kriengsak Lirdprapamongkol and 3 Jisnuson Svasti Pharmaceutical Technology (International Program), Department of Food and Pharmaceutical Chemistry, Faculty of Pharmaceutical Sciences. *Am. J. Appl. Sci.* **2010**, *7*, 1038–1042.
45. Cho, Y.; Yoon, J.-H.; Yoo, J.-J.; Lee, M.; Lee, D.H.; Cho, E.J.; Lee, J.-H.; Yu, S.J.; Kim, Y.J.; Kim, C.Y. Fucoidan protects hepatocytes from apoptosis and inhibits invasion of hepatocellular carcinoma by up-regulating p42/44 MAPK-dependent NDRG-1/CAP43. *Acta Pharm. Sin. B* **2015**, *5*, 544–553. [CrossRef] [PubMed]
46. Sun, J.; Sun, J.; Song, B.; Zhang, L.; Shao, Q.; Liu, Y.; Yuan, D.; Zhang, Y.; Qu, X. Fucoidan inhibits CCL22 production through NF-κB pathway in M2 macrophages: A potential therapeutic strategy for cancer. *Sci. Rep.* **2016**, *6*, 35855. [CrossRef]
47. Hsu, H.; Lin, T.; Hu, C.; Ta, D.; Shu, F.; Lu, M. Fucoidan upregulates TLR4/CHOP-mediated caspase-3 and PARP activation to enhance cisplatin-induced cytotoxicity in human lung cancer cells. *Cancer Lett.* **2018**, *432*, 112–120. [CrossRef]
48. Qiu, W.L.; Tseng, A.J.; Hsu, H.Y.; Hsu, W.H.; Lin, Z.H.; Hua, W.J.L.T. Fucoidan increased the sensitivity to gefitinib in lung cancer cells correlates with reduction of TGFβ-mediated Slug expression. *Int. J. Biol. Macromol.* **2020**, *153*, 796–805. [CrossRef]
49. Li, W.; Xue, D.; Xue, M.; Zhao, J.; Liang, H.U.I.; Liu, Y.; Sun, T. Fucoidan inhibits epithelial-to-mesenchymal transition via regulation of the HIF-1 α pathway in mammary cancer cells under hypoxia. *Oncol. Lett.* **2019**, *18*, 330–338. [CrossRef]

50. Burney, M.; Mathew, L.; Gaikwad, A.; Nugent, E.K.; Gonzalez, A.O.; Smith, J.A. Evaluation Fucoidan Extracts From Undaria pinnatifida and Fucus vesiculosus in Combination With Anticancer Drugs in Human Cancer Orthotopic Mouse Models. *Integr. Cancer Ther.* **2017**, *17*, 755–761. [CrossRef]
51. Pawar, V.K.; Singh, Y.; Sharma, K.; Shrivastav, A.; Sharma, A.; Singh, A.; Meher, J.G.; Singh, P.; Raval, K.; Kumar, A.; et al. Improved chemotherapy against breast cancer through immunotherapeutic activity of fucoidan decorated electrostatically assembled nanoparticles bearing doxorubicin. *Int. J. Biol. Macromol.* **2019**, *122*, 1100–1114. [CrossRef]
52. Zhang, Y.; Zhao, D.; Yang, S.; Yao, H.; Li, M.; Zhao, C.; Zhang, J.; Xu, G.-T.; Li, H.; Wang, F. Protective Effects of Fucoidan on Epithelial-Mesenchymal Transition of Retinal Pigment Epithelial Cells and Progression of Proliferative Vitreoretinopathy. *Cell. Physiol. Biochem.* **2018**, *46*, 1704–1715. [CrossRef]
53. Kim, I.H.; Kwon, M.J.; Nam, T.J. Differences in cell death and cell cycle following fucoidan treatment in high-density HT-29 colon cancer cells. *Mol. Med. Rep.* **2017**, *15*, 4116–4122. [CrossRef]
54. Yun, C.W.; Yun, S.; Lee, J.H.; Han, Y.-S.; Yoon, Y.M.; An, D.; Lee, S.H. Silencing Prion Protein in HT29 Human Colorectal Cancer Cells Enhances Anticancer Response to Fucoidan. *Anticancer. Res.* **2016**, *36*, 4449–4458. [CrossRef] [PubMed]
55. Hsu, H.-Y.; Hwang, P.-A. Clinical applications of fucoidan in translational medicine for adjuvant cancer therapy. *Clin. Transl. Med.* **2019**, *8*, 15. [CrossRef] [PubMed]
56. Shin, S.-W.; Jung, W.; Choi, C.; Kim, S.-Y.; Son, A.; Kim, H.; Lee, N.; Park, H.C. Fucoidan-Manganese Dioxide Nanoparticles Potentiate Radiation Therapy by Co-Targeting Tumor Hypoxia and Angiogenesis. *Mar. Drugs* **2018**, *16*, 510. [CrossRef] [PubMed]
57. Rui, X.; Pan, H.-F.; Shao, S.-L.; Xu, X.-M. Anti-tumor and anti-angiogenic effects of Fucoidan on prostate cancer: Possible JAK-STAT3 pathway. *BMC Complement. Altern. Med.* **2017**, *17*, 378. [CrossRef] [PubMed]
58. Zhang, Z.; Teruya, K.; Yoshida, T.; Eto, H.; Shirahata, S. Fucoidan Extract Enhances the Anti-Cancer Activity of Chemotherapeutic Agents in MDA-MB-231 and MCF-7 Breast Cancer Cells. *Mar. Drugs* **2013**, *11*, 81–98. [CrossRef] [PubMed]
59. Thakur, V.; Lu, J.; Roscilli, G.; Aurisicchio, L.; Cappelletti, M. The natural compound fucoidan from New Zealand Undaria pinnatifida synergizes with the ERBB inhibitor lapatinib enhancing melanoma growth inhibition Fucoidan extracted from New Zealand. *Oncotarget* **2017**, *8*, 17887–17896. [CrossRef]
60. Tsai, H.-L.; Tai, C.-J.; Huang, C.-W.; Chang, F.-R.; Wang, J.-Y. Efficacy of Low-Molecular-Weight Fucoidan as a Supplemental Therapy in Metastatic Colorectal Cancer Patients: A Double-Blind Randomized Controlled Trial. *Mar. Drugs* **2017**, *15*, 122. [CrossRef]
61. Foley, S.; Szegezdi, E.; Mulloy, B.; Samali, A.; Tuohy, M.G. An Unfractionated Fucoidan fromAscophyllum nodosum: Extraction, Characterization, and Apoptotic Effects in Vitro. *J. Nat. Prod.* **2011**, *74*, 1851–1861. [CrossRef]
62. Riou, D.; Colliec-Jouault, S.; Du Sel, D.P.; Bosch, S.; Siavoshian, S.; Le Bert, V.; Tomasoni, C.; Sinquin, C.; Durand, P.; Roussakis, C. Antitumor and antiproliferative effects of a fucan extracted from ascophyllum nodosum against a non-small-cell bronchopulmonary carcinoma line. *Anticancer Res.* **1996**, *16*, 1213–1218.
63. Deslandes, E.; Pondaven, P.; Auperin, T.; C, C.R.; Guezennec, J.; Stiger-Pouvreau, V.; Payri, C. Preliminary study of the in vitro antiproliferative effect of a hydroethanolic extract from the subtropical seaweed Turbinaria ornata (Turner) J. Agardh on a human non-small-cell bronchopulmonary carcinoma line (NSCLC-N6). *Environ. Biol. Fishes* **2000**, *12*, 257–262. [CrossRef]
64. Thanh, T.T.T.; Tran, V.T.T.; Yuguchi, Y.; Bui, L.M.; Nguyen, T.T. Structure of Fucoidan from Brown Seaweed Turbinaria ornata as Studied by Electrospray Ionization Mass Spectrometry (ESIMS) and Small Angle X-ray Scattering (SAXS) Techniques. *Mar. Drugs* **2013**, *11*, 2431–2443. [CrossRef] [PubMed]
65. Lim, S.J.; Mustapha, W.A.W.; Schiehser, S.; Rosenau, T.; Böhmdorfer, S. Structural elucidation of fucoidan from Cladosiphon okamuranus (Okinawa mozuku). *Food Chem.* **2019**, *272*, 222–226. [CrossRef] [PubMed]
66. Kang, S.; Kang, K.; Chae, A.; Kim, Y.-K.; Jang, H.; Min, D.-H. Fucoidan-coated coral-like Pt nanoparticles for computed tomography-guided highly enhanced synergistic anticancer effect against drug-resistant breast cancer cells. *Nanoscale* **2019**, *11*, 15173–15183. [CrossRef] [PubMed]
67. National Cancer Institute Home Page. Types of Cancer Treatment. Available online: https://www.cancer.gov/about-cancer/treatment/types (accessed on 3 April 2020).

68. Alfarouk, K.; Stock, C.-M.; Taylor, S.; Walsh, M.; Muddathir, A.K.; Verduzco, D.; Bashir, A.; Mohammed, O.Y.; ElHassan, G.O.; Harguindey, S.; et al. Resistance to cancer chemotherapy: Failure in drug response from ADME to P-gp. *Cancer Cell Int.* **2015**, *15*, 71. [CrossRef] [PubMed]
69. Shi, W.-J.; Gao, J.-B. Molecular mechanisms of chemoresistance in gastric cancer. *World J. Gastrointest. Oncol.* **2016**, *8*, 673–681. [CrossRef]
70. Sun, S.; Cai, J.; Yang, Q.; Zhu, Y.; Zhao, S.; Wang, Z. Prognostic Value and Implication for Chemotherapy Treatment of ABCB1 in Epithelial Ovarian Cancer: A Meta-Analysis. *PLoS ONE* **2016**, *11*, e0166058. [CrossRef]
71. Balch, C.; Huang, T.H.-M.; Brown, R.; Nephew, K.P. The epigenetics of ovarian cancer drug resistance and resensitization. *Am. J. Obstet. Gynecol.* **2004**, *191*, 1552–1572. [CrossRef]
72. Niero, E.L.; Rocha-Sales, B.; Lauand, C.; Cortez, B.A.; De Souza, M.M.; Rezende-Teixeira, P.; Urabayashi, M.; Martens, A.A.; Neves, J.H.; Machado-Santelli, G.M. The multiple facets of drug resistance: One history, different approaches. *J. Exp. Clin. Cancer Res.* **2014**, *33*, 37. [CrossRef]
73. Szakács, G.; Jakab, K.; Antal, F.; Sarkadi, B. Diagnostics of multidrug resistance in cancer. *Pathol. Oncol. Res.* **1998**, *4*, 251–257.
74. Rabik, C.; Dolan, M.E. Molecular mechanisms of resistance and toxicity associated with platinating agents. *Cancer Treat. Rev.* **2006**, *33*, 9–23. [CrossRef] [PubMed]
75. Johnstone, R.W.; Ruefli, A.A.; Tainton, K.M.; Smyth, M.J. A Role for P-Glycoprotein in Regulating Cell Death. *Leuk. Lymphoma* **2000**, *38*, 1–11. [CrossRef] [PubMed]
76. Harfe, B.D. MicroRNAs in vertebrate development. *Curr. Opin. Genet. Dev.* **2005**, *15*, 410–415. [CrossRef] [PubMed]
77. Hwang, W.; Hwang, Y.; Lee, S.; Lee, D.S. Rule-based multi-scale simulation for drug effect pathway analysis. *BMC Med. Inform. Decis. Mak.* **2013**, *13*, S4. [CrossRef]
78. Galluzzi, L.; Senovilla, L.; Vitale, I.; Michels, J.; Martins, I.; Kepp, O.; Castedo, M.; Kroemer, G. Molecular mechanisms of cisplatin resistance. *Oncogene* **2011**, *31*, 1869–1883. [CrossRef]
79. Lee, J.H.; Yun, C.W.; Lee, S.H. Cellular Prion Protein Enhances Drug Resistance of Colorectal Cancer Cells via Regulation of a Survival Signal Pathway. *Biomol. Ther.* **2017**, *26*, 313–321. [CrossRef]
80. Jones, V.S.; Huang, R.-Y.; Chen, L.-P.; Chen, Z.-S.; Fu, L.; Huang, R.-P. Cytokines in cancer drug resistance: Cues to new therapeutic strategies. *Biochim. Biophys. Acta (BBA)-Bioenerg.* **2016**, *1865*, 255–265. [CrossRef]
81. Aldinucci, D.; Colombatti, A. The Inflammatory Chemokine CCL5 and Cancer Progression. *Mediat. Inflamm.* **2014**, *2014*, 292376. [CrossRef]
82. Salgado, R.; Junius, S.; Benoy, I.; Van Dam, P.A.; Vermeulen, P.; Van Marck, E.; Huget, P.; Dirix, L. Circulating interleukin-6 predicts survival in patients with metastatic breast cancer. *Int. J. Cancer* **2002**, *103*, 642–646. [CrossRef]
83. Bar-Eli, M. Role of interleukin-8 in tumor growth and metastasis of human melanoma. *Pathobiology* **1999**, *67*, 12–18. [CrossRef]
84. Benoy, I.; Salgado, R.; Van Dam, P.A.; Geboers, K.; Van Marck, E.; Scharpe, S.; Vermeulen, P.B.; Dirix, L. Increased Serum Interleukin-8 in Patients with Early and Metastatic Breast Cancer Correlates with Early Dissemination and Survival. *Clin. Cancer Res.* **2004**, *10*, 7157–7162. [CrossRef] [PubMed]
85. Kornienko, A.E.; Guenzl, P.M.; Barlow, D.P.; Pauler, F.M. Gene regulation by the act of long non-coding RNA transcription. *BMC Biol.* **2013**, *11*, 59. [CrossRef] [PubMed]
86. Schneider, G.; Salcedo, R.; Welniak, L.; Howard, O.; Murphy, W. The diverse role of chemokines in tumor progression: Prospects for intervention (Review). *Int. J. Mol. Med.* **2001**, *8*, 235–244. [CrossRef] [PubMed]
87. Carreno-Gomez, B.; Duncan, R. Compositions with Enhanced Oral Bioavailability. U.S. Patent 20030211072A1, 13 November 2003.
88. Hwang, P.-A.; Lin, X.-Z.; Kuo, K.-L.; Hsu, F.-Y. Fabrication and Cytotoxicity of Fucoidan-Cisplatin Nanoparticles for Macrophage and Tumor Cells. *Mater.* **2017**, *10*, 291. [CrossRef]
89. Tocaciu, S.; Oliver, L.J.; Lowenthal, R.M.; Peterson, G.M.; Patel, R.; Shastri, M.; McGuinness, G.; Olesen, I.; Fitton, J.H. The Effect of Undaria pinnatifida Fucoidan on the Pharmacokinetics of Letrozole and Tamoxifen in Patients With Breast Cancer. *Integr. Cancer Ther.* **2016**, *17*, 99–105. [CrossRef]
90. Ikeguchi, M.; Yamamoto, M.; Arai, Y.; Maeta, Y.; Ashida, K.; Katano, K.; Miki, Y.; Kimura, T. Fucoidan reduces the toxicities of chemotherapy for patients with unresectable advanced or recurrent colorectal cancer. *Oncol. Lett.* **2011**, *2*, 319–322. [CrossRef]

91. Nagamine, T.; Kadena, K.; Tomori, M.; Nakajima, K.; Iha, M. Activation of NK cells in male cancer survivors by fucoidan extracted from Cladosiphon okamuranus. *Mol. Clin. Oncol.* **2019**, *12*, 81–88. [CrossRef]
92. Takahashi, H.; Kawaguchi, M.; Kitamura, K.; Narumiya, S.; Kawamura, M.; Tengan, I.; Nishimoto, S.; Hanamure, Y.; Majima, Y.; Tsubura, S.; et al. An Exploratory Study on the Anti-inflammatory Effects of Fucoidan in Relation to Quality of Life in Advanced Cancer Patients. *Integr. Cancer Ther.* **2017**, *17*, 282–291. [CrossRef]
93. Nishimoto, S. Clinical Improvement in Cancer Patients through Integrated Medicine, Mainly Using Low Molecular Weight Fucoidan Supplements. *J. Int. Soc. Life Inf. Sci.* **2015**, *33*, 25–37.

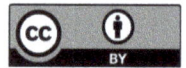

© 2020 by the authors. Licensee MDPI, Basel, Switzerland. This article is an open access article distributed under the terms and conditions of the Creative Commons Attribution (CC BY) license (http://creativecommons.org/licenses/by/4.0/).

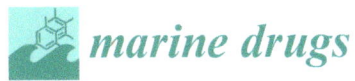

Article

Are *Helicobacter pylori* Infection and Fucoidan Consumption Associated with Fucoidan Absorption?

Makoto Tomori [1,*], Takeaki Nagamine [2] and Masahiko Iha [1]

[1] South Product Co. Ltd., Uruma 904-2234, Okinawa, Japan; miha.south@nifty.com
[2] Department of Nutrition, Takasaki University of Health and Welfare, Takasaki 370-0036, Gunma, Japan; nagamine-t@kendai-clinic.jp
* Correspondence: m-tomori@south-p.co.jp; Tel.: +81-98-982-1272; Fax: +81-98-921-3038

Received: 18 March 2020; Accepted: 28 April 2020; Published: 30 April 2020

Abstract: We examined the associations of *Helicobacter pylori* and mozuku consumption with fucoidan absorption. Overall, 259 Japanese volunteers consumed 3 g fucoidan, and their urine samples were collected to measure fucoidan values and *H. pylori* titers before and 3, 6, and 9 h after fucoidan ingestion. Compared to the basal levels (3.7 ± 3.4 ng/mL), the urinary fucoidan values significantly increased 3, 6, and 9 h (15.3 ± 18.8, 24.4 ± 35.1, and 24.2 ± 35.2 ng/mL, respectively) after fucoidan ingestion. The basal fucoidan levels were significantly lower in *H. pylori*-negative subjects who rarely ate mozuku than in those who regularly consumed it. Regarding the ΔMax fucoidan value (highest value − basal value) in *H. pylori*-positive subjects who ate mozuku at least once a month, those aged ≥40 years exhibited significantly lower values than <40 years old. Among subjects ≥40 years old who regularly consumed mozuku, the ΔMax fucoidan value was significantly lower in *H. pylori*-positive subjects than in *H. pylori*-negative ones. In *H. pylori*-positive subjects who ate mozuku at least once monthly, basal fucoidan values displayed positive correlations with *H. pylori* titers and ΔMax fucoidan values in subjects <40 years old. No correlations were found in *H. pylori*-positive subjects who ate mozuku once every 2–3 months or less. Thus, fucoidan absorption is associated with *H. pylori* infection and frequency of mozuku consumption.

Keywords: fucoidan; *Helicobacter pylori*; mozuku; *Cladosiphon okamuranus* Tokida; urinalysis

1. Introduction

Fucoidan is a complex sulfated polysaccharide that is mostly found in brown marine algae. Fucoidan exhibits a broad spectrum of biological activities, including anti-inflammatory, immunomodulatory, anti-oxidant, anti-tumor, and anti-infection effects [1–5]. Several investigators have reported a potential role of fucoidan as an anti-*Helicobacter pylori* (*H. pylori*) agent based on its ability to disrupt the adhesion of the microbe to the gastric epithelium in vivo and in vitro [6–9]. The inhibitory effect of fucoidan derived from *Cladosiphon okamuranus* (Okinawa mozuku) on *H. pylori* was demonstrated in vitro by Shibata et al. [6]. Their study showed that the *H. pylori* binding to human gastric cell lines was inhibited more by *Cladosiphon* fucoidan than by fucoidan procured from *Fucus*. In addition, fucoidan blocked both Leb- and sulfatide-mediated attachment of *H. pylori* to gastric cells. They concluded that the inhibitory effect of *Cladosiphon* fucoidan on the binding of *H. pylori* and gastric cells might be caused by the coating with this component of the bacterial surface. However, no bacteriostatic or bactericidal activity was observed against *H. pylori* for any fucoidan preparation [9].

Fucoidan is reported to be absorbed across the intestinal tract via energy-dependent processes and pinocytosis [10–12]. In Japanese volunteers, fucoidan was detected in the majority of urine following oral administration [13]. Because the rate of fucoidan absorption through the small intestine was highly variable among the participants, various factors were suggested to influence its absorption. For example, the consumption of Okinawa mozuku (*Cladosiphon okamuranus* Tokida), a brown seaweed containing fucoidan, is an important factor associated with fucoidan absorption. Based on a previous report by Hehemann et al. [14], we speculated that the gastrointestinal microbiota can influence the absorption of fucoidan.

H. pylori is a Gram-negative, spiral-shaped, microaerophilic bacterium. It colonizes the entire gastric mucosa in approximately half of the world's human population, and a poor socioeconomic condition is an important risk factor for infection [15–18]. *H. pylori* causes peptic ulcer disease and atrophic gastritis, and it is associated with primary gastric B-cell lymphoma and gastric adenocarcinoma. The host immune system cannot clear the infection, and it persists without treatment.

Many studies have focused on the modification of the gastric environment induced by *H. pylori* infection. For example, *H. pylori* infection can lead to the deficiency of vitamins, such as vitamin C, vitamin A, α-tocopherol, vitamin B_{12}, and folic acid, as well as essential minerals [19–21]. Moreover, gastric *H. pylori* infection affects local and distant microbial populations and host responses.

Because fucoidan can bind to *H. pylori* and disrupt its attachment to the gastric epithelium [6–8], *H. pylori* infection is assumed to affect fucoidan absorption. In this study, we examined the effects of *H. pylori* infection on the absorption of fucoidan extracted from Okinawa mozuku in Japanese volunteers. Although fucoidan absorption is extremely low in humans, the fucoidan concentration after oral administration is approximately 10-fold higher in urine than in serum [22]. Therefore, urinary fucoidan concentrations were measured before and after the oral administration of mozuku fucoidan.

2. Results

2.1. Prevalence of H. Pylori Infection AccordingTo the Frequency of Mozuku Consumption and Age

The relevance of mozuku consumption and age to *H. pylori* infection is shown in Table 1. Regarding age, *H. pylori* infection was detected in 60.0%, 58.7%, 61.9%, 77.8%, and 88.5% of participants aged 20–29, 30–39, 40–49, 50–59, and ≥60 years old, respectively.

According to logistic regression analysis, age was a significant risk factor for *H. pylori* infection, as the risk of infection was significantly higher in patients ≥40 years old than in those <40 years old. Mozuku consumption was not a significant risk factor for *H. pylori* infection (Table 2).

Table 1. *Helicobacter pylori* infection according to the frequency of mozuku consumption and age.

Age Group	1–3 Times Weekly		Once Every 2 Weeks		Once Monthly		Once Every 2–3 Months		Hardly Eat	
	H. Pylori		H. Pylori		H. Pylori		H. Pylori		H. Pylori	
	(-)	(+)	(-)	(+)	(-)	(+)	(-)	(+)	(-)	(+)
20's (n = 50)	2	5	6	7	5	5	4	5	3	8
30's (n = 75)	2	3	3	10	6	11	10	11	9	10
40's (n = 63)	3	4	2	10	6	11	10	7	3	7
50's (n = 45)	2	6	2	7	2	11	3	4	1	7
≥60's (n = 26)	0	6	0	2	2	7	1	5	0	3

20's: 20–29 years old, 30's: 30–39 years old, 40's: 40–49 years old, 50's: 50–59 years old, ≥60's: over 60 years old. n = number of subjects.

Table 2. Relevance of age and mozuku consumption to *Helicobacter pylori* infection: logistic regression analysis.

		Odds Ratio	95%CI
Habit of eating mozuku		1.12	0.89–1.42
Age	40y.o.<	1.00	
	≥40y.o.	1.70	1.01–2.85

y.o.: years old.

2.2. Urinary Fucoidan Values before and after Fucoidan Ingestion

In all subjects, the urinary fucoidan values significantly increased 3, 6, and 9 h after fucoidan ingestion compared to the basal values (Table 3). The urinary fucoidan values were significantly higher at 6 and 9 h than those at 3 h. A significant difference was not observed in the urinary fucoidan values between the group that regularly ate mozuku and group that rarely ate mozuku.

Table 3. Time course of urinary fucoidan.

	0	3 h	6 h	9 h
		ng/mL		
Subjects (n = 259)	3.7 ± 3.4	15.3 ± 18.8 [a]	24.4 ± 35.1 [a,b]	24.2 ± 35.2 [a,b]

All data are presented as mean ± SD. Different letters indicate a significant difference as follows: [a] compared to the basal value ($p < 0.01$). [b] Compared to the fucoidan values at 3 h ($p < 0.01$). n = number of subjects.

2.3. Basal Levels (before Ingestion) of Fucoidan

Among subjects who rarely ate mozuku, the basal fucoidan levels were significantly lower in the *H. pylori*-negative group than in the *H. pylori*-positive group. Among *H. pylori*-negative subjects, the basal fucoidan levels were significantly lower in those who rarely ate mozuku than in those who ate mozuku 1–3 times weekly, once monthly, or once every 2–3 months. Conversely, the basal fucoidan levels were not affected by the frequency of mozuku consumption or age in *H. pylori*-positive subjects (Table 4).

Table 4. Basal fucoidan levels according to the frequency of mozuku consumption in *Helicobacter pylori*-negative and *Helicobacter pylori*-positive subjects.

Habit of Eating Mozuku	*H. pylori* (-)	*H. pylori* (+)	P-Value *H. pylori* (-) vs *H. pylori* (+)
1–3 times weekly	4.1 ± 1.3 (n =9) [a]	3.2 ± 3.0 (n = 24)	0.29
Once every 2 weeks	2.7 ± 3.2 (n = 14)	3.2 ± 2.6 (n = 35)	0.58
Once monthly	3.1 ± 3.0 (n = 21) [b]	2.8 ± 2.8 (n = 44)	0.69
Once every 2–3 months	3.3 ± 3.3 (n = 28) [c]	4.3 ± 5.7 (n = 33)	0.40
hardly eat	1.4 ± 1.5 (n = 16)	3.3 ± 3.4 (n = 35)	0.01

All data are presented as mean ± SD. Different letters indicate a significant difference as follows: [a] compared to *H. pylori*-negative subjects who hardly ate mozuku ($p = 0.01$); [b] compared to *H. pylori*-negative subjects who hardly ate mozuku ($p = 0.03$); [c] compared to *H. pylori*-negative subjects who hardly ate mozuku ($p = 0.03$). n = number of subjects.

2.4. Relationship between H. pylori Titers and Basal Fucoidan Levels

Among *H. pylori*-positive subjects, a significant positive correlation existed between *H. pylori* titers and basal fucoidan levels in participants <40 years old who ate mozuku at least once monthly. A significant correlation between *H. pylori* titers and basal fucoidan levels was not found in participants aged ≥40 years irrespective of the frequency of mozuku consumption (Figure 1).

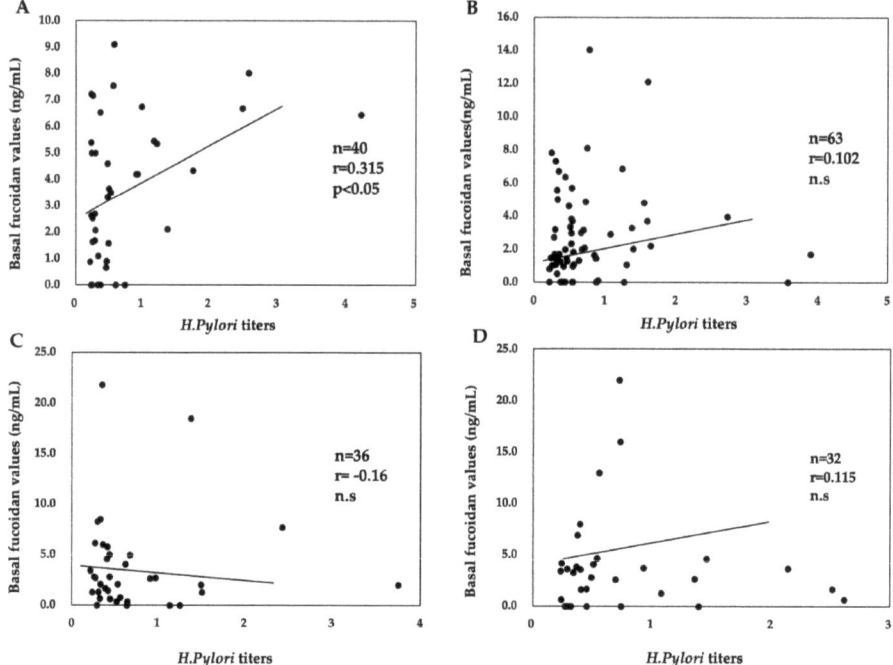

Figure 1. Relationship between *Helicobacter pylori* titers and basal fucoidan levels according to the frequency of mozuku consumption and age in among *H. pylori*-positive subjects. (**A**) Subjects aged <40 years who ate mozuku at least once a month. (**B**) Subjects aged ≥40 years who ate mozuku at least once a month. (**C**) Subjects aged <40 years who ate mozuku once every 2–3 months or less. (**D**) Subjects aged ≥40 years who ate mozuku once every 2–3 months or less. n = number of subjects, r = correlation coefficient, n.s = not significant.

2.5. Maximum Absorption of Fucoidan (ΔMax Fucoidan Value)

Urinary fucoidan was detected in 252 of 259 subjects following a single oral dose of 3 g. The ΔMax fucoidan values exhibited a wide distribution, ranging from 0 to 273.6 ng/mL. Among the participants in whom urinary fucoidan was not detected, three rarely ate mozuku, one ate mozuku once every 2–3 months, and three ate mozuku once monthly.

Table 5 shows the relevance of *H. pylori* infection and age to the ΔMax fucoidan values. The ΔMax fucoidan values in all subjects were similar between *H. pylori*-positive and *H. pylori*-negative subjects. Compared with the values in *H. pylori-negative* subjects, the ΔMax fucoidan values of *H. pylori*-positive subjects tended to be higher in subjects in their 20s and 30s and lower in those in their 40s and 50s (data not shown). To determine relevance of age to fucoidan absorption, the subjects were divided into two age groups (<40 and ≥40 years).

ΔMax fucoidan values were significantly lower in subjects aged ≥40 years than in younger subjects among *H. pylori*-positive participants. No effect of age on ΔMax fucoidan values was observed among *H. pylori*-negative subjects. No significant difference of ΔMax fucoidan values was found according to the presence of *H. pylori* infection in either age group.

Table 5. Comparison of ΔMax fucoidan values by age.

	H.pylori (-)	H.pylori (+)	H.pylori (-) vs H.pylori (+)
Total	29.4 ± 40.1 (n = 88)	24.2 ± 37.1 (n = 171)	$P = 0.300$
40 y.o.<	26.4 ± 38.8 (n = 52)	35.3 ± 47.6 (n = 76)	$P = 0.323$
≥40 y.o.	33.8 ± 59.8 (n = 36)	21.9 ± 35.3 (n = 95) [a]	$P = 0.135$

All data were presented as mean ± SD. [a] There is a significant difference ($p < 0.01$) compared to H. pylori-positive subjects aged <40 years. n = number of subjects, y.o.: years old; $P = P$ value.

2.6. Relevance of H. Pylori Infection and Mozuku Consumption to Fucoidan Absorption

In a comparison between participants aged ≥40 years and those aged <40 years, the ΔMax fucoidan values were decreased by regular mozuku consumption in *H. pylori*-positive subjects but not in *H. pylori*-negative subjects (Table 6). Specifically, ΔMax fucoidan values were lower in *H. pylori*-positive subjects aged ≥40 years who ate mozuku at least once a month than in those who ate mozuku less frequently. Subsequently, the subjects were divided into groups based on the frequency of mozuku consumption, and the relevance of mozuku consumption to ΔMax fucoidan values was elucidated (Table 7).

Table 6. Relevance of *Helicobacter pylori* infection, frequency of mozuku consumption, and age to ΔMax fucoidan values.

Habit of Eating Mozuku	H.pylori (-)		H.pylori (+)		P-Value
	40 y.o.<	≥40 y.o.	40 y.o.<	≥40 y.o.	H. pylori(+) Aged <40 y.o. vs. H. pylori(+) Aged ≥40 y.o.
1–3 times weekly	25.0 ± 8.2 (n = 4)	37.8 ± 20.3 (n = 5)	20.4 ± 16.1 (n = 8)	17.4 ± 25.6 (n = 16)	n.s
Once every 2 weeks	24.5 ± 25.2 (n = 10)	36.4 ± 14.8 (n = 4) [a]	34.8 ± 52.7 (n = 17)	12.9 ± 14.7 (n = 18)	0.08
Once monthly	29.1 ± 71.6 (n = 11)	27.7 ± 17.8 (n = 10)	41.9 ± 54.5 (n = 16)	18.9 ± 21.4 (n = 28)	0.06
Once every 2-3 months	31.1 ± 31.8 (n = 15)	39.3 ± 67.0 (n = 13)	36.2 ± 46.7 (n = 18)	42.5 ± 73.1 (n = 15)	n.s
hardly eat	24.4 ± 22.0 (n = 12)	15.8 ± 22.9 (n = 4)	38.1 ± 53.3 (n = 18)	22.2 ± 17.9 (n = 17)	n.s

All data are presented as mean ± SD. [a] Compared to H. pylori-negative subjects aged ≥40 years who hardly ate mozuku ($p < 0.01$). n = number of subjects, n.s: not significant; y.o.: years old.

Table 7. Relevance of *Helicobacter pylori* infection and age to ΔMax fucoidan values according to the frequency of mozuku consumption.

Habit of Eating Mozuku	H.pylori (-)		H.ylori (+)	
	40 y.o <	≥40 y.o	40 y.o <	≥40 y.o
Regularly consumed mozuku [1)]	26.6 ± 48.7 (n = 25)	32.1 ± 17.6 (n = 19)	34.5 ± 48.1 (n = 40)	16.8 ± 20.8 [a,b,c] (n = 63)
Rarely ate mozuku [2)]	28.1 ± 27.6 (n = 27)	33.8 ± 59.8 (n = 17)	33.9 ± 47.7 (n = 36)	30.5 ± 51.9 (n = 32)

All data are presented as mean ± SD. [1)] Regularly consumed mozuku: 1–3 times weekly + once every 2 weeks + once monthly; [2)] rarely ate mozuku: once every 2–3 months + hardly ate. [a] Compared to H. pylori-positive subjects aged <40 years who ate mozuku at least once monthly ($p = 0.03$). [b] Compared to H. pylori-positive subjects aged ≥40 years who ate mozuku once every 2–3 months or less ($p = 0.01$). [c] Compared to H. pylori-negative subjects aged ≥40 years who ate mozuku at least once monthly ($p = 0.01$). n = number of subjects, y.o = years old.

Among *H. pylori*-positive subjects who ate mozuku at least once a month, ΔMax fucoidan values were significantly lower in those aged ≥40 years than in those aged <40 years. In addition, among *H. pylori*-positive subjects aged ≥40 years, the ΔMax fucoidan values were significantly lower in those who regularly consumed mozuku than in those who rarely ate mozuku. In addition, the ΔMax fucoidan values were significantly different between *H. pylori*-positive (16.8 ± 20.8) and *H. pylori*-negative subjects (32.1 ± 17.6) among those who ate mozuku at least once a month. However, no difference in ΔMax fucoidan values was noted according to age or frequency of mozuku consumption among *H. pylori*-negative participants.

2.7. Relationship between the Basal and Δmax Fucoidan Values in H. Pylori-Positive Subjects

Among *H. pylori*-positive subjects who regularly consumed mozuku, a significant positive correlation between the basal and ΔMax fucoidan values was found for those aged <40 years but not those aged ≥40 years. No significant correlation was found between the basal and ΔMax fucoidan levels among participants who rarely ate mozuku (Figure 2).

In addition, no significant correlations were found between the basal and ΔMax fucoidan levels in *H. pylori*-negative subjects regardless of the frequency of mozuku consumption (data not shown).

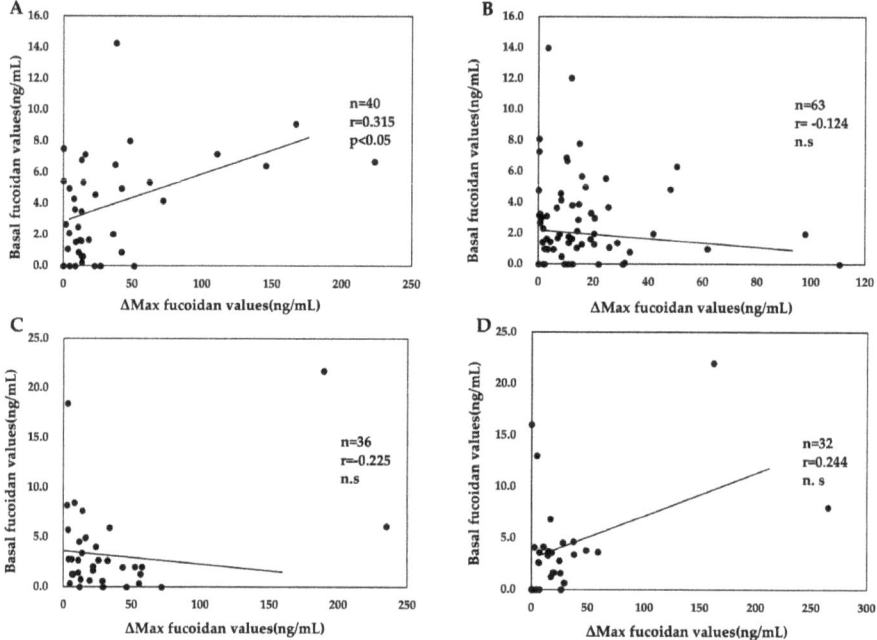

Figure 2. Relationship between basal fucoidan values and the maximum absorption of fucoidan (ΔMax fucoidan values) according to the frequency of mozuku consumption and age in *Helicobacter pylori*-positive subjects. (**A**) Consumption of mozuku at least once monthly among subjects aged <40 years (**B**) Consumption of mozuku at least once monthly among subjects aged ≥40 years (**C**) Consumption of mozuku once every 2–3 months or less among subjects aged <40 years (**D**) Consumption of mozuku once every 2–3 months or less among subjects aged ≥40 years. n = number of subjects, r = correlation coefficient, n.s = not significant.

3. Discussion

The present study revealed an association between *H. pylori* infection and the absorption of fucoidan. Specifically, fucoidan absorption was significantly diminished among *H. pylori*-positive subjects aged ≥40 years who ate mozuku at least once monthly, whereas no association was found among *H. pylori*-negative subjects irrespective of the frequency of mozuku consumption and age. In addition, fucoidan absorption was not diminished among *H. pylori*-positive subjects who ate mozuku once every 2–3 months or less; therefore, mozuku consumption affects the absorption of fucoidan.

Although the precise mechanisms by which *H. pylori* infection and mozuku consumption reduce fucoidan absorption have not been determined, a few possibilities have been postulated.

As ΔMax fucoidan values were similar between *H. pylori*-negative and *H. pylori*-positive subjects among participants aged ≥40 years, *H. pylori* was less likely to directly diminish the absorption of fucoidan in this age group. Excluding *H. pylori*-positive participants aged ≥40 years who ate mozuku regularly, ΔMax fucoidan values were similar between *H. pylori*-positive and *H. pylori*-negative subjects. In addition, the frequency of mozuku consumption among *H. pylori*-positive participants was similar between subjects aged <40 years and those aged ≥40 years; therefore, the frequency of mozuku consumption is not directly associated with the absorption of fucoidan. Given that *H. pylori* positivity and regular mozuku consumption were associated with diminished fucoidan absorption among subjects aged ≥40 years but not among younger subjects, the duration of *H. pylori* infection and the frequency of mozuku appear important for fucoidan absorption.

How do frequent mozuku consumption and *H. pylori* infection disturb fucoidan absorption in subjects aged ≥40 years? *H. pylori* can change the secretion and acidification functions of the stomach because it penetrates into this organ. Although nutrient absorption does not occur in the stomach, *H. pylori* infection can affect the digestion and absorption of nutrients such as vitamin B_{12}, vitamin C, vitamin A, vitamin E, and folate [19–21]. Shibata et al. [7] reported that mozuku fucoidan can bind to *H. pylori* and inhibit its attachment to the gastric mucosa at pH 2.0 and 4.0, but not at pH 7.4. It is well known that *H. pylori* rarely causes atrophic gastritis in young people (<40 years old), whereas *H. pylori*-induced atrophic gastritis tends to be rather common in the elderly [15–18]. When hypochlorhydria occurs after *H. pylori*-induced atrophic gastritis, intragastric pH increases, consequently inhibiting the ability of *H. pylori* to bind to fucoidan. However, fucoidan absorption was not diminished in *H. pylori*-positive subjects aged ≥40 years who rarely ate mozuku, suggesting the influence of a long duration of mozuku ingestion on fucoidan absorption. Amornlerdpison et al. reported that fucoidan present in mozuku acts as an antagonist of the H_2 receptor (similar to cimetidine), decreasing the acidity of gastric acid and raising the pH in the stomach [23]. Taken together, *H. pylori*-induced atrophic gastritis and a long duration of mozuku ingestion may markedly decrease acid secretion, consequently leading to the failure of *H. pylori* to bind fucoidan and reductions of its absorption in the small intestine in people aged ≥40 years. Thus, the possible mechanism by which *H. pylori* infection leads to reduced gastric acid secretion and fucoidan absorption has not been sufficiently investigated to draw definite conclusions, and other mechanisms other than hypochlorhydria following *H. pylori* infection are possible.

Of note, significant positive correlations of the basal fucoidan levels with both *H. pylori* titers and ΔMax fucoidan values were revealed in *H. pylori*-positive subjects aged <40 years who frequently consumed fucoidan. Such correlations were not found in the corresponding group of participants aged ≥40 years, nor were they observed in *H. pylori*-positive subjects who rarely ate mozuku or in *H. pylori*-negative subjects. Because the significance of the positive correlation observed in *H. pylori*-positive subjects aged <40 years who frequently consumed fucoidan is unclear, further research is necessary to clarify the relevance of *H. pylori* infection and mozuku intake to fucoidan absorption using a large number of subjects.

Interestingly, basal fucoidan levels were significantly increased by *H. pylori* infection and mozuku consumption. As *H. pylori* is known to affect the absorption of various nutrients, this stomach bacterium may participate in basal fucoidan absorption. In recent years, "the nutrition-gut microbiome-physiology axis" has attracted substantial attention [24–28]. Because *H. pylori* can induce drastic alterations in the variety of the gastrointestinal microbiota [29–31], the microbe is speculated to increase basal fucoidan levels by modifying the gastrointestinal microbiota. Basal fucoidan levels were also significantly higher in *H. pylori*-negative subjects who regularly consumed mozuku than in their counterparts who rarely ate mozuku, which confirmed our previous findings [13]. We speculated that Japanese people may have acquired digestive enzymes from mozuku because the seaweed is extensively consumed within this area. Because of the limited evidence, the overall significance of *H. pylori* infection and mozuku consumption to basal fucoidan levels is unclear.

This study had several limitations. First, subjects who received eradication therapy for *H. pylori* and underwent gastrectomy prior to the study were not excluded. The study also did not exclude subjects who used complementary and alternative medicines, which can affect the absorption of fucoidan.

Second, a urine-based ELISA kit (URINELISA) was used to assay *H. pylori* infection, and the high accuracy of this test was certified by several investigators [32,33]. A disadvantage of this test is that proteinuria can cause false-positive results; therefore, urine protein levels should be measured in future research. We plan to study the relationship of *H. pylori* infection with fucoidan absorption using serum-based ELISA kits or the ^{13}C urea breath test (^{13}C-UBT) in future research.

In addition, the specificity of our fucoidan ELISA was limited. We assayed urinary fucoidan levels using a polyclonal antibody for Okinawa mozuku fucoidan, which weakly cross-reacted with *Fucus vesiculosus* fucoidan [22]. Because the brown seaweeds of kombu (*Laminaria japonica*) and wakame (*Undaria pinnatifida*) are traditional foodstuffs in Japan, fucoidan contained in these seaweeds may cross-react with our antibody. Further studies are necessary to elucidate the effects of mozuku consumption on the intestinal absorption of fucoidan using ELISA with a monoclonal antibody.

4. Materials and Methods

4.1. Subjects

We published pamphlets describing the purpose, methods, and exclusion items of our research titled "The reference of *H. pylori* infection to absorption of mozuku fucoidan" on the Internet and recruited volunteer participants. Two hundred sixty-two Japanese people submitted applications from April 2014 to June 2016. They completed a questionnaire assessing gender, age, and mozuku consumption. We enrolled 259 volunteers who completed questionnaires and collected urine samples as planned. Subjects were divided into five age groups: 20–29, 30–39, 40–49, 50–50, and ≥60 years old.

The frequency of mozuku consumption was divided into five groups as follows: approximately 1–3 times weekly, approximately once every 2 weeks, approximately once monthly, approximately once every 2–3 months, and rarely (Table 1).

This study was conducted according to the Declaration of Helsinki. The protocol of the study was approved by the Ethics Committee of South Product Co., Ltd. (UMIN000039117). Following an explanation of the study and its aim, all subjects provided informed consent.

4.2. Oral Intake of Fucoidan and Collection of Urine Samples

Subjects refrained from marine algae and fucoidan supplementation on the day before the test and on the day of the test to avoid the effects of diet. Subjects orally consumed two fucoidan drinks (1500 mg/bottle) at 9:00 in the morning. Urine samples were extracted four times, namely, before (0) and 3, 6, and 9 h after fucoidan ingestion. Urine samples were collected by a parcel delivery service.

In this study, the subjects orally consumed 3 g of mozuku fucoidan. The drink was prepared by South Product Co., Ltd.

4.3. Assay for Fucoidan Levels in Urine Samples

Urine fucoidan levels were assayed using a sandwich ELISA method developed by our laboratory [22]. The reproducibility of the fucoidan ELISA method was as follows. The intra- and inter-assay CVs for serum, plasma, and urine, using high and low concentrations of fucoidan, were in the range of 1.5–13.4%. The detection limit concentration of our ELISA was less than 1 ng/mL.

4.4. Assay for Anti-H. pylori Antibody Titers in Urine

Single-void urine samples were obtained and stored at 2–8 °C until use. Urinary IgG antibodies to *H. pylori* were measured using a urine-based ELISA kit (URINELISA®, Otsuka Pharmaceutical Co.,

Ltd.) that utilizes a VacA- and CagA-positive *H. pylori* strain isolated from a Japanese patient with gastritis as the antigen source. This ELISA-based test result was considered positive when a cutoff index of 1.0 (optical density = 0.218) or greater was obtained after measurement of the optical density according to the manufacturer's instructions [32–34].

The ΔMax fucoidan value was calculated by subtracting the basal value (before ingestion) from the highest level of urinary fucoidan following fucoidan ingestion. If the basal fucoidan level was higher than that after fucoidan ingestion, then the ΔMax fucoidan value was recorded as 0.

4.5. Statistical Analysis

The urinary fucoidan values after fucoidan ingestion were analyzed using two-way analysis of variance (ANOVA) or one-way ANOVA followed by Tukey's test for multiple comparisons. SAS version 9.4 (Statistical Analysis Software 9.4, SAS Institute Inc., Cary, NC, USA) was used to perform statistical analyses.

The Mann–Whitney U-test was used to analyze between-group differences. Statistical correlations were analyzed using Spearman's rank correlation coefficient. In addition, multiple regression analysis was performed with *H. pylori* infection as the dependent variable and age and mozuku consumption as the independent variables. The results were expressed as the hazard ratio and 95% confidence interval. Data are expressed as the mean ± SD. $P < 0.05$ indicated a statistically significant difference.

5. Conclusions

The present data illustrated that fucoidan absorption is associated with *H. pylori* infection and mozuku consumption. Fucoidan absorption in *H. pylori*-positive subjects who regularly consumed mozuku differed by age, being significantly lower in subjects aged ≥40 years than in their younger counterparts. A significant positive correlation between the basal fucoidan level and ΔMax fucoidan value was found among subjects aged <40 who regularly consumed mozuku but not among their older counterparts. Further studies are needed to elucidate the precise mechanisms influencing fucoidan absorption.

Author Contributions: T.N. designed the experiments and wrote the manuscript, M.T. wrote the manuscript; M.I. reviewed the manuscript. All authors have read and agreed to the published version of the manuscript.

Funding: This research received no external funding.

Acknowledgments: We would like to thank Kizuku Kadena for assistance with all experiments. In addition, we would like to thank Assistant Professor Kenji Nakamura (Takasaki University of Health and Welfare) for his helpful advice regarding the statistical analysis.

Conflicts of Interest: The authors declare no conflicts of interest.

References

1. Cumashi, A.; Ushakova, N.A.; Preobrazhenskaya, M.E.; D'Incecco, A.; Piccoli, A.; Totani, L.; Tinari, N.; Morozevich, G.E.; Berman, A.E.; Bilan, M.I.; et al. A comparative study of the anti-inflammatory, anticoagulant, antiangiogenic, and antiadhesive activities of nine different fucoidans from brown seaweeds. *Glycobiology* **2007**, *17*, 541–552. [CrossRef]
2. Wu, L.; Sun, J.; Su, X.; Yu, Q.; Yu, Q.; Zhang, P.; Suna, J. A review about the development of fucoidan in antitumor activity: Progress and challenges. *Carbohydr. Polym.* **2016**, *10*, 96–111. [CrossRef]
3. Fitton, J.H.; Park, A.Y.; Stringer, D.N.; Karpiniec, S.S. Therapies from fucoidan: New developments. *Mar. Drugs* **2019**, *17*, 571. [CrossRef]
4. Van Weelden, G.; Bobiński, M.; Okła, K.; Van Weelden, W.J.; Romano, A.; Pijnenborg, J.M.A. Fucoidan structure and activity in relation to anti-cancer mechanisms. *Mar. Drugs* **2019**, *17*, 32. [CrossRef]
5. Wang, Y.; Xing, M.; Cao, Q.; Ji, A.; Liang, H.; Song, S. Biological activities of fucoidan and the factors mediating its therapeutic effects: A Review of Recent Studies. *Mar. Drugs* **2019**, *17*, 183. [CrossRef]

6. Shibata, H.; Kimura-Takagi, I.; Nagaoka, M.; Hashimoto, S.; Sawada, H.; Ueyama, S.; Yokokura, T. Inhibitory effect of cladosiphon fucoidan on the adhesion of helicobacter pylori to human gastric cells. *J. Nutr. Sci. Vitaminol. (Tokyo)* **1999**, *45*, 325–336. [CrossRef]
7. Shibata, H.; Iimuro, M.; Uchiya, N.; Kawamori, T.; Nagaoka, M.; Ueyama, S.; Hashimoto, S.; Yokokura, T.; Sugimura, T.; Wakabayashi, K. Preventive effects of cladosiphon fucoidan against Helicobacter pylori infection in mongolian gerbils. *Helicobacter* **2003**, *8*, 59–65. [CrossRef]
8. Besednova, N.N.; Zaporozhets, T.S.; Somova, L.M.; Kuznetsova, T.A. Review: Prospects for the use of extracts and polysaccharides from marine algae to prevent and treat the diseases caused by Helicobacter pylori. *Helicobacter* **2015**, *20*, 89–97. [CrossRef]
9. Chua, E.G.; Verbrugghe, P.; Perkins, T.T.; Tay, C. Fucoidans disrupt adherence of Helicobacter pylori to AGS cells in vitro. *Evid.-Based Complement. Altern. Med.* **2015**, *2015*, 1–6. [CrossRef]
10. Nagamine, T.; Hayakawa, K.; Nakazato, K.; Iha, M. Determination of the active transport of fucoidan derived from Okinawa Mozuku across the human intestinal Caco-2 cells as assessed by size-exclusion chromatography. *J. Chromatogr. B Analyt. Technol. Biomed. Life Sci.* **2015**, *997*, 187–193. [CrossRef]
11. Zhang, E.; Chu, F.; Xu, L.; Liang, H.; Song, S.; Ji, A. Use of fluorescein isothiocyanate isomer I to study the mechanism of intestinal absorption of fucoidan sulfate in vivo and in vitro. *Biopharm. Drug. Dispos.* **2018**, *39*, 298–307. [CrossRef]
12. Imbs, T.I.; Zvyagintseva, T.N.; Ermakova, S.P. Is the transformation of fucoidans in human body possible? *Int. J. Biol. Macromol.* **2020**, *142*, 778–781. [CrossRef]
13. Kadena, K.; Tomori, M.; Iha, M.; Nagamine, T. Absorption study of Mozuku Fucoidan in Japanese volunteers. *Mar. Drugs* **2018**, *16*, 254. [CrossRef]
14. Hehemann, J.-H.; Correc, G.; Barbeyron, T.; Helbert, W.; Czjzek, M.; Michel, G. Transfer of carbohydrate-active enzymes from marine bacteria to Japanese gut microbiota. *Nature* **2010**, *464*, 908–912. [CrossRef]
15. Sipponen, P.; Helske, T.; Järvinen, P.; Hyvarinen, H.; Seppälä, K.; Siurala, M. Fall in the prevalence of chronic gastritis over 15 years: Analysis of outpatient series in Finland from 1977, 1985, and 1992. *Gut* **1994**, *35*, 1167–1171. [CrossRef]
16. Kamada, T.; Haruma, K.; Akiyama, T.; Tanaka, S.; Shiotani, A.; Graham, D.Y.; Ito, M.; Inoue, K.; Manabe, N.; Matsumoto, H.; et al. Time trends in Helicobacter pylori infection and atrophic gastritis over 40 Years in Japan. *Helicobacter* **2015**, *20*, 192–198. [CrossRef]
17. Pichon, M.; Burucoa, C. Impact of the gastro-intestinal bacterial microbiome on Helicobacter-associated diseases. *Healthcare* **2019**, *7*, 34. [CrossRef]
18. Pero, R.; Brancaccio, M.; Laneri, S.; Biasi, M.; Lombardo, B.; Scudiero, O. A novel view of human Helicobacter pylori infections: Interplay between microbiota and beta-defensins. *Biomolecules* **2019**, *9*, 237. [CrossRef]
19. Franceschi, F.; Annalisa, T.; Teresa, D.R.; Giovanna, D.; Ianiro, G.; Franco, S.; Viviana, G.; Valentina, T.; Riccardo, L.L.; Antonio, G. Role of Helicobacter pylori infection on nutrition and metabolism. *World J. Gastroenterol.* **2014**, *20*, 12809–12817. [CrossRef]
20. Aditi, A.; Graham, D.Y. Vitamin C, Gastritis, and gastric disease: A historical review and update. *Dig. Dis. Sci.* **2012**, *57*, 2504–2515. [CrossRef]
21. Ackam, M. Helicobacter pylori and micronutrients. *Indian Pediatr.* **2010**, *47*, 119–126.
22. Tokita, Y.; Nakajima, K.; Mochida, H.; Iha, M.; Nagamine, T. Development of a fucoidan-specific antibody and measurement of fucoidan in serum and urine by Sandwich ELISA. *Biosci. Biotechnol. Biochem.* **2010**, *74*, 350–357. [CrossRef]
23. Amornlerdpison, D.; Peerapompisal, Y.; Taesoticul, T.; Noiraraksar, T.; Kanjanapothi, D. Gastroprotective activity of Padina minor Yamada. *Chiang Mai J. Sci.* **2009**, *36*, 92–103.
24. Biesalski, H.K. Nutrition meets the microbiome: Micronutrients and the microbiota. *Ann. N. Y. Acad. Sci.* **2016**, *1372*, 53–64. [CrossRef]
25. Ticinesi, A.; Lauretani, F.; Milani, C.; Nouvenne, A.; Tana, C.; Del Rio, D.; Maggio, M.; Ventura, M.; Meschi, T. Aging gut microbiota at the cross-road between nutrition, physical frailty, and sarcopenia: Is there a gut-muscle axis? *Nutrients* **2017**, *9*, 1303. [CrossRef]
26. Sandhu, K.V.; Sherwin, E.; Schellekens, H.; Stanton, C.; Dinan, T.G.; Cryan, J.F. Feeding the microbiota-gut-brain axis: Diet, microbiome, and neuropsychiatry. *Transl. Res.* **2017**, *179*, 223–244. [CrossRef]
27. Valdes, A.M.; Walter, J.; Segal, E.; Spector, T.D. Role of the gut microbiota in nutrition and health. *BMJ* **2018**, *361*, k2179. [CrossRef]

28. Moschen, A.R.; Wieser, V.; Tilg, H. Dietary factors: Major regulators of the gut's microbiota. *Gut Liver* **2012**, *6*, 411–416. [CrossRef]
29. Das, A.; Pereira, V.; Saxena, S.; Ghosh, T.S.; Anbumani, D.; Bag, S.; Das, B.; Nair, G.B.; Abraham, P.; Mande, S.S. Gastric microbiome of Indian patients with Helicobacter pylori infection, and their interaction networks. *Sci. Rep.* **2017**, *7*, 15438. [CrossRef] [PubMed]
30. Maldonado-Contreras, A.; Goldfarb, K.C.; Godoy-Vitorino, F.; Karaoz, U.; Contreras, M.; Blaser, M.J.; Brodie, E.L.; Dominguez-Bello, M.G. Structure of the human gastric bacterial community in relation to Helicobacter pylori status. *ISME J.* **2010**, *5*, 574–579. [CrossRef]
31. Schulz, C.; Schütte, K.; Koch, N.; Vilchez-Vargas, R.; Wos-Oxley, M.L.; Oxley, A.P.A.; Vital, M.; Malfertheiner, P.; Pieper, D.H. The active bacterial assemblages of the upper GI tract in individuals with and withoutHelicobacterinfection. *Gut* **2016**, *67*, 216–225. [CrossRef] [PubMed]
32. Kato, M.; Asaka, M.; Saito, M.; Sekine, H.; Ohara, S.; Toyota, T.; Akamatsu, T.; Kaneko, T.; Kiyosawa, K.; Nishizawa, O.; et al. Clinical usefulness of urine-based enzyme-linked immunosorbent assay for detection of antibody to Helicobacter pylori: A collaborative study in nine medical institutions in Japan. *Helicobacter* **2000**, *5*, 109–119. [CrossRef] [PubMed]
33. Miwa, H.; Hirose, M.; Kikuchi, S.; Terai, T.; Iwazaki, R.; Kobayashi, O.; Takei, Y.; Ogihara, T.; Sato, N. How useful is the detection kit for antibody to Helicobacter pylori in urine (URINELISA) in clinical practice? *Am. J. Gastroenterol.* **1999**, *94*, 3460–3463. [CrossRef] [PubMed]
34. Katsuragi, K.; Noda, A.; Tachikawa, T.; Azuma, A.; Mukai, F.; Murakami, K.; Fujioka, T.; Kato, M.; Asaka, M. Highly sensitive urine-based enzyme-linked immunosorbent assay for detection of antibody to Helicobacter pylori. *Helicobacter* **1998**, *3*, 289–295. [CrossRef]

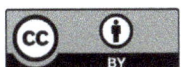

© 2020 by the authors. Licensee MDPI, Basel, Switzerland. This article is an open access article distributed under the terms and conditions of the Creative Commons Attribution (CC BY) license (http://creativecommons.org/licenses/by/4.0/).

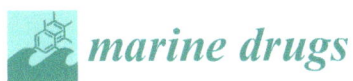

Article

Effects of a Newly Developed Enzyme-Assisted Extraction Method on the Biological Activities of Fucoidans in Ocular Cells

Philipp Dörschmann [1],*, Maria Dalgaard Mikkelsen [2], Thuan Nguyen Thi [2], Johann Roider [1], Anne S. Meyer [2] and Alexa Klettner [1]

- [1] Department of Ophthalmology, University Medical Center, University of Kiel, Arnold-Heller-Str. 3, Haus 25, 24105 Kiel, Germany; johann.roider@uksh.de (J.R.); alexakarina.klettner@uksh.de (A.K.)
- [2] Department of Biotechnology and Biomedicine, Technical University of Denmark, Søltofts Plads, 2800 Kongens Lyngby, Denmark; mdami@dtu.dk (M.D.M.); thuthi@dtu.dk (T.N.T.); asme@dtu.dk (A.S.M.)
- * Correspondence: philipp.doerschmann@uksh.de; Tel.: +49-431-500-13712

Received: 30 April 2020; Accepted: 25 May 2020; Published: 26 May 2020

Abstract: Fucoidans from brown seaweeds are promising substances as potential drugs against age-related macular degeneration (AMD). The heterogeneity of fucoidans requires intensive research in order to find suitable species and extraction methods. Ten different fucoidan samples extracted enzymatically from *Laminaria digitata* (LD), *Saccharina latissima* (SL) and *Fucus distichus* subsp. *evanescens* (FE) were tested for toxicity, oxidative stress protection and VEGF (vascular endothelial growth factor) inhibition. For this study crude fucoidans were extracted from seaweeds using different enzymes and SL fucoidans were further separated into three fractions (SL_F1-F3) by ion-exchange chromatography (IEX). Fucoidan composition was analyzed by high performance anion exchange chromatography (HPAEC) after acid hydrolysis. The crude extracts contained alginate, while two of the fractionated SL fucoidans SL_F2 and SL_F3 were highly pure. Cell viability was assessed with an 3-(4,5-dimethylthiazol-2-yl)-5-(3-carboxymethoxyphenyl)-2-(4-sulfophenyl)-2H-tetrazolium (MTS) assay in OMM-1 and ARPE-19. Protective effects were investigated after 24 h of stress insult in OMM-1 and ARPE-19. Secreted VEGF was analyzed via ELISA (enzyme-linked immunosorbent assay) in ARPE-19 cells. Fucoidans showed no toxic effects. In OMM-1 SL_F2 and several FE fucoidans were protective. LD_SiAT2 (Cellic®CTec2 + Sigma-Aldrich alginate lyase), FE_SiAT3 (Cellic® CTec3 + Sigma-Aldrich alginate lyase), SL_F2 and SL_F3 inhibited VEGF with the latter two as the most effective. We could show that enzyme treated fucoidans in general and the fractionated SL fucoidans SL_F2 and SL_F3 are very promising for beneficial AMD relevant biological activities.

Keywords: fucoidan; fucose; enzymatic purification; age-related macular degeneration; VEGF; oxidative stress; *Laminaria digitata*; *Fucus distichus* subsp. *evanescens*; *Saccharina latissima*; retinal pigment epithelium

1. Introduction

AMD (age-related macular degeneration) as main cause of central vision loss in the elderly is an irreversible disease with the number of patients annually increasing [1]. In the late phase of the disease, two forms exist which both lead to a degeneration of retinal components in the macula lutea. In the early form of AMD oxidized lipid protein molecules are deposited, terminating in accumulated drusen, which may interfere with retinal pigment epithelium (RPE) function. RPE cells are important for the maintenance of the photoreceptors. In the late stages of the disease geographic atrophies can occur, with large areas of RPE and photoreceptor degeneration [2,3]. In the exudative ("wet") late form, an excessive production of the vascular endothelial growth factor (VEGF) leads to the formation of new blood vessels growing under and into the retina, causing edema and bleeding which ruptures the retina [2]. The pathology and causes of AMD development are not completely understood, but factors like complement activation, oxidative stress, inflammatory milieu and the excess VEGF are correlated with the development of AMD [2,4–6]. Up until now, the only treatment available are VEGF inhibiting agents, which need to be regularly injected in the human eye and slow down the deterioration but cannot cure the disease [7].

Brown seaweeds produce numerous very promising chemical compounds that are interesting for medical research, because of their beneficial effects for human health. An example are fucoidans, also designated as sulfated fucans, which are marine polysaccharides mainly composed of sulfated fucosyl moieties and sulfate ester groups. Minor constituents in fucoidans include other sugar moieties like galactose, mannose, xylose and glucuronic acids. Fucoidans are cell wall components and serve mainly as protective agent against pathogens and other environmental influences in the ocean [8]. In addition, they are also important as structural component and protect against dehydration [9]. Fucoidans exert many additional biological effects. These biological activities depend on the structure and this in turn depends on factors like algal species [10], harvest place and harvest time [11]. Among the different biological effects are the capability to lower inflammatory cytokines, to reduce oxidative burden and to inhibit VEGF as well as blood lipids [12]. These effects pave the way for a possible treatment option for AMD and other diseases in the human eye [13]. However, the activities of the fucoidans are highly dependent on the biological systems they are applied to. Therefore, appropriate testing systems are vital for investigating its potential and furthermore, the extraction method, as this effects the structure and the purity of the tested extracts are of high importance for reproducible beneficial effects.

In order to properly elucidate structure-function relationships of fucoidans for prevention of AMD or other degenerative diseases, it is essential to focus on the extraction technology. In particular, to obtain pure fucoidans, while maintaining the relevant structural features required for specific biological activities. Early work on fucoidans relied on several steps of acidic extraction at elevated temperatures (70–100 °C), but such extractions may affect the chemical composition and size of the extracted fucoidans [14]. Instead, we have developed several targeted enzymatic assisted extraction procedures that gently and precisely loosens up the cell wall matrix, releasing fucoidans in a gentle way, obtaining crude fucoidan extracts, containing also low molecular weight alginates In previous work one of these new enzymatic treatments were used and followed by ion-exchange chromatographic (IEX) purification obtaining well-defined, pure fucoidans from *Saccharina latissima* (SL) [15].

We showed already promising effects of different fucoidans on ocular cells. In brief, fucoidans from past studies were extracted with hot water, followed by precipitation with $CaCl_2$ and ultrafiltration or dialysis [16–19]. *Fucus vesiculosus* fucoidan from Sigma-Aldrich can reduce angiogenesis and VEGF of RPE [13]. Fucoidans from *Fucus serratus*, *Laminaria digitata* (LD) and *Fucus distichus* subsp. *evanescens* (FE) were protective against oxidative stress in the uveal melanoma cell line OMM-1 and could inhibit ARPE-19 VEGF production [19] exactly like a other *Saccharina latissima* fucoidan, which was protective in ARPE-19 and lowered VEGF of primary RPE [19]. Different sized fucoidans from *Laminaria hyperborea* showed that the large, non-degraded fucoidan is most suitable for oxidative stress protection and VEGF inhibition [17]. Moreover, the tested fucoidans are not antiproliferative for ocular cells in general [16], which is necessary for use in medical treatments. However, the biological effects of fucoidan differ strongly in relation to their chemical characteristics, which are influenced by the extraction method, and activities may be confounded by contaminants in the extracts [20,21].

The objective of this work was to examine fucoidans from three different algal species (LD, SL, FE), which were extracted with four different enzymatic treatments, followed by alginate precipitation with either HCl or $CaCl_2$. Additionally, crude fucoidan from SL was further purified and separated by ion-exchange chromatographic (IEX). In our previous studies related to fucoidans and their effect on ocular cells, we focused on the comparison of different algal species, fucoidans with different molecular weights or the effects on cell viability in tumor and non-tumor cell lines. In this study we tested fucoidans from different species, extracted from the seaweeds by different enzymatic methods. In addition, SL extracts were further purified and fractionated by IEX thereby removing contaminating compounds like alginate and polyphenols and achieving a higher fucose content. This study focuses on investigating whether the biological activity of fucoidans can be improved by different enzyme assisted purification methods. We compare fucoidans from different brown algal species and different enzymatically assisted treatments as well as IEX fractionation, to choose the most promising combination for further AMD research. Performed tests include detection of toxic effects, the ability to protect ocular cells against oxidative stress and to inhibit VEGF secretion. Furthermore, molecular weights and monosaccharide composition was determined to make a connection to the biological effects. Taken together, this study is well equipped to compare the bioactivity of fucoidans in relation to enzymatic extraction methods (different FE enzymatic purified extracts), further isolating steps (fractionated SL extracts), and also different species of origin (LD, SL, FE) in relation to the molecular weight and monosaccharide composition.

2. Results

2.1. Chemical Characterization of the Fucoidans

All tested fucoidans and the used extraction and purification methods were designated according to a code as seen in Table 1 In brief, the dried seaweed material was enzymatically extracted with commercial cellulase preparations Cellic®CTec2 or Cellic®CTec3 mixes ("2" or "3" in extraction code) and additional alginate lyase from Sigma-Aldrich SigmALy (SiAT) or alginate lyase SALy expressed from *Sphingomonas* sp. (SAT) were added (making the extracts SiAT2, SiAT3 as well as SAT2 and SAT3). The extracts with an additional "ad" in the code were precipitated with acid (HCl). Other extracts were precipitated with $CaCl_2$. F1–F3 stands for an additional three-step fractionation process with chromatographic isolation (IEX).

Table 1. Overview of the used fucoidans, including algae species, extraction method and code used in this manuscript. For the explanation of the extraction methods refer to Section 2.1.

Fucoidan Code	Extraction Method	Algal Species
LD_SiAT2	SigmALY_CTECH2_crude	*Laminaria digitata*
SL_SiAT2	SigmAly_CTECH2_crude	*Saccharina latissima*
FE_SiAT2	SigmAly_CTECH2_crude	*Fucus distichus* subsp. *evanescens*
FE_SiAT2ad	SigmAly_CTECH2_acid_dialysis	*Fucus distichus* subsp. *evanescens*
FE_SiAT3ad	SigmAly_CTECH3_acid_dialysis	*Fucus distichus* subsp. *evanescens*
FE_SAT2ad	Saly_CTECH2_acid_dialysis	*Fucus distichus* subsp. *evanescens*
FE_SAT3ad	Saly_CTECH3_acid_dialysis	*Fucus distichus* subsp. *evanescens*
SL_F1	SALy_CTECH2_$CaCl_2$_IEX_filtering_Fraction 1 *	*Saccharina latissima*
SL_F2	SALy_CTECH2_$CaCl_2$_IEX_filtering_Fraction 2 *	*Saccharina latissima*
SL_F3	SALy_CTECH2_$CaCl_2$_IEX_filtering_Fraction 3 *	*Saccharina latissima*

* Nguyen et al., 2020 [15].

Three crude extracts were made with Cellic®CTec2 and SigmALy from the three different algae (LD_SiAT2, SL_SiAT2 and FE_SiAT2). The residual alginate was not precipitated in these extracts and the alginate content was high (mannuronic acid plus guluronic acid) 87.2%, 80.3% and 67.5% and the fucose content was low 3.9, 12.3 and 15.5% respectively, as determined by high performance anion exchange chromatography (HPAEC) with pulsed amperometric detection (PAD) (Table 2; [22]) (chemical composition with standard deviations in Table A1).

Table 2. Overview of monosaccharide and uronic acid composition in mol%. (Fuc-Fucose, Ara/Rham-Arabinose/Rhamnose, Gal-Galactose, Glc-Glucose, Xyl-Xylose, Man-Mannose, GuluA-guluronic acid, GluA-glucoronic acid, ManA-mannonic acid); GuluA + ManA was calculated together and equals mol% alginates; the highest values are marked in bold.

Sample	Fuc	GuluA	ManA	GuluA + ManA	Mannitol	Ara/Rham	Gal	Glc	Xyl	Man	GluA	Total	Sulfate (SO_4^{2-}), %
LD_SiAT2	3.9	12.4	74.8	87.2	**1.2**	0.1	1.4	2.3	1.5	1.2	1.2	100.0	9.3
SL_SiAT2	12.3	**32.2**	48.1	80.3	0.2	0.2	1.3	2.6	0.9	0.8	1.5	100.0	14.4
FE_SiAT2	15.5	18.7	48.8	67.5	0.0	0.3	2.5	2.1	3.6	1.8	6.5	100.0	20.2
FE_SiAT2ad	36.1	7.1	30.0	37.1	0.1	0.6	6.6	**5.7**	**10.2**	1.8	2.0	100.0	30.1
FE_SiAT3ad	35.9	10.0	40.4	50.4	0.1	0.4	2.8	2.2	4.1	2.0	2.2	100.0	29.4
FE_SAT2ad	52.2	8.8	12.5	21.3	0.0	**1.2**	4.8	2.7	9.3	**4.7**	3.9	100.0	31.7
FE_SAT3ad	48.3	11.6	16.4	28.0	0.1	0.7	5.0	2.0	8.3	4.0	3.7	100.0	29.9
SL_F1 *	5.4	8.5	**82.4**	**90.9**	0.0	0.1	0.5	0.4	0.8	0.8	1.1	100.0	6.6
SL_F2 *	**64.7**	0.0	6.9	6.9	0.1	0.3	12.2	0.6	4.8	3.5	**6.9**	100.0	35.6
SL_F3 *	63.3	0.0	0.8	0.8	0.0	0.3	**26.9**	0.4	3.4	2.1	2.8	100.0	**46.4**

* Nguyen et al., [15]. To extract fucoidans in a more gentle way in order to retain the molecule as intact as possible, enzymes were employed in the extraction procedure. Crude fucoidan extracts were prepared using different enzyme cocktails, with either the cell wall degrading enzyme mix Cellic®CTec2 or 3 from Novozymes A/S, enzyme cocktails developed to degrade polysaccharides from terrestrial plant cell walls. In addition, alginate lyases were also added, since alginate is a brown seaweed specific polysaccharide that is not degraded by the Cellic®CTec2 or 3 [23]. Two different alginate lyases were used (refer Section 4.2.2), which have different specificities [15]. Fucoidans have previously been purified using different enzymes, including the cellulase enzyme Celluclast [25] The Cellic®CTec2 used here contains extra β-glucosidases and lytic cellulose monooxygenases (1.14.99.54, 1.14.99.56, AA9) as well as other proprietary proteins compared to Celluclast. In addition, it has specifically been shown that Cellic®CTec2 can degrade laminarin [23]. Furthermore, this new method includes the novel use of two different alginate lyases for purification of fucoidans.

In order to see the highest values of each substance instantly, we marked these values in bold. Not all alginate was degraded by the alginate lyase SigmALy, therefore the following extracts were prepared with different enzyme mixes and with further alginate precipitation with acid followed by neutralization of pH and dialysis (FE_SiAT2ad, FE_SiAT3ad, FE_SAT2ad, FE_SAT3ad). Since it contains the highest amount of fucoidan FE was used for these extractions. The resulting extracts had a comparable lower content of alginates 37.1, 50.4, 21.3 and 28.0% and higher content of fucose 36.1, 35.9, 52.2, 48.3%, respectively, compared to the previous extract FE_SiAT2. Furthermore, it was evident that the use of the alginate lyase SALy was more efficient in degrading the alginate than SigmALy, in particular the mannuronic acids (Table 2). These optimizations of using SALy and alginate precipitation was used to prepare highly pure and fractionated fucoidans from *S. latissima* by ion-exchange chromatography (IEX), the purification method was described previously [15], while the bioactivity is tested here. SL was chosen, since previous work has shown that SL fucoidan has biological effects [19]. A further optimization was used, were the alginate was precipitated by $CaCl_2$ instead of acid, this method is believed to be gentler and is therefore likely to preserve the fucoidan structure better than the use of acid. Crude extracts from SL and FE using this method contained comparable total fucose yields and sulfate content, compared to a mild chemical extraction using acid [15]. In comparison to the LD extract three fractions of fucoidans were obtained by IEX, SL_F1, SL_F2 and SL_F3. The first elution SL_F1 contained almost exclusively alginates (90.9%) of lower molecular weight (4 kDa; [15]) while the fucose content was 5%. The SL_F2 and SL_F3 extracts contained very low amounts of alginates (6.9% and 0.8%) and high fucose content (64.7 and 63.3%), respectively. Furthermore, the SL_F2 and SL_F3 extracts contained a considerable amount of galactose, which is a likely constituent of SL fucoidan (12.2 and 26.9%) [15].

The sulfate content was previously determined for the SL fractions and corresponds well to the high amount of fucoidan present in the F2 and F3 fractions. The sulfate content for SL_F1, F2 and F3 was 6.6 ± 3.6, 35.6 ± 2.5 and 46.4 ± 3.5% respectively [15].

The size of the fucoidans was determined using high performance size-exclusion chromatography (HP-SEC). The calculated size of the fucoidans was between ~250 to over 800 kDa, with a general broad estimated size distribution (Table 3). Fucoidans from FE were generally around 350 kDa with an estimated distribution from 200–500 kDa, while the crude extracts of SL and LD were smaller, with a size around 250 and 320 kDa, respectively. The SL_F1 fraction contained mostly low molecular weight alginates with a size around 10 kDa, a peak which was also present in all crude extracts. The comparably low amount of fucoidans made it hard to determine the size in the SL_F1 extract. The size distribution was comparable and very large for SL_F2 and F3, and ranged from 100–1000 kDa, with a calculated size of over 800 kDa.

Table 3. Size and size-distribution of fucoidans determined by HP-SEC.

Fucoidan Code	Fucoidan Size Calculated (kDa)	Fucoidan Size-Distribution Estimated (kDa)
LD_SiAT2	322	250–450
SL_SiAT2	251	100–400
FE_SiAT2	322	100–500
FE_SiAT2ad	366	200–500
FE_SiAT3ad	416	200–500
FE_SAT2ad	366	200–500
FE_SAT3ad	366	200–500
SL_F1 *	Not determined	Not determined
SL_F2 *	>800	100–1000
SL_F3 *	>800	100–1000

* Nguyen et al., 2020 [15].

2.2. Effects on Cell Viability

Cell viability of the uveal melanoma cell line OMM-1 was determined after treatment with the different fucoidans for 24 h using the commercially available 3-(4,5-dimethylthiazol-2-yl)-5-(3-carboxymethoxyphenyl)-2-(4-sulfophenyl)-2H-tetrazolium (MTS) assay (Figure 1). None of the tested fucoidans significantly lowered cell viability, but some significantly increased the viability, for instance 100 µg/mL LD_SiAT2 increased viability up to 113% ± 6% ($p < 0.001$) and the SL fucoidan SL_SiAT2 increased viability to 115% ± 4% ($p < 0.001$). This might be related to the SiAT2 extraction method (in case of SL and LD fucoidan), which perhaps leads to fucoidans with beneficial effects for the cell viability of OMM-1 cells.

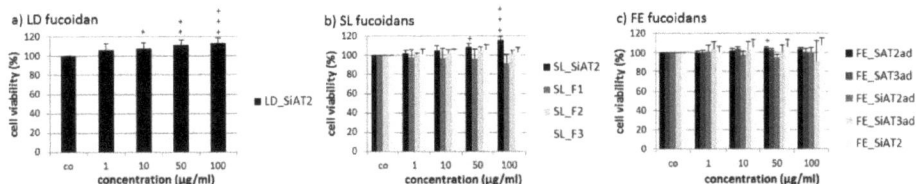

Figure 1. The cell viability of the uveal melanoma cell line OMM-1 was assessed after treatment for 24 h with *Laminaria digitata* (LD) fucoidan (**a**), *Saccharina latissima* (SL) fucoidans (**b**) and *Fucus distichus* subsp. *evanescens* (FE) fucoidans (**c**) extracted with SiAT2/3 or SAT2/3 (SiAT2/3 = Cellic®CTec2 or 3 enzyme mix + Sigma-Aldrich alginate lyase (SigmALy), SAT2/3 = Cellic®CTec2 or 3 enzyme mix + alginate lyase expressed from *Sphingomonas* sp. (SALy), ad = acid treatment and dialysis). Also, three SL ion-exchange chromatography (IEX) fractions (SL_F1, SL_F2 and SL_F3) were invastigated. Cell viability was analyzed with a MTS (3-(4,5-Dimethylthiazol-2-yl)-5-(3-carboxymethoxyphenyl)-2-(4-sulfophenyl)-2H-tetrazolium) assay and is shown as the mean and standard deviation in relation to the 100% control. Significance was determined with ANOVA; + $p < 0.05$, ++ $p < 0.01$, +++ $p < 0.001$ compared to control ($n \geq 4$; number of independent experiments). No fucoidan exhibited antiproliferative effects.

The same procedure was performed for the human RPE cell line ARPE-19 (Figure 2). Cell viability was determined after 24 h with the MTS assay. Again, none of the fucoidan displayed significant antiproliferative effects. SiAT2 extracts from all three seaweed species, increased cell viability slightly at 100 µg/mL, again, although under 10% difference compared to control and therefore not biological relevant.

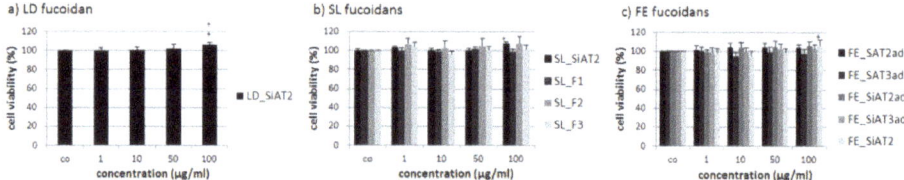

Figure 2. The cell viability of the human RPE cell line ARPE-19 was assessed after treatment for 24 h with LD fucoidan (**a**), SL fucoidans (**b**) and FE fucoidans (**c**). Cell viability was analyzed with a MTS assay and is shown as the mean and standard deviation in relation to the 100% control. Significance was determined with ANOVA; + $p < 0.05$, ++ $p < 0.01$ compared to control ($n \geq 4$, number of independent experiments). No fucoidan showed antiproliferative effects.

2.3. Effects on Oxidative Stress Protection

The LD fucoidan showed no significant protective effects against any tested concentration of H_2O_2, in the melanoma cell line OMM-1 (Figure 3). From SL, only the SL_F2 increased cell viability significantly at all concentrations tested with 10 µg/mL and 50 µg/mL showing the best protection (both 51% ± 1, $p < 0.001$ against 39% ± 1 stress control). FE fucoidans showed heterogeneous results depending on the tested concentration and used extraction method. FE_SAT2ad showed significant protective effects (49% ± 4%, $p < 0.01$; 49% ± 5%, $p < 0.01$; 47% ± 3%, $p < 0.05$ against 37% ± 2% stress control) at different concentrations 10 µg/mL, 50 µg/mL and 100 µg/mL, respectively In addition, 10 µg/mL FE_SAT3ad and FE_SiAT2 increased cell viability up to 61% ± 2%, $p < 0.01$ and 60% ± 8%, $p < 0.01$. It seems that the protective effects are more dependent on the tested FE fucoidan concentration then on the extraction method.

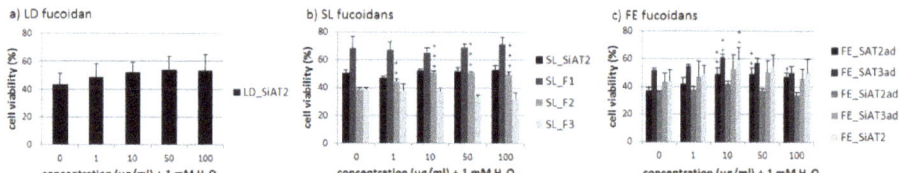

Figure 3. OMM-1 cell survival after 30 min treatment with LD fucoidan (**a**), SL fucoidans (**b**) and FE fucoidans (**c**) and 24 h stress insult with 1 mM H_2O_2, which reduced cell viability to at least 60% in all cases. Viability was determined with MTS assay. Values are pictured as the mean and standard deviation in relation to an untreated control (100%). Significance was evaluated via ANOVA; + $p < 0.05$, ++ $p < 0.01$, +++ $p < 0.001$ versus 0 µg/mL fucoidan + 1 mM H_2O_2 ($n \geq 4$, number of independent experiments).

One role of RPE cells is to limit the oxidative stress in the human retina [4]. ARPE-19 cells as an RPE cell line are very resistant against hydrogen peroxide [26]. Therefore we used 0.5 mM *tert*-butyl hydroperoxide (TBHP) to lower the cell viability of ARPE-19 significantly after 24 h, as previously shown [19]. Again, the LD fucoidan showed no significant effect (Figure 4). Some of the FE fucoidans also had a slight additional toxic effect at 50 and 100 µg/mL, while 10 µg/mL FE_SAT2ad, FE_SiAT2ad and FE_SiAT3ad had a minimal protective effect. FE fucoidan at 10 µg/mL seems to be the best concentration concerning oxidative stress protection, but the effects are small and not relevant, corresponding to the fact that ARPE-19 are rather resistant against oxidative stress on their own and are hardly affected by fucoidan extracts [17,19]. SL_F2 and SL_F3 at concentrations of 50 µg/mL slightly decreased cell viability significantly down to 47% ± 3, $p < 0.05$ and 49% ± 2%, $p < 0.05$, respectively compared to 54% ± 3% stress control, but this not likely to be biological relevant. Otherwise, there were no significant effects for the SL fucoidans.

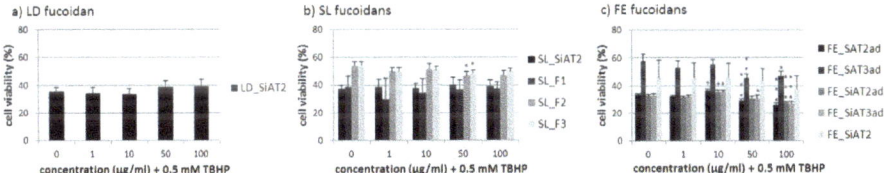

Figure 4. ARPE-19 cell survival after 30 min treatment with LD fucoidan (**a**), SL fucoidans (**b**) and FE fucoidans (**c**) and 24 h stress insult with 0.5 mM TBHP (*tert*-butyl hydroperoxide), which reduced cell viability below 60% in all cases. Viability was determined with MTS assay. Values are pictured as the mean and standard deviation in relation to an untreated control (100%). Significance was evaluated via ANOVA; + / * $p < 0.05$, ** $p < 0.01$, *** $p < 0.001$ versus 0 µg/mL fucoidan + 0.5 mM TBHP ($n \geq 4$, number of independent experiments).

2.4. VEGF Secretion of ARPE-19

We tested the influence of the ten different fucoidans on the VEGF secretion of the human RPE cell line ARPE-19. The optimal parameters for VEGF determination after fucoidan treatment were determined in a previous study [11]. In brief, cells were incubated for three days with the fucoidans and media exchange was done 24 h before taking of the supernatant for a subsequent ELISA analysis. VEGF in % was set in relation to cell viability in % both compared to untreated control (in arbitrary units [arb. unit]. The cell viability of both cell types was essentially unaffected by treatment with any sulfated fucans and at any tested concentrations (data not shown).

LD_SiAT2 lowered secreted VEGF at 10, 50 and 100 µg/mL to 0.92 ± 0.08 [arb. unit (arbitrary unit)] ($p < 0.05$), 0.88 ± 0.04 [arb. unit] ($p < 0.01$) and 0.81 ± 0.07 [arb. unit] ($p < 0.001$), respectively (Figure 5). SL_F2 and SL_F3 reduced VEGF significantly at all tested concentration, in contrast to the first fraction SL_F1 and the unfractionated SL_SiAT2 with the highest effect at 100 µg/mL (SL_F2 with 0.40 ± 0.07 [arb. unit], $p < 0.001$ and SL_F3 with 0.37 ± 0.04 [arb. unit], $p < 0.001$). The FE extracts did not show any significant VEGF reducing effects, which could be also due to the high standard deviation and heterogeneous results, with the only exception of FE_SiAT2, which lowered VEGF significant at 10 µg/mL to 0.80 ± 0.21 [arb. unit], $p < 0.05$ and at 100 µg/mL to 0.72 ± 0.10 [arb. unit], $p < 0.001$.

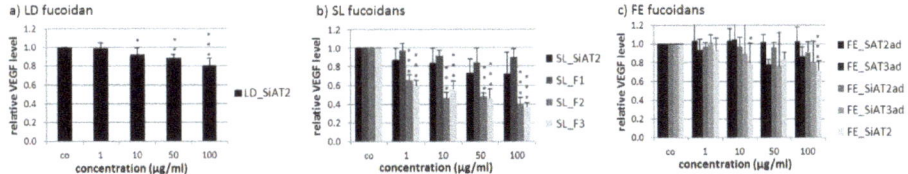

Figure 5. Secreted VEGF (vascular endothelial growth factor) of ARPE-19 after three days of incubation with 1, 10, 50 and 100 µg/mL LD fucoidan (**a**), SL fucoidans (**b**) and FE fucoidans (**c**). VEGF amount was determined with ELISA and normalized to cell survival, making a quotient of VEGF and cell viability. 10–100 µg/mL LD_SiAT2 and 1–100 µg/mL SL_F2 and SL_F3 decreased VEGF significantly. Significant values were analyzed with ANOVA, * $p < 0.05$, ** $p < 0.01$, *** $p < 0.001$ compared to the control ($n \geq 4$, number of independent experiments).

3. Discussion

3.1. Integration in Previous Studies

This study is the continuation of fucoidan research within the EU FucoSan project in regards to finding a possible treatment for AMD [16–19]. One main goal of this international project is to characterize different fucoidans to choose the best fucoidan for a potential medical application. Factors like algae species, extraction method, purity, chemical composition, harvest place and time are important to define fucoidans with the best beneficial effects for further treatment development in AMD. In previous studies, factors like algae species and molecular weight were in focus. We could show that fucoidans from SL and LH (extracted with hot water extraction followed by $CaCl_2$ precipitation and ultrafiltration or dialysis) showed the most promising effects of the species tested so far. In addition, high-molecular weight correlates with beneficial activities relevant for AMD [17,19]. Another study, testing fucoidan of FE, gave first indication that purity is an important factor for the relevant biological activities [18]. It has been suspected that in addition to the algae species the extraction method is a huge influencing factor concerning the biological activity, because it influences the structure and overall composition of the extract, leading to differential effects dependent on the method of extraction. Therefore, we investigated fucoidans purified by a novel technique using different enzymes. Additionally, we compared the effects in the three species LD, SL and FE, with different molecular weights and different monosaccharide compositions, to elucidate the best suited extraction method and algal species.

3.2. Slightly Increased Cell Viability in OMM-1 and ARPE-19 Relation to Uronic Acids, Molecular Weight and Concentration

Toxicity was not found after treatment with any extracts, which corresponds to previously published studies [16–19]. Crude LD_SiAT2 and SL_SiAT2 improved the cell viability of the OMM-1 cell line slightly. Our data indicate that further fractionation could attenuate this effect, as can be seen for the SL fractions in this work, suggesting that this effect may be due to contaminating agents. Glucose, mannitol or guluronic acid were reduced by fractionation. In addition, other not investigated agents like phenols, could have been diminished by purification. Mak et al., 2014 described that crude fucoidans from *Undaria pinnatifida* have a higher toxicity on tumor cells because of the higher yield of uronic acids [27]. However, while the crude fucoidans of this work also have higher amounts of uronic acids compared to the fractions, there were protective for OMM-1. Our fractions have although high molecular weights, which could influence the protective properties [27] and in addition different species may exert different effects.

We also gathered some data indicating that fucoidans can increase the cell viability of ARPE-19 in higher concentrations. It is unknown whether this is due to an actual protective effect of the fucoidan (which is not the case for the oxidative stress protection in ARPE-19, here only 10 µg/mL FE fucoidans had a small protective effect). It could be speculated that fucoidans in higher concentration starting with 100 µg/mL increase the cell metabolism and leads to an increased proliferation rate. It was also reported that 100 µg/mL of commercially available fucoidan from Sigma Aldrich can reduce the apoptosis of ARPE-19 cells via different cellular pathways [28].

3.3. Effects on Oxidative Stress Protection-Heterogeneous Results, Dependency on Alginates and Galactose

We also tested the influence of oxidative stress protection of H_2O_2 treated OMM-1 and TBHP treated ARPE-19. FE_SAT2ad, FE_SiAT2ad and FE_SiAT3ad at 10 µg/mL showed a small protective effect in ARPE-19, which was also seen in OMM-1 cells. However, the effects of FE was highly heterogeneous as for the FE_SiAT2 extract (no acid precipitation) and also FE_SAT3ad displaying no effect at all. Furthermore, the measured protective effects were small and their biological relevance questionable. This corresponds to early studies, which showed no protective effects of FE fucoidans on oxidative stress toxicity in ARPE-19 [17,19]. As described above, FE_SiAT2 has the highest yield of guluronic and mannonic acid the main component of alginates and lowest mol% of fucose. FE_SAT3ad has the second highest content of guluronic acid. Mannuronic acid yield of FE_SiAT2 is rather high in these samples due to lack of alginate precipitation. It could be speculated that alginates are cumbersome for the protective effects. FE-SAT3ad has the lowest glucose content, an important nutrient for the growth of tumor cells, which could lower the metabolism of cancer cells and interferes with the protective effects on OMM-1 cells. The SL_F2 extract showed the best protective effects in OMM-1 and this is in contrast to the other three SL extracts. The SL_F2 extract had the highest amount of fucose, the main component of fucoidans, with 64.7 mol%. However, SL_F3 had nearly the same content (63.3 mol%), so the loss of the protective effect and overall biological activity against H_2O_2 is not due to the fucose content. Also the size and sulfation content between these two SL extracts is similar [15]. It could be suspected that the overall antioxidative effects are due to accompanying substances like phenols [21,29]. The molecular weight and the monosaccharide composition are similar, with the exception that SL_F3 had a higher amount of galactose. It could be speculated that the amount of galactose plays an important role regarding the antioxidative effects, because it is much higher in SL_F3. In relation to heart aging, galactose is described as antioxidants reducing as well as oxidative stress and inflammation inducing [30], so it could interfere with the protective effects. SL_F1 has nearly no fucose but consists of high amounts of alginates. This extract showed no biological activity in any of the tests in this study, which leads us to the conclusion, that algae extracts with lower contents of alginates are recommended for obtaining protective effects.

3.4. Effects on VEGF-Acid Precipitation Lowers and Higher Molecular Weight Improves VEGF Inhibition

Several extracts reduced the VEGF secretion after three days of stimulation. FE_SiAT2 was the only FE extract, which inhibited VEGF significantly. This extract has the highest amount of fucose, arabinose/rhamnose and the lowest amount of glucuronic acid, compared to LD_SiAT2 and SL_SiAT2. All other FE extracts were treated with acid and did not lower VEGF significantly. This strongly indicates that acid may alter the structure of FE fucoidan, interfering with VEGF interaction. Indeed, in this study, no fucoidan treated with acid displayed any VEGF reduction effects. The LD extract showed a VEGF inhibiting effect. It had the lowest fucose content out of all extracts, but the highest mannitol content. VEGF inhibition could be caused by mannitol, although this has not yet been investigated no literature regarding the effect of mannitol and VEGF secretion can currently be found. In contrast to the crude SL_SiAT2 and the first fraction SL_F1, the extracts SL_F2 and SL_F3 lowered VEGF very efficiently in comparison to all other extracts. They had both a much higher fucose content and were the purest extracts. The fucose content alone seems not to be the only biological factor contributing to VEGF inhibition, since the FE extracts also had higher fucose content and was not causing VEGF reduction. In addition to fucose content, molecular weight could be of high importance. The two SL fractions SL_F2 and SL_F3 had a significant higher molecular weight (>800 kDa (Table 3)) than all other tested extracts, which supports our findings that bigger fucoidans from *Laminaria hyperborea* were more effective regarding VEGF inhibition [17]. This could be due to a steric interference with the VEGF molecules. This corresponds with previous findings, which suggested that fucoidans with higher molecular weight are generally more anti-angiogenic, while fucoidans with low molecular weight are considered more pro-angiogenic [31].

3.5. Comparison of Cellic®CTec2 and 3, Alginate Lyases as Well as Precipitation Technique

The Cellic®CTec2 vs. Cellic®CTec3 relates to different enzyme-mixes added in the first step of the purification procedure. They are both enzyme mixes made for degradation of land plant cell walls. They were applied to degrade the brown algal cell wall cellulose and hemicelluloses as well as the storage compound laminarin. In addition, two different alginate lyases (SigmALy and SALy) were used to degrade the cell wall alginate and together these enzymes release the fucoidans gently from the cell wall matrix. FE extracts of this study can be utilized to compare the biological effects after application of these four enzyme purification techniques. Regarding VEGF inhibition they showed no significant effects with the exception of FE_SiAT2 which was VEGF inhibiting. The use of an additional acid precipitation step seems to be more important for this function than the enzyme mix applied, because only the fraction not treated with acid, FE_SiAT2, exhibited VEGF inhibition. The effects on oxidative stress protection were rather heterogeneous and seem to be more related to the concentration applied. The influence on cell viability of ARPE-19 and OMM-1 were rather similar. Overall, we cannot determine a significant biological difference between the extracts treated with the four enzymatic techniques, suggesting that all methods can be used to purify fucoidans resulting in a slightly different amount of monosaccharide and uronic acid compositions only. Overall, acid precipitation is not recommended, because beneficial biological effects important to AMD could be lost due to a possible removal of sidechains or sulfates from the fucoidans. or perhaps more importantly, reduce the size of the fucoidans by partial hydrolysis of the fucoidan backbone. Since, high molecular weight fucoidans are considered antiangiogenic and of great importance when using fucoidans against AMD [17,31]. $CaCl_2$ precipitation of alginate is preferred. Indeed, fucoidans with very high molecular weight of over 800 kDa were obtained in the SL_F2 and F3 fractions treated with $CaCl_2$, and these extracts showed the most promising biological effects.

3.6. Different Fucoidan Structures between Algal Species Lead to the Described Biological Effects

It is well known that the biological properties of the fuciodans are highly dependent on the fucoidan structure and composition. While no structural data of fucoidan from LD can currently be found in literature, the structure of SL and FE fucoidans is different. FE fucoidan consists of alternating α-(1-3)- and α-(1-4)-linked L-fucopyranose unit with sulfate group primarily at C2 [10,32,33] while sulfate groups have been found at C2 and C4 of some fucose residues [34]. Fucoidans from SL are very diverse. Their structure is depending on the overall harvest time, extraction method and further fractionation, which could lead to mixture of different low-sulfated heteropolysaccharides with proteins and uronic acids [29]. Four partial structures of fucoidans from SL have been reported: fucan sulfate, fucogalactan, fucoglucuronomannan, and fucoglucuronan [29,35]. It can be speculated that the different algal origins with very heterogeneous structural compositions, leads to the different biological effects that we described.

3.7. Conclusive Words

This study was well equipped to compare the biological activities of ten fucoidans, with several extract variables. We investigated three different species, from which SL seems most promising. We could demonstrate that the use of acid for alginate precipitation is not recommended and $CaCl_2$ should be used. In the four different tested enzymatic treatments, no significant difference could be determined in the biological activities, but the used SAT2 enzyme mix seems very promising considering the activities of the SL_F2 and SL_F3 fractions, that were purified with these enzymes. Also a three-step fractionation after the enzyme treatment with IEX was conducted and we could clearly show that fractionation is recommended to achieve fucoidan extracts with high fucose and low alginate content. The extract SL_F2 which resulted from IEX fractionation after an enzyme assisted extraction with $CaCl_2$ precipitation is the most promising extract regarding oxidative stress protection and VEGF inhibition. Considering all tested brown seaweed extracts so far, fractionated SL extracts SL_F2 and SL_F3 are the most efficient regarding VEGF inhibiting effect in ARPE-19. They lowered VEGF nearly to 40%. In previous studies we could determine inhibitory effects of a pure LH fucoidan with nearly 50% at 50 and 100 µg/mL [17] and another SL extract which also lowered the VEGF secretion to nearly 50% at 100 µg/mL [19]. The latter extract contained a very high fucose content of 83.8% and only 6% uronic acids [21] (comparable to SL_F2/F3). Surprisingly, the SL extracts from this study lowered VEGF in all concentrations, already very efficiently at 1 µg/mL. So we can conclude that SL is a promising fucoidan source besides *Laminaria hyperborea* [17] regarding potential treatment of AMD. The enzymatically-assisted extraction method, followed by IEX fractionation seem very promising to obtain highly pure and large sized fucoidans with high content of fucose and low content of alginates. With this novel method fucoidans were produced that showed promising VEGF reducing and anti-oxidative properties. Further research is warranted to confirm the beneficial effects in primary in vitro, ex vivo and in vivo models.

4. Material and Methods

4.1. Cell Culture

OMM-1, a uveal melanoma cell line [36] was kindly donated by Dr. Sarah Coupland. The cultivation mediumRPMI 1640 (Merck, Darmstadt, Germany) was added with 10% fetal calf serum (Linaris GmbH, Wertheim-Bettingen, Germany) and 1% penicillin/streptomycin (Merck). The human RPE cell line ARPE-19 [37] was bought from ATCC and cultivated in HyClone DMEM (GE Healthcare, München, Germany), supplemented with 1% penicillin/streptomycin, 2.5% HEPES (Merck), 1% non-essential amino acids (Merck) and 10% fetal calf serum. ARPE-19 cells were treated at confluence and OMM-1 cells were treated at subconfluence.

4.2. Used Fucoidans, Extraction and Purification Process

4.2.1. Fucoidan Origin

Dried flakes of the brown algae SL were obtained from Icelandic Blue Mussel & Seaweed (Bláskel, Iceland) in June 2017. LD (June 2017) and FE (March 2016) were collected by Coastal Research & Management (Kiel, Germany) in the Kiel Canal. LD and FE seaweeds were washed in demineralized water, lyophilized and grround to a size of approximately 0.25–3 mm.

4.2.2. Alginate Lyase Expression and Purification

The alginate lyase SigmALy was purchased from Sigma-Aldrich (Steinheim, Germany). The alginate lyase SALy A1-II′ from *Sphingomonas* sp. was expressed and purified in *Escherichia coli*, as previously described in Manns et al. [24] with modifications described in Nguyen et al. [15].

4.2.3. Enzyme Assisted Extraction of Brown Seaweed Polysaccharides

The enzymatic extraction of fucoidan was performed in 55 mM phosphate, 15 mM citrate buffer pH 6 with 5% substrate concentration. The enzymes were added with ratio 5% (v/w) for Cellic®CTec2/3 (Novozymes A/S, Bagsværd, Denmark), 0.35% (w/w) for alginate lyases. The treatment was performed at 40 °C at 100 rpm. The reaction was stopped by boiling at 90 °C for 10 min and cooling on ice. The supernatant was collected by centrifugation 10 min at 19000 rpm. The fucoidans were precipitated and isolated by addition of 96% EtOH to a final concentration of 72% (except for the SL_F1-F3, where this step was performed after the alginate precipitation). Residual high molecular weight alginates were precipitated either by a two-step acid precipitation (pH 4 followed by pH 2 adjustment with HCl and neutralization with NaOH to pH 7 followed by dialysis in demineralized water using a 3 kDa membrane) or by precipitation with 2% $CaCl_2$ (except the LD_SiAT2, FE_SiAT2 and SL_SiAT2 crude extract alginate was not further precipitated). The fucoidans were isolated by centrifugation and lyophilized.

4.2.4. SL Fucoidan Fractionation by Anion-Exchange Chromatography

The SL fucoidans were fractionated as previously described in Nguyen et al. [15]. The fucoidan solution (5 g in 100 mL) was applied to a DEAE-Macroprep column (2.6 cm × 40 cm) in Cl⁻ form. The unbound materials were washed from the column with NaCl 0.1 M and the fucoidans were eluted in concentration gradient of NaCl from 0.1–2 M. The eluates were combined into fractions based on the results of total carbohydrate analysis by phenol-sulfuric acid method [38]. The fractions were passed through a 10 kDa membrane to up-concentrate and remove salt, followed by lyophilization.

Fucoidans were solved in Ampuwa bidest (Fresenius, Schweinfurt, Germany) at concentrations of 1 mg/mL with exception of the three SL fraction SL_F1, SL_F2 and SL_F3 which were soluble at 5 mg/mL. Right before stimulation, used extracts were filtered with 0.2 µm Sarstedt filter (Nümbrecht, Germany) and a dilution series with appropriate medium was performed to get the final concentrations of 1, 10, 50 and 100 µg/mL.

4.3. Chemical Composition and Size Distribution Analysis

The monosaccharide composition of the fucoidans was determined as previously described [22]. The size distribution of the fucoidans was determined by HP-SEC as previously described in Nguyen et al. [15] and the pullulan standard was fitted with a Weibull decay model by the following equation: $y = a * (1 - EXP(-(x/b)^{\wedge}(c)))$. The sulfate content of the crude extracts were determined as previously described [15] and sulfate content of the SL_F1, F2 and F3 extracts was performed as previously described [15].

4.4. Oxidative Stress

4.4.1. OMM-1

Oxidative stress in the uveal melanoma cell line OMM-1 was induced by treatment with 1 mM H_2O_2 as previously shown [39]. The appropriate H_2O_2 concentration to lower cell viability of OMM-1 cells to nearly 50% after 24 h was previously determined [19] and applied for the assessment of protective effects of fucoidans (1, 10, 50 and 100 µg/mL). Fucoidans were applied 30 min before stress insult. In parallel, cells were treated with the extracted fucoidans only (1, 10, 50 and 100 µg/mL) to determine possible anti-proliferative effects. To measure cell viability, a MTS-assay was performed as described below.

4.4.2. ARPE-19

The appropriate TBHP concentration to lower cell viability of ARPE-19 cells to nearly 50% after 24 h (0.5 mM TBHP) was previously determined [19] and applied for the assessment of protective effects of fucoidans (1, 10, 50 and 100 µg/mL). Fucoidans were applied 30 min before stress insult. In parallel, cells were treated with only the extracted fucoidans (1, 10, 50 and 100 µg/mL) to determine anti-proliferative effects. To measure cell viability the MTS-Assay was performed as described below.

4.5. Methyl Thiazolyl Tetrazolium (MTT)-Assay

The established cell viability assay MTT [40] was performed as previously described [13,19] and was applied after three days of stimulation with fucoidans, after collection of the supernatant for VEGF-content assessment. The biological material was washed with PBS and cultivated with 0.5 mg/mL MTT for 2 h. After removal of MTT, cells were treated with dimethyl sulfoxide. Color formation was measured at 550 nm with an Elx800 instrument (BioTek Instruments Inc., Bad Friedrichshall, Germany).

4.6. MTS-Assay

For the cell viability and protection assays after 24 h a commercially proliferation assay named "CellTiter 96® AQueous One Solution Cell Proliferation Assay" from Promega Corporation (Mannheim, Germany) was applied as described in the instructions of the supplier. Twenty µL of the MTS solution was added to each treated well of a 96 well plates for 1 h. For the prior treatment of cells, media without phenol red was used.

4.7. VEGF ELISA

Secreted VEGF in ARPE-19 supernatant was determined with the Human VEGF DuoSet ELISA Kit from R&D Systems (Wiesbaden, Germany) according to manufacturer's protocol. Supernatants were collected after three days of stimulation with different fucoidan extracts and an MTT assay was conducted to set the VEGF effect in relation to the cell viability as previously described [19]. The medium was exchanged 24 h before collecting of supernatant.

4.8. Statistics

At least four independent experiments per assay have been performed. Statistics have been made with Microsoft Excel (Excel 2010, Microsoft, Redmond, WA, USA) and GraphPad PRISM 7 (GraphPad Software, Inc., San Diego, CA, USA, 2017). One-Way ANOVA was conducted to determine significances. *P* values lower than 0.05 are considered significant. The diagram bars stand for mean and the attached lines for standard deviations.

5. Conclusions

Fucoidans or sulfated fucans are very promising marine polysaccharides for a possible new treatment development for AMD. With this study we wanted to test the influence of a new enzymatic purification method on the biological activity of fucoidans from different algal species. We tested ten different fucoidans, from the brown seaweed species LD, SL and FE and compared them with regards to toxicity, oxidative stress protection against H_2O_2 or TBHP and VEGF secretion. Furthermore, we assessed which enzymatic purification method (testing five different FE extracts) and how IEX fractionation (testing four different SL extracts) were most promising for these biological activities. No fucoidan displayed a negative effect on viability after 24 h. Some FE fucoidans were slightly (but not relevantly) protective in ARPE-19 cells. SL_F2 and some of the FE extracts showed protective effects in the melanoma cell line OMM-1. Effective extracts reducing VEGF were LD_SiAT2, FE_SiAT2 and SL_F2 and SL_F3 fucoidans. The enzymatic method SAT2 without acid dialysis seems most promising for biological effects, which could be confirmed for with the SL fractions SL_F2 and F3. They were the most effective fucoidans regarding VEGF inhibition, which correlated with a high fucose and low alginate content. SL fucoidans, which were treated with SAT2 enzymes and further processed with ion-exchange chromatography, are the most promising extracts for a potential application in AMD.

Author Contributions: Conceptualization, A.K., A.S.M.; Methodology, A.K., M.D.M., P.D., T.N.T.; Validation, M.D.M., P.D., T.N.T.; Formal Analysis, P.D.; Investigation, M.M., P.D., T.T.; Resources, A.K., A.M., J.R.; Data Curation, A.K., M.M., P.D.; Writing—Original Draft Preparation, M.D.M., P.D.; Writing—Review and Editing, A.K., A.S.M., M.D.M., P.D.; Visualization, M.D.M., P.D.; Supervision, A.K., A.S.M., J.R. All authors have read and agreed to the published version of the manuscript.

Funding: This study is part of the FucoSan-Health from the Sea Project and is supported by EU InterReg-Deutschland-Denmark and the European Fund of Regional Development. This work was part of the BioValue SPIR Platform funded by Innovation Fund Denmark, case no. 0603-00522B.

Acknowledgments: We thank the Coastal Research & Management for the provision of the algae.

Conflicts of Interest: The authors declare no conflict of interest.

Appendix A

Table A1. Monosaccharide composition of fucoidans determined by HPAEC, including standard deviations (%mol).

Sample	Fuc	Mannitol	Ara/Rham	Gal	Glc	Xyl	Man	GuluA	GluA	ManA	Total	Sulfate (SO_4^{2-}) mol%
LD_SiAT2	3.9 ± 0.1	1.2 ± 0.1	0.1 ± 0.0	14 ± 0.2	2.3 ± 0.1	1.5 ± 0.1	1.2 ± 0.1	12.4 ± 1.4	1.2 ± 0.1	74.8 ± 1.5	100	9.3 ± 2.4
SL_SiAT2	12.3 ± 0.8	0.2 ± 0.0	0.2 ± 0.0	1.3 ± 1.1	2.6 ± 0.2	0.9 ± 0.0	0.8 ± 0.0	32.2 ± 1.2	1.5 ± 0.2	48.1 ± 0.7	100	14.4 ± 0.6
FE_SiAT2	15.5 ± 0.9	0.0 ± 0.0	0.3 ± 0.0	2.5 ± 0.0	2.1 ± 0.0	3.6 ± 0.1	1.8 ± 0.2	18.7 ± 0.8	6.5 ± 5.5	48.8 ± 3.5	100	20.2 ± 1.5
FE_SiAT2ad	36.1 ± 3.1	0.1 ± 0.1	0.6 ± 0.6	6.6 ± 1.9	5.7 ± 1.5	10.2 ± 3.2	1.8 ± 1.5	7.1 ± 0.7	2.0 ± 0.4	30.0 ± 2.0	100	30.1 ± 0.6
FE_SiAT3ad	35.9 ± 1.2	0.1 ± 0.0	0.4 ± 0.3	2.8 ± 0.7	2.2 ± 0.1	4.1 ± 0.3	2.0 ± 0.1	10.0 ± 0.2	2.2 ± 0.0	40.4 ± 0.5	100	29.4 ± 1.7
FE_SAT2ad	52.2 ± 1.9	0.0 ± 0.0	1.2 ± 0.2	4.8 ± 0.5	2.7 ± 0.5	9.3 ± 1.1	4.7 ± 0.7	8.8 ± 1.2	3.9 ± 0.3	12.5 ± 0.8	100	31.7 ± 2.0
FE_SAT3ad	48.3 ± 0.6	0.1 ± 0.1	0.7 ± 0.6	5.0 ± 0.7	2.0 ± 0.1	8.3 ± 0.5	4.0 ± 0.7	11.6 ± 0.1	3.7 ± 0.2	16.4 ± 0.3	100	29.9 ± 1.4
SL_F1 *	5.4 ± 1.2	0.0 ± 0.0	0.1 ± 0.0	0.5 ± 0.0	0.4 ± 0.0	0.8 ± 0.1	0.8 ± 0.1	8.5 ± 4.7	1.1 ± 0.1	82.4 ± 4.3	100	6.6 ± 3.6
SL_F2 *	64.7 ± 0.3	0.1 ± 0.0	0.3 ± 0.0	12.2 ± 0.1	0.6 ± 0.1	4.8 ± 0.0	3.5 ± 0.2	0.0 ± 0.0	6.9 ± 0.3	6.9 ± 0.1	100	35.6 ± 2.5
SL_F3 *	63.3 ± 0.7	0.0 ± 0.0	0.3 ± 0.0	26.9 ± 0.3	0.4 ± 0.1	3.4 ± 0.2	2.1 ± 0.1	0.0 ± 0.0	2.8 ± 0.2	0.8 ± 0.1	100	46.4 ± 3.5

* Nguyen et al. 2020 [15].

References

1. Wong, W.L.; Su, X.; Li, X.; Cheung, C.M.G.; Klein, R.; Cheng, C.-Y.; Wong, T.Y. Global prevalence of age-related macular degeneration and disease burden projection for 2020 and 2040: A systematic review and meta-analysis. *Lancet Glob. Health* **2014**, *2*, e106–e116. [CrossRef]
2. Miller, J.W. Age-related macular degeneration revisited–piecing the puzzle: The LXIX Edward Jackson memorial lecture. *Am. J. Ophthalmol.* **2013**, *155*, 1–35.e13. [CrossRef] [PubMed]
3. Ding, X.; Patel, M.; Chan, C.-C. Molecular pathology of age-related macular degeneration. *Prog. Retin. Eye Res.* **2009**, *28*, 1–18. [CrossRef] [PubMed]
4. Klettner, A. Oxidative stress induced cellular signaling in RPE cells. *Front. Biosci.* **2012**, *4*, 392–411. [CrossRef]
5. Hageman, G.S.; Anderson, D.H.; Johnson, L.V.; Hancox, L.S.; Taiber, A.J.; Hardisty, L.I.; Hageman, J.L.; Stockman, H.A.; Borchardt, J.D.; Gehrs, K.M.; et al. A common haplotype in the complement regulatory gene factor H (HF1/CFH) predisposes individuals to age-related macular degeneration. *Proc. Natl. Acad. Sci. USA* **2005**, *102*, 7227–7232. [CrossRef]
6. McHarg, S.; Clark, S.J.; Day, A.J.; Bishop, P.N. Age-related macular degeneration and the role of the complement system. *Mol. Immunol.* **2015**, *67*, 43–50. [CrossRef]
7. Schmidt-Erfurth, U.; Chong, V.; Loewenstein, A.; Larsen, M.; Souied, E.; Schlingemann, R.; Eldem, B.; Monés, J.; Richard, G.; Bandello, F. Guidelines for the management of neovascular age-related macular degeneration by the European Society of Retina Specialists (EURETINA). *Br. J. Ophthalmol.* **2014**, *98*, 1144–1167. [CrossRef]
8. Deniaud-Bouët, E.; Kervarec, N.; Michel, G.; Tonon, T.; Kloareg, B.; Hervé, C. Chemical and enzymatic fractionation of cell walls from Fucales: Insights into the structure of the extracellular matrix of brown algae. *Ann. Bot.* **2014**, *114*, 1203–1216. [CrossRef]
9. Catarino, M.D.; Silva, A.M.S.; Cardoso, S.M. Phycochemical Constituents and Biological Activities of Fucus spp. *Mar. Drugs* **2018**, *16*, 249. [CrossRef]
10. Ale, M.T.; Meyer, A.S. Fucoidans from brown seaweeds: An update on structures, extraction techniques and use of enzymes as tools for structural elucidation. *RSC Adv.* **2013**, *3*, 8131–8141. [CrossRef]
11. Li, B.; Lu, F.; Wei, X.; Zhao, R. Fucoidan: Structure and bioactivity. *Molecules* **2008**, *13*, 1671–1695. [CrossRef] [PubMed]
12. Klettner, A. Fucoidan as a Potential Therapeutic for Major Blinding Diseases–A Hypothesis. *Mar. Drugs* **2016**, *14*, 31. [CrossRef] [PubMed]
13. Dithmer, M.; Fuchs, S.; Shi, Y.; Schmidt, H.; Richert, E.; Roider, J.; Klettner, A. Fucoidan reduces secretion and expression of vascular endothelial growth factor in the retinal pigment epithelium and reduces angiogenesis in vitro. *PLoS ONE* **2014**, *9*, e89150. [CrossRef] [PubMed]
14. Ale, M.T.; Mikkelsen, J.D.; Meyer, A.S. Important determinants for fucoidan bioactivity: A critical review of structure-function relations and extraction methods for fucose-containing sulfated polysaccharides from brown seaweeds. *Mar. Drugs* **2011**, *9*, 2106–2130. [CrossRef] [PubMed]
15. Nguyen, T.T.; Mikkelsen, M.D.; Ha, V.T.N.; Dieu, T.V.T.; Rhein-Knudsen, N.; Holck, J.; Rasin, A.B.; Cao, H.T.T.; Van, T.T.T.; Meyer, A.S. Enzyme assisted fucoidan extraction from the brown macroalgae. *Mar. Drugs* **2020**, *18*, 168.
16. Bittkau, K.S.; Dörschmann, P.; Blümel, M.; Tasdemir, D.; Roider, J.; Klettner, A.; Alban, S. Comparison of the Effects of Fucoidans on the Cell Viability of Tumor and Non-Tumor Cell Lines. *Mar. Drugs* **2019**, *17*, 441. [CrossRef]
17. Dörschmann, P.; Kopplin, G.; Roider, J.; Klettner, A. Effects of Sulfated Fucans from Laminaria hyperborea Regarding VEGF Secretion, Cell Viability, and Oxidative Stress and Correlation with Molecular Weight. *Mar. Drugs* **2019**, *17*, 548. [CrossRef]
18. Rohwer, K.; Neupane, S.; Bittkau, K.S.; Galarza Pérez, M.; Dörschmann, P.; Roider, J.; Alban, S.; Klettner, A. Effects of Crude Fucus distichus Subspecies evanescens Fucoidan Extract on Retinal Pigment Epithelium Cells-Implications for Use in Age-Related Macular Degeneration. *Mar. Drugs* **2019**, *17*, 538. [CrossRef]
19. Dörschmann, P.; Bittkau, K.S.; Neupane, S.; Roider, J.; Alban, S.; Klettner, A. Effects of fucoidans from five different brown algae on oxidative stress and VEGF interference in ocular cells. *Mar. Drugs* **2019**, *17*, 258. [CrossRef]
20. Schneider, T.; Ehrig, K.; Liewert, I.; Alban, S. Interference with the CXCL12/CXCR4 axis as potential antitumor strategy: Superiority of a sulfated galactofucan from the brown alga Saccharina latissima and fucoidan over heparins. *Glycobiology* **2015**, *25*, 812–824. [CrossRef]

21. Bittkau, K.S.; Neupane, S.; Alban, S. Initial evaluation of six different brown algae species as source for crude bioactive fucoidans. *Algal Res.* **2020**, *45*, 101759. [CrossRef]
22. Manns, D.; Deutschle, A.L.; Saake, B.; Meyer, A.S. Methodology for quantitative determination of the carbohydrate composition of brown seaweeds (Laminariaceae). *RSC Adv.* **2014**, *4*, 25736–25746. [CrossRef]
23. Manns, D.; Andersen, S.K.; Saake, B.; Meyer, A.S. Brown seaweed processing: Enzymatic saccharification of Laminaria digitata requires no pre-treatment. *J. Appl. Phycol.* **2016**, *28*, 1287–1294. [CrossRef]
24. Manns, D.; Nyffenegger, C.; Saake, B.; Meyer, A.S. Impact of different alginate lyases on combined cellulase–lyase saccharification of brown seaweed. *RSC Adv.* **2016**, *6*, 45392–45401. [CrossRef]
25. Alboofetileh, M.; Rezaei, M.; Tabarsa, M. Enzyme-assisted extraction of Nizamuddinia zanardinii for the recovery of sulfated polysaccharides with anticancer and immune-enhancing activities. *J. Appl. Phycol.* **2019**, *31*, 1391–1402. [CrossRef]
26. Karlsson, M.; Kurz, T. Attenuation of iron-binding proteins in ARPE-19 cells reduces their resistance to oxidative stress. *Acta Ophthalmol.* **2016**, *94*, 556–564. [CrossRef]
27. Mak, W.; Wang, S.K.; Liu, T.; Hamid, N.; Li, Y.; Lu, J.; White, W.L. Anti-Proliferation Potential and Content of Fucoidan Extracted from Sporophyll of New Zealand Undaria pinnatifida. *Front. Nutr.* **2014**, *1*, 9. [CrossRef]
28. Li, X.; Zhao, H.; Wang, Q.; Liang, H.; Jiang, X. Fucoidan Protects Arpe-19 Cells from Oxidative Stress via Normalization of Reactive Oxygen Species Generation Through the Ca^{2+}-Dependent Erk Signaling Pathway. *Mol. Med. Rep.* **2015**, *11*, 3746–3752. [CrossRef]
29. Ehrig, K.; Alban, S. Sulfated galactofucan from the brown alga Saccharina latissima–variability of yield, structural composition and bioactivity. *Mar. Drugs* **2014**, *13*, 76–101. [CrossRef]
30. Bo-Htay, C.; Palee, S.; Apaijai, N.; Chattipakorn, S.C.; Chattipakorn, N. Effects of d-galactose-induced ageing on the heart and its potential interventions. *J. Cell. Mol. Med.* **2018**, *22*, 1392–1410. [CrossRef]
31. Van Weelden, G.; Bobiński, M.; Okła, K.; van Weelden, W.J.; Romano, A.; Pijnenborg, J.M.A. Fucoidan Structure and Activity in Relation to Anti-Cancer Mechanisms. *Mar. Drugs.* **2019**, *17*, 32. [CrossRef] [PubMed]
32. Bilan, M.I.; Grachev, A.A.; Ustuzhanina, N.E.; Shashkov, A.S.; Nifantiev, N.E.; Usov, A.I. Structure of a fucoidan from the brown seaweed Fucus evanescens C.Ag. *Carbohydr. Res.* **2002**, *337*, 719–730. [CrossRef]
33. Zvyagintseva, T.N.; Shevchenko, N.M.; Chizhov, A.O.; Krupnova, T.N.; Sundukova, E.V.; Isakov, V.V. Water-soluble polysaccharides of some far-eastern brown seaweeds. Distribution, structure, and their dependence on the developmental conditions. *J. Exp. Mar. Biol. Ecol.* **2003**, *294*, 1–13. [CrossRef]
34. Menshova, R.V.; Shevchenko, N.M.; Imbs, T.I.; Zvyagintseva, T.N.; Malyarenko, O.S.; Zaporoshets, T.S.; Besednova, N.N.; Ermakova, S.P. Fucoidans from Brown Alga Fucus evanescens: Structure and Biological Activity. *Front. Mar. Sci.* **2016**, *3*, 7. [CrossRef]
35. Bilan, M.I.; Grachev, A.A.; Shashkov, A.S.; Kelly, M.; Sanderson, C.J.; Nifantiev, N.E.; Usov, A.I. Further studies on the composition and structure of a fucoidan preparation from the brown alga Saccharina latissima. *Carbohydr. Res.* **2010**, *345*, 2038–2047. [CrossRef] [PubMed]
36. Luyten, G.P.; Naus, N.C.; Mooy, C.M.; Hagemeijer, A.; Kan-Mitchell, J.; van Drunen, E.; Vuzevski, V.; de Jong, P.T.; Luider, T.M. Establishment and characterization of primary and metastatic uveal melanoma cell lines. *Int. J. Cancer* **1996**, *66*, 380–387. [CrossRef]
37. Dunn, K.C.; Aotaki-Keen, A.E.; Putkey, F.R.; Hjelmeland, L.M. ARPE-19, a human retinal pigment epithelial cell line with differentiated properties. *Exp. Eye Res.* **1996**, *62*, 155–169. [CrossRef]
38. DuBois, M.; Gilles, K.A.; Hamilton, J.K.; Rebers, P.A.; Smith, F. Colorimetric Method for Determination of Sugars and Related Substances. *Anal. Chem.* **1956**, *28*, 350–356. [CrossRef]
39. Dithmer, M.; Kirsch, A.-M.; Richert, E.; Fuchs, S.; Wang, F.; Schmidt, H.; Coupland, S.E.; Roider, J.; Klettner, A. Fucoidan Does Not Exert Anti-Tumorigenic Effects on Uveal Melanoma Cell Lines. *Mar. Drugs.* **2017**, *15*, 193. [CrossRef]
40. Riss, T.L.; Moravec, R.A.; Niles, A.L.; Duellman, S.; Benink, H.A.; Worzella, T.J.; Minor, L. Cell Viability Assays. In *Assay Guidance Manual [Internet]*; Sittampalam, G.S., Coussens, N.P., Brimacombe, K., Grossman, A., Arkin, M., Auld, D., Austin, C., Baell, J., Bejcek, B., Caaveiro, J.M.M., et al., Eds.; Eli Lilly & Company and the National Center for Advancing Translational Sciences: Indianapolis, IN, USA, 2016.

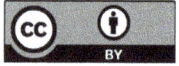

© 2020 by the authors. Licensee MDPI, Basel, Switzerland. This article is an open access article distributed under the terms and conditions of the Creative Commons Attribution (CC BY) license (http://creativecommons.org/licenses/by/4.0/).

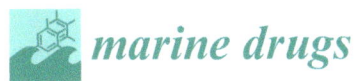

Article

Protective Effect of a Fucose-Rich Fucoidan Isolated from *Saccharina japonica* against Ultraviolet B-Induced Photodamage In Vitro in Human Keratinocytes and In Vivo in Zebrafish

Wanchun Su [1], Lei Wang [2,3], Xiaoting Fu [1,*], Liying Ni [1], Delin Duan [4,5], Jiachao Xu [1] and Xin Gao [1]

1. College of Food Science & Engineering, Ocean University of China, 5th Yushan Road, Qingdao 266003, China; suwanccchun@163.com (W.S.); niliying12@163.com (L.N.); xujia@ouc.edu.cn (J.X.); xingao@ouc.edu.cn (X.G.)
2. Department of Marine Life Sciences, Jeju National University, Jeju Self-Governing Province 63243, Korea; comeonleiwang@163.com
3. Marine Science Institute, Jeju National University, Jeju Self-Governing Province 63333, Korea
4. State Key Lab of Seaweed Bioactive Substances, 1th Daxueyuan Road, Qingdao 266400, China; dlduan@qdio.ac.cn
5. Key Laboratory of Experimental Marine Biology, Institute of Oceanology, Chinese Academy of Sciences, No. 7 Nanhai Road, Qingdao 266071, China
* Correspondence: xiaotingfu@ouc.edu.cn; Tel.: +86-532-82032182

Received: 14 May 2020; Accepted: 8 June 2020; Published: 15 June 2020

Abstract: A fucose-rich fucoidan was purified from brown seaweed *Saccharina japonica*, of which the UVB protective effect was investigated in vitro in keratinocytes of HaCaT cells and in vivo in zebrafish. The intracellular reactive oxygen species levels and the viability of UVB-irradiated HaCaT cells were determined. The results indicate that the purified fucoidan significantly reduced the intracellular reactive oxygen species levels and improved the viability of UVB-irradiated HaCaT cells. Furthermore, the purified fucoidan remarkably decreased the apoptosis by regulating the expressions of Bax/Bcl-xL and cleaved caspase-3 in UVB-irradiated HaCaT cells in a dose-dependent manner. In addition, the in vivo UV protective effect of the purified fucoidan was investigated using a zebrafish model. It significantly reduced the intracellular reactive oxygen species level, the cell death, the NO production, and the lipid peroxidation in UVB-irradiated zebrafish in a dose-dependent manner. These results suggest that purified fucoidan has a great potential to be developed as a natural anti-UVB agent applied in the cosmetic industry.

Keywords: ROS; Phaeophyta; carbohydrate; UVB irradiation; HaCaT cells; zebrafish

1. Introduction

Human skin is one of the most fundamental organs which is directly exposed to the external environment. It acts as a barrier to prevent the body from external damage, including ultraviolet (UV) irradiation exposure [1]. Although UV is beneficial to the human body to a certain extent, the excessive exposure to UV will damage the ability of basal keratinocytes, which are responsible for maintaining skin homeostasis to resist UV-induced damage, which can lead to different skin diseases such as accelerated degradation of collagen, inflammatory reaction, epidermal hyperplasia and skin cancers [2,3]. Solar UV irradiation contains wavelengths from approximately 100 to 400 nm, but only UVB (280–315 nm) and UVA (315–400 nm) reach the terrestrial surface [4]. It is now commonly known that the exposure to solar UVB is the major factor causing keratinocyte damage, causing DNA mutations, which can induce photo-aging and skin cancer [5].

The UVB damages skin through stimulating the production of reactive oxygen species (ROS) [6,7]. The expression of apoptosis-related cytokines induced by excessive ROS can lead to skin oxidative damage, and cause apoptosis [8]. Therefore, inhibiting the excessive ROS generation and eliminating potential cancer-causing cells are important strategies that constitute photoprotection and inhibit apoptosis [9].

Currently, researchers are focusing on developing natural compounds to explore their protective effects on UVB-induced photodamage. Seaweed is a plant abundantly growing in the sea and is broadly distributed all over the world. It can endure strong sunlight without any structural damage, which indicates that seaweed can protect itself from photodynamic damage, including UVB irradiation [10]. Thus, many studies have been conducted to find bioactive extracts or active ingredients derived from seaweed, such as polyphenol, polysaccharide, fucoxanthin, by which the generation of UVB-induced ROS can be modulated [11–13].

Saccharina japonica (*S. japonica*), a brown seaweed, used to be known as *Laminaria japonica* (*L. japonica*), which is plentifully produced in Asian countries and used as a traditional Chinese medicine and functional food [14,15]. In addition, it contains plenty of biological compounds, including fucoidan. Previous studies have reported that fucoidan isolated from *S. japonica* has a variety of bioactivities, such as neuroprotective, anti-inflammation, antioxidant, antiviral, immunomodulatory, atherosclerosis mitigation and anticoagulant activities [16–21]. Some researchers have investigated the anti-UVB ability of fucoidan from brown seaweed, such as *Costaria costata*, *Fucus evanescens* and *Undaria pinnatifida* [22–24]; however, this is the first study on the anti-UVB activities of fucoidan extracted from *S. japonica*.

In our latest work, the structure and anti-inflammatory activities of a fucoidan fraction of LJSF4 from *S. japonica* were studied [25]. In this study, we further investigated its photo-protective activity. The possible mechanisms against UVB-induced photodamage were examined in vitro using human keratinocyte (HaCaT) cells and in vivo in a zebrafish model in order to provide evidence for its application as an anti-UVB agent in cosmetics.

2. Results and Discussion

2.1. Purification and Monosaccharide Determination of Fucoidan Fractions

Fucoidan fractions of LJSF1-LJSF4 were purified from *S. japonica* (Figure 1A), among which LJSF4 has the highest sulfate content of 30.72%. As shown in Figure 1B, its monosaccharide compositions were determined to be 79.49% of fucose and 16.76% of galactose, thus it is a fucose-rich fucoidan. In our recently published work, the structures of LJSF4 were analyzed by different spectroscopic methods and its excellent anti-inflammatory activities were studied in vitro and in vivo [25]. In order to achieve the application of this fucoidan, knowledge of its various bioactivities is required. Thus, its anti-UVB activity and mechanism both in vitro and in vivo were investigated in this study.

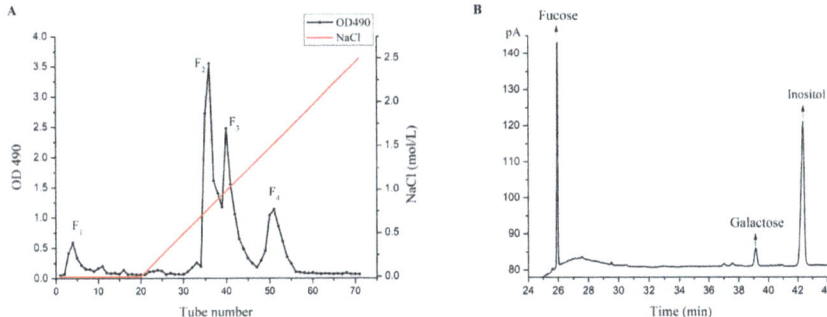

Figure 1. Purification and monosaccharide determination of fucoidan fractions: (**A**) elution profile of *S. japonica* crude fucoidan on DEAE-Sepharose Fast Flow anion exchange chromatography; (**B**) monosaccharide compositions of LJSF4 determined by gas chromatography.

2.2. Effect of LJSF4 on UVB-Irradiated HaCaT Cells

2.2.1. Effect of LJSF4 on Intracellular ROS Generation and Cell Death in UVB-Irradiated HaCaT Cells

Prior to evaluate the anti-UVB effect of LJSF4 on HaCaT cells, we detected its potential toxicity on HaCaT cells through the MTT viability assay. As shown in Figure 2A, the viability of HaCaT cells without LJSF4 treatment was 100%, and those treated with LJSF4 were above 90%. In addition, compared with the control group, cells treated with 50 µg/mL of LJSF4 even had higher cell viability. These results indicate that LJSF4 had no cytotoxicity on HaCaT cells and even exhibited positive effect on the cells at the concentration of 50 µg/mL.

Exposure of cells to UVB irradiation results in ROS excessive production and cellular damage, which is the cause of skin cancer and photoaging [26]. Therefore, suppressing the excessive production of ROS can protect the skin from the damage of UVB [27]. In this study, the HaCaT cell damage induced by UVB irradiation was examined by measuring the intracellular ROS generation and cell death. As shown in Figure 2B, the ROS level of UVB-irradiated cells was significantly increased compared to those of non-irradiated cells, while the ROS levels of those treated with different concentrations of LJSF4 were significantly decreased in a dose-dependent manner. In addition, the viability of cells irradiated by UVB was significantly decreased, and dose-dependently increased in LJSF4 treated cells (Figure 2C). These results indicate that LJSF4 possessed a protective effect against UVB-induced HaCaT cell damage. The anti-UVB activities of fucoidan extracted from other brown seaweed of *Costaria costata*, *Fucus evanescens* and *Undaria pinnatifida* have been investigated [22–24]. However, these seaweed resources are not as rich as *S. japonica*, which is the most abundant economic seaweed around the world [28]. In addition, fucoidan extracted from *C. costata* increase the cell viability by 1.77% and 4.94% at concentrations of 0.01 and 0.1 µg/mL, respectively, while the fucoidan was mildly cytotoxic at the concentration of 1 µg/mL [24]. However, LJSF4 was able to increase the cell viability by 16.14% at the concentration of 100 µg/mL with no cytotoxic effect. Therefore, LJSF4 possessed an excellent anti-UVB activity on HaCaT cells.

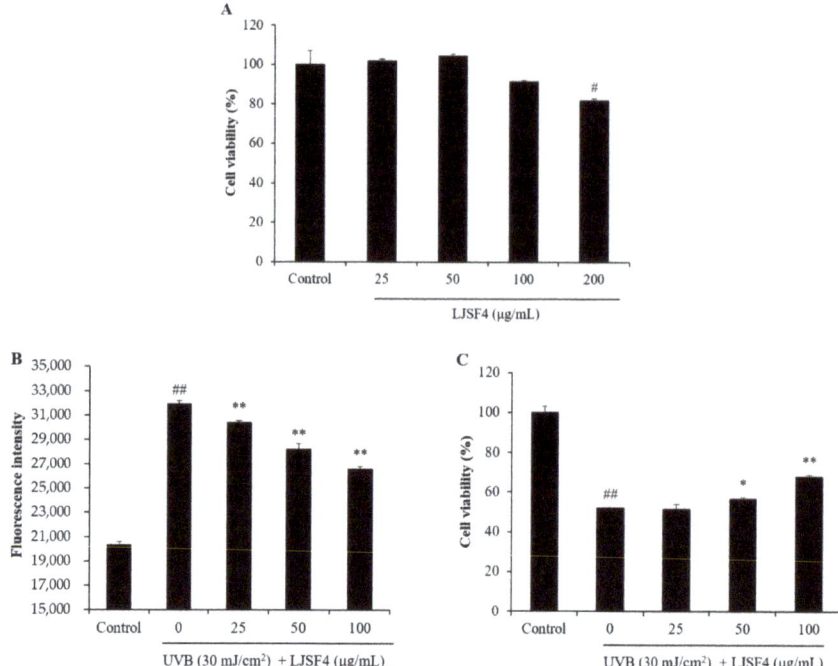

Figure 2. Protective effect of LJSF4 on UVB-induced HaCaT cells: (**A**) cytotoxicity of LJSF4 on HaCaT cells; (**B**) intracellular ROS level of UVB-irradiated HaCaT cells; (**C**) the viability of UVB-irradiated HaCaT cells. All experiments were performed in triplicate. Data are expressed as means ± standard error of the means (S.E.M). * $p < 0.05$, ** $p < 0.01$ as compared to the UVB-treated group and # $p < 0.05$, ## $p < 0.01$ as compared to the control group.

2.2.2. Effect of LJSF4 on Apoptosis in UVB-Irradiated HaCaT Cells

Apoptosis is a strong response of cells to UVB-induced damage. Cells eventually undergo apoptosis to eliminate severely damaged cells. However, even if serious damage occurs, some cells can still escape apoptosis, then turn into cancer cells. Studies have found that inhibiting apoptosis plays an important part in the formation of cancer [29].

In order to measure the protective effect of LJSF4 from UVB irradiation, HaCaT cells were stained with Hoechst 33342, which is a cell-permeable DNA dye. Later, the nuclear morphology of cells was observed by fluorescence microscopy. The cell images are shown in Figure 3. We found that the amount of apoptotic body of cells with UVB irradiation was almost 2.5 fold greater than that of cells without UVB irradiation, while those of cells pre-treated with 25 to 100 µg/mL of LJSF4 were decreased in a dose-dependent manner significantly. Masaki et al. reported that UVB-induced apoptosis was related to the increase in intracellular ROS generation. Inhibiting the production of ROS contributed to improving the intracellular defense against oxidative stress, thereby reducing cell apoptosis [27]. Our study evaluated the levels of ROS and apoptosis with or without LJSF4 treatment, and intervened with different concentrations of LJSF4. This result indicates that LJSF4 possessed excellent protective effect against UVB-induced HaCaT cell apoptosis.

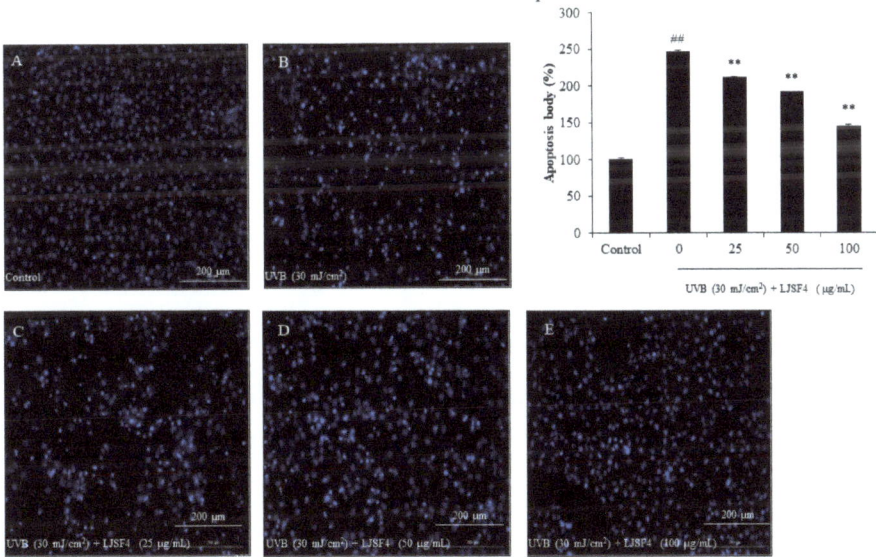

Figure 3. The apoptotic body formation levels in UVB-irradiated HaCaT cells: (**A**) nuclear morphology of non UVB-irradiated HaCaT cells; (**B**) nuclear morphology of UVB-irradiated HaCaT cells; (**C**) nuclear morphology of cells treated with 25 of µg/mL LJSF4 and irradiated with UVB; (**D**) nuclear morphology of cells treated with 50 of µg/mL LJSF4 and irradiated with UVB; (**E**) nuclear morphology of cells treated with 100 of µg/mL LJSF4 and irradiated with UVB; (**F**) reactive apoptotic body formation. Apoptosis levels were measured using Image J software. All experiments were performed in triplicate. Data are expressed as means ± standard error of the means (S.E.M). ** $p < 0.01$ as compared to the UVB-treated group and ## $p < 0.01$ as compared to the control group.

2.2.3. Effect of LJSF4 on Bax/Bcl-xL and Cleaved Caspase-3 Levels in UVB-Irradiated HaCaT Cells

Apoptosis is a regulated mechanism of cell suicide, usually manifested as nuclear condensation, wrinkling, membrane foaming as well as chromosomal DNA fragmentation [29–31]. According to the previous studies, the formation of apoptosome is an intrinsic apoptotic signaling pathway which could activated by oxidative stress [32–34]. Excessive ROS production as a second messenger regulates apoptotic signaling pathway following UV irradiation. In this case, the balance of anti-apoptotic molecules of Bcl-xL and pro-apoptotic molecules of Bax indicated whether apoptosis is promoted or suppressed [35]. Eventually, their imbalance triggered the caspase cascade [36]. In addition, cleaved caspase-3 directly induces cell death as a critical executor of apoptosis [37].

The Bax/Bcl-xL and cleaved caspase-3 levels of UVB-irradiated HaCaT cells were measured by Western blot analysis. As shown in Figure 4, the UVB irradiation increased the Bax level and decreased the Bcl-xL level, while pre-treatment with LJSF4 significantly increased the Bcl-xL level and decreased the Bax level in a dose-dependent manner. Moreover, LJSF4 reduced UVB-induced cleaved caspase-3 activation in UVB-irradiated HaCaT cells. These results indicate that LJSF4 inhibited UVB-induced apoptosis by the regulation of Bax, Bcl-xL and cleaved caspase-3 levels. The anti-UVB activity of Sargachromenol extracted from the brown seaweed of *Sargassum micracanthum* has been investigated, and the similar pathway by regulation of Bax, Bcl-xL and cleaved caspase-3 levels has been reported [38]. In addition, fucoidans isolated from different brown algae have been reported to inhibit UVB-induced photoaging through other signaling pathways, such as by inhibiting the MAPK pathways related to NF-κB and AP-1, by inhibiting MMP-1 expression via blocking the signal pathways of p38, JNK, and ERK [23,39]. Thus, the *S. japonica* fucoidan showed a different anti-UVB pathway to those of other reported fucoidan via regulating the expression of Bax, Bcl-xL and cleaved caspase-3.

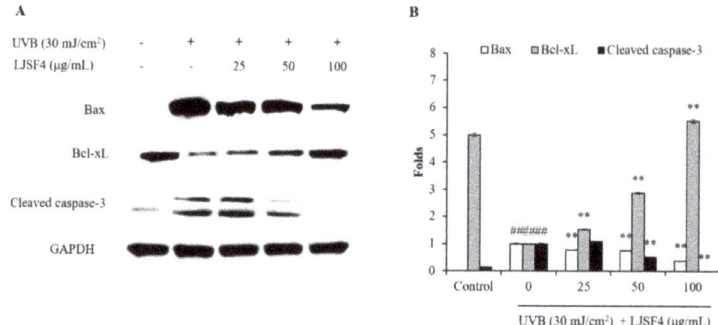

Figure 4. Effect of LJSF4 on Bax/Bcl-xL, and cleaved caspase-3 levels in UVB-irradiated HaCaT cells: (**A**) the effect of LJSF4 on UVB-induced apoptosis related protein expression; (**B**) the relative amounts of Bax/Bcl-xL and cleaved caspase-3 levels compared with GAPDH. The Bax level of control group and the cleaved caspase-3 level of experimental group treated with 100μg/mL of LJSF4 were not detected. All experiments were performed in triplicate. Data are expressed as means ± standard error of the means (S.E.M). ** $p < 0.01$ as compared to the UVB-treated group and ## $p < 0.01$ as compared to the control group.

2.3. Effect of LJSF4 on UVB-Irradiated Zebrafish

Zebrafish has become a popular animal model in the field of biological activity, due to the fact that its tissues and organs are very similar to mammals at the genetic, physiological, behavioral, and anatomical levels [40]. In previous reports, researchers have successfully used the zebrafish model to explore the protective effects of natural compounds on UVB-induced oxidative stress [41]. Therefore, we chose the same model to evaluate the protective effect of LJSF4 on UVB-irradiated photoaging in vivo. Zebrafish were pre-treated with LJSF4 of 25 to 100 μg/mL, respectively, and subsequently exposed to 50 mJ/cm^2 of UVB.

Excessive ROS produced by UVB stimulation plays a critical role in destroying keratinocytes through cell damage. ROS can be detected by using 2′, 7′-dichlorodihydrofluorescein diacetate (DCFH-DA) staining in living embryos. As shown in Figure 5A, the control group without exposure to UVB had no fluorescent generation, whereas that with exposure to UVB generated fluorescence, which indicated the generation of ROS on UVB-irradiated zebrafish. However, the zebrafish treated with different concentrations of LJSF4 showed a dose-dependent reduction in the production of ROS before being exposed to UVB irradiation. This result indicates that ROS levels decreased by 237.64% in zebrafish treated with 100 μg/mL of LJSF4. Then, cell death was determined by staining the embryos with acridine orange. The result indicates that the fluorescence intensity of the LJSF4 pretreatment group at the concentration of 100 μg/mL was decreased to almost the same level to that of the control group (Figure 5B). In addition, the protective effect of the fucoidan on zebrafish was determined against ROS-activated NO generation. As shown in Figure 5C, compared to that of the control group with no UVB irradiation, the production of NO was significantly increased 3.64 fold, while the pretreatment with LJSF4 inhibited the production of NO in a dose-dependent manner significantly. A similar result of dose-dependent inhibition for lipid peroxidation by LJSF4 treatment was also obtained (Figure 5D). This is similar to the results of previous studies, which reported that zebrafish exposed to UVB increased ROS generation, cell death levels, NO generation, and lipid peroxidation levels compared to that without UVB irradiation [12,42]. Furthermore, Wang et al. (2017) demonstrated that DPHC, isolated from *I. okamurae*, could decrease ROS levels by 85.21% with the concentration of 100 μM [41]. In short, the results show that LJSF4 extracted from *S. japonica* could excellently inhibit the generation of inflammation and reduce the destruction of cellular components by decreasing ROS levels, thereby further indicating the photoprotective effect of LJSF4 in zebrafish.

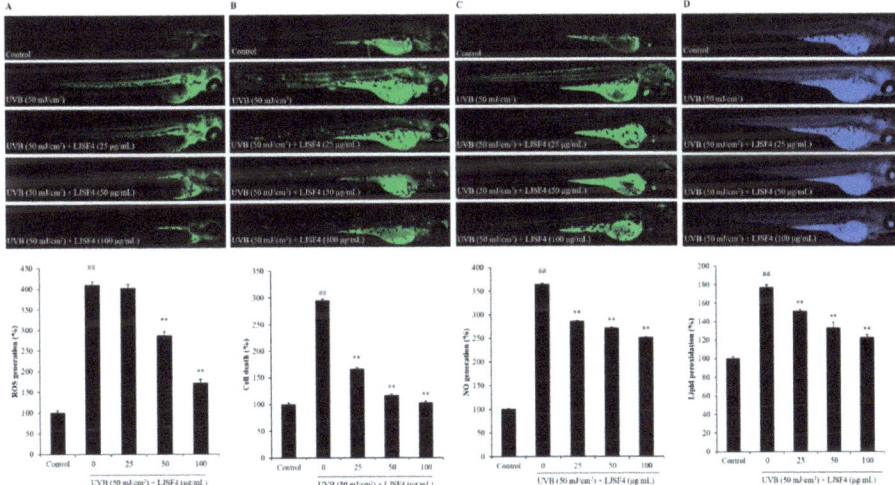

Figure 5. The effect of LJSF4 on UVB-irradiated zebrafish: (**A**) effect of LJSF4 on UVB-irradiated ROS generation in zebrafish; (**B**) effect of LJSF4 on UVB-irradiated cell death levels in zebrafish; (**C**) effect of LJSF4 on UVB-irradiated NO level in zebrafish; (**D**) effect of LJSF4 on UVB-irradiated lipid peroxidation levels in zebrafish. Zebrafish embryos at 2 days post-fertilization (dpf) were used for the anti-UVB study. Data are expressed as means ± standard error of the means (S.E.M). ** $p < 0.01$ as compared to the UVB-treated group and ## $p < 0.01$ as compared to the control group.

3. Materials and Methods

3.1. Reagents and Chemicals

S. japonica was harvested in Xiapu coastal area, Fujian province, China. Phosphate-buffered saline (PBS) and fetal bovine serum (FBS) were purchased from Solarbio (Beijing, China). The dimethyl sulfoxide (DMSO), DCFH-DA, 1,3-Bis (diphenylphosphino) propane (DPPP), dimethyl sulfoxide (DMSO), diaminofluorophore 4-amino-5-methylamino-2′, 7′-difluorofluorescein diacetate (DAF-FM-DA), bovine serum albumin (BSA), 3-(4, 5)-dimethylthiazol-2-yl)-2, 5-diphenyltetrazolium bromide (MTT), acridine orange, and Hoechst 33342 were purchased from Sigma Co. (St. Louis, MO, USA). Penicillin/streptomycin (P/S) and Dulbecco's modified Eagle's medium (DMEM) were purchased from Gibco (Rockville, MD, USA). Antibodies against GAPDH (clone number of ARC0205, catalog number of MA5-35235), Bax (clone number of ARC0164, catalog number of MA5-35342), Bcl-xL (clone number of C.85.1, catalog number of MA5-15142), and cleaved caspase-3 (clone number of ARC0133, catalog number of MA5-35333) were purchased from Thermo Scientific (Waltham, MA, USA). All other reagents used in this study were of analytical grade and purchased from Solarbio (Beijing, China).

3.2. Purification and Monosaccharide Determination of Fucoidan Fractions

3.2.1. Extraction and Purification of Polysaccharides

LJSF4 was prepared according to the method described in our previous study [25]. In brief, the defatted sample of *S. japonica* was extracted by triple volume of distilled water at 120 °C for 2 h, and then the supernatant was collected. Then, via adding an equal volume of 2% $CaCl_2$ solution in order to remove the alginate in the supernatant, and the resulting supernatant was finally lyophilized to gain crude fucoidan of LJS. The crude LJS was further purified by an anion exchange chromatography (AKTA Purifier UPC100, GE healthcare, Pittsburgh, PA, USA) to obtain the four fractions of LJSF1, LJSF2, LJSF3, LJSF4. The sulfate content and total sugar of each fraction were determined according to our published work [25]. LJSF4 was collected for further assays in this work.

3.2.2. Determination of Monosaccharide Composition

Monosaccharide composition of LJSF4 was analyzed by a 6890 N gas chromatographic system (Agilent 6890 N, Agilent, Santa Clara, CA, USA) after hydrolysis and acetylation according to the method described by Zha et al. [43].

3.3. Effect of LJSF4 on UVB-Irradiated HaCaT Cells

3.3.1. HaCaT Cells Culture and UVB Irradiation

HaCaT cell line was obtained from Korean Cell Line Bank (Seoul, Korea). Cells were cultured in DMEM supplemented with 100 µg/mL of streptomycin, 100 unit/mL of penicillin, and 10% FBS at 37 °C in humidified atmosphere with 5% CO_2.

Cells were exposed to UVB irradiation at wavelength of 280–320 nm by a UVB meter (UV Lamp, VL-6LM, Vilber Lourmat, Paris, France). Cells were irradiated by UVB at a dose of 30 mJ/cm^2 [40,42] and incubated until analysis.

3.3.2. Cell Viability Assay

The cytotoxicity of LJSF4 on HaCaT cells were determined by MTT assay. In brief, HaCaT cells were seeded in a 96-well plate at a density of 3×10^4 cells per well. After 24 h, the supernatant was discarded and wells were treated with 25, 50, 100 µg/mL of LJSF4, respectively. Then, after being further incubated for 24 h, the MTT solution was applied into the wells for 4 h. At last, the formazan crystals were dissolved in DMSO, and the absorbance were measured at 540 nm by an ELISA plate reader (BioTek PowerWave XS, Winooski, VT, USA) [10].

3.3.3. Measurement of Intracellular ROS Generation and Cell Viability in UVB-Irradiated HaCaT Cells

Intracellular ROS generation of LJSF4 on UVB-irradiated HaCaT cells was determined by the DCFH-DA method [44]. Briefly, after incubation for 24 h, cells were treated with LJSF4 for 30 min. Then, 500 µg/mL of DCFH-DA was added into each well and incubated for 30 min. Subsequently, cells were exposed to 30 mJ/cm^2 of UVB and measured according to the reported procedure of Wang et al. [42].

In order to measure the cell viability of LJSF4 on UVB-induced HaCaT cells, cells were treated with LJSF4 (25, 50, 100 µg/mL). After being cultured for 2 h, cells were exposed to 30 mJ/cm^2 of UVB and incubated for 24 h. Subsequently, cell viability was examined by the MTT assay described previously [10,45].

3.3.4. Measurement of Apoptosis in UVB-Irradiated HaCaT Cells

As in the procedure described by Naito et al., the apoptosis body formation was assessed by nuclear staining [46]. After being seeded in 24-well plates for 24 h, cells were treated with LJSF4 and incubated for another 2 h. Then, cells were exposed to 30 mJ/cm^2 of UVB and incubated with serum-free DMEM solution for 6 h. After incubation, cells were treated with Hoechst 33342 (stock, 10 mg/mL) for 10 min. At last, the stained cells were photographed by a fluorescence microscope equipped with a Cool SNAP-Procolor digital camera (Olympus, Tokyo, Japan). Apoptosis levels were measured using Image J software automatically.

3.3.5. Western Blot Analysis

To investigate the effect of LJSF4 on the expression of apoptosis-related proteins, Western blot analysis was performed by the method described by Wijesinghe et al. [47]. Briefly, cells exposing to 30 mJ/cm^2 of UVB were pretreated with different concentrations of LJSF4. After incubation for 24 h, cells were harvested in lysis buffer. The total protein levels of the supernatant were measured using a BCATM kit. A gradient 10% SDS-PAGE was used to separate the total protein extracts (50 µg), which were then electrophoretically transferred onto nitrocellulose membranes. The membranes were then blocked with skim milk (5%), and the immunoblotting procedure, including incubation with primary antibodies, washing, and incubation with secondary antibodies, was carried out as previously reported [47]. Finally, the target bands were observed by enhanced chemiluminescence (ELC), and detected by Tanon-5200 detection system (Tanon Science, Shanghai, China).

3.4. Effect of LJSF4 on UVB-Irradiated Zebrafish

3.4.1. Origin and Maintenance of Parental Zebrafish

This study work was approved by the ethical committee of experimental animal care of Ocean University of China at College of Food Science and Engineering, (Approval No. 2019-05). Adult zebrafish were obtained from the Molecular Medicine Laboratory (Ocean University of China, Qingdao, China) and kept in an automatic circulation culture system (ESEN, Beijing, China) at 28.5 ± 1 °C with a cycle of 14/10 h of light/dark. Live brine shrimps were fed twice a day to the parental zebrafish. Embryos were obtained from natural spawning according to the method reported by Zou et al. [48]. Fertilized embryos were collected in petri dishes completely within 30 min.

3.4.2. Measurement of Effect of LJSF4 Against UVB-Irradiation in Zebrafish

At 2 dpf, the zebrafish were transferred to a 24-well plate and treated with LJSF4 with final concentrations of 25, 50, and 100 μg/mL, respectively. The incubation, UVB-irradiation process and determination of ROS level, cell death, and NO production were carried out according to the reported procedure of Ko et al. [12]. The zebrafish larvae were photographed under the microscope Cool SNAP-Procolor digital camera, and the individual zebrafish larvae fluorescence intensity was quantified using an Image J program (National Institutes of Health, Bethesda, MD, US).

3.5. Statistical Analysis

Three independent experiments were carried out for each assay. Data were expressed as means ± standard error of the means (S.E.M) and analyzed by one-way ANOVA followed by the least significant differences test using SPSS 20.0 (SPSS Inc., Chicago, IL, USA). Turkey's multiple-range test was used to assess the significant differences of the means. In all cases, the *p*-value ($p < 0.05$) was indicated as statistically significant differences.

4. Conclusions

In this study, we evaluated the protective effect of LJSF4 against UVB-induced photodamage by in vitro and in vivo models. Treatment with LJSF4 prior to UVB exposure considerably protected the HaCaT cells against ROS generation. In addition, the ROS, the cell death, the nitric oxide, and the lipid peroxidation induced by UVB radiation in zebrafish were reduced by the addition of LJSF4. This study suggested the potential use of LJSF4 from *S. japonica* for the treatment of UVB-caused skin damage, which indicated that LJSF4 has a great potential to be used in cosmetic products as an effective natural anti-UVB agent.

Author Contributions: Conceptualization, funding acquisition and Supervision, X.F.; methodology, investigation, data curation, W.S., L.W. and L.N.; project administration, X.F., J.X. and X.G.; sample preparation and collection, D.D.; formal analysis and writing, W.S. All authors have read and agreed to the published version of the manuscript.

Funding: This research was funded by National Key R&D Program of China (Grant No. 2018YFD0901104), and the Major Scientific and Technological Innovation Project of Shandong Province (Grant No. 2019JZZY020613).

Conflicts of Interest: The authors declare no conflict of interest.

References

1. Hwang, P.-A.; Yan, M.-D.; Kuo, K.-L.; Phan, N.N.; Lin, Y.-C. A mechanism of low molecular weight fucoidans degraded by enzymatic and acidic hydrolysis for the prevention of UVB damage. *J. Appl. Phycol.* **2017**, *29*, 521–529. [CrossRef]
2. Tanaka, K.; Hasegawa, J.; Asamitsu, K.; Okamoto, T. *Magnolia ovovata* extract and its active component magnolol prevent skin photoaging via inhibition of nuclear factor kappa B. *Eur. J. Pharmacol.* **2007**, *565*, 212–219. [CrossRef] [PubMed]
3. Marrot, L.; Belaidi, J.P.; Chaubo, C.; Meunier, J.R.; Perez, P.; Agapakis-Causse, C. Fluoroquinolones as chemical tools to define a strategy for photogenotoxicity in vitro assessment. *Toxicol. Vitro* **2001**, *15*, 131–142. [CrossRef]
4. Svobodova, A.; Psotova, J.; Walterova, D. Natural phenolics in the prevention of UV-induced skin damage. A review. *Biomed. Pap.* **2003**, *147*, 137–145. [CrossRef]
5. Katiyar, S.K.; Pal, H.C.; Prasad, R. Dietary proanthocyanidins prevent ultraviolet radiation-induced non-melanoma skin cancer through enhanced repair of damaged DNA-dependent activation of immune sensitivity. *Semin. Cancer Biol.* **2017**, *46*, 138–145. [CrossRef] [PubMed]
6. Pallela, R.; Na-Young, Y.; Kim, S.-K. Anti-photoaging and photoprotective compounds derived from marine organisms. *Mar. Drugs* **2010**, *8*, 1189–1202. [CrossRef]
7. Tomaino, A.; Cristani, M.; Cimino, F.; Speciale, A.; Trombetta, D.; Bonina, F.; Saija, A. In vitro protective effect of a Jacquez grapes wine extract on UVB-induced skin damage. *Toxicol. Vitro* **2006**, *20*, 1395–1402. [CrossRef]
8. Hseu, Y.-C.; Chou, C.-W.; Kumar, K.J.S.; Fu, K.-T.; Wang, H.-M.; Hsu, L.-S.; Kuo, Y.-H.; Wu, C.-R.; Chen, S.-C.; Yang, H.-L. Ellagic acid protects human keratinocyte (HaCaT) cells against UVA-induced oxidative stress and apoptosis through the upregulation of the HO-1 and Nrf-2 antioxidant genes. *Food Chem. Toxicol.* **2012**, *50*, 1245–1255. [CrossRef]
9. Kim, S.; You, D.H.; Han, T.; Choi, E.M. Modulation of viability and apoptosis of UVB-exposed human keratinocyte HaCaT cells by aqueous methanol extract of laver (*Porphyra yezoensis*). *J. Photochem. Photobiol. B Biol.* **2014**, *141*, 301–307. [CrossRef]
10. Heo, S.J.; Ko, S.C.; Cha, S.H.; Kang, D.H.; Park, H.S.; Choi, Y.U.; Kim, D.; Jung, W.K.; Jeon, Y.J. Effect of phlorotannins isolated from *Ecklonia cava* on melanogenesis and their protective effect against photo-oxidative stress induced by UV-B radiation. *Toxicol. Vitro* **2009**, *23*, 1123–1130. [CrossRef]
11. Hu, S.; Huang, J.; Pei, S.; Ouyang, Y.; Ding, Y.; Jiang, L.; Lu, J.; Kang, L.; Huang, L.; Xiang, H.; et al. *Ganoderma lucidum* polysaccharide inhibits UVB-induced melanogenesis by antagonizing cAMP/PKA and ROS/MAPK signaling pathways. *J. Cell. Physiol.* **2019**, *234*, 7330–7340. [CrossRef] [PubMed]
12. Ko, S.-C.; Cha, S.-H.; Heo, S.-J.; Lee, S.-H.; Kang, S.-M.; Jeon, Y.-J. Protective effect of *Ecklonia cava* on UVB-induced oxidative stress: In vitro and in vivo zebrafish model. *J. Appl. Phycol.* **2010**, *23*, 697–708. [CrossRef]
13. Heo, S.J.; Jeon, Y.J. Protective effect of fucoxanthin isolated from *Sargassum siliquastrum* on UV-B induced cell damage. *J. Photochem. Photobiol. B Biol.* **2009**, *95*, 101–107. [CrossRef] [PubMed]
14. Liu, F.; Wang, X.; Yao, J.; Fu, W.; Duan, D. Development of expressed sequence tag-derived microsatellite markers for *Saccharina* (*Laminaria*) *japonica*. *J. Appl. Phycol.* **2009**, *22*, 109–111. [CrossRef]
15. Zha, X.-Q.; Xiao, J.-J.; Zhang, H.-N.; Wang, J.-H.; Pan, L.-H.; Yang, X.-F.; Luo, J.-P. Polysaccharides in *Laminaria japonica* (LP): Extraction, physicochemical properties and their hypolipidemic activities in diet-induced mouse model of atherosclerosis. *Food Chem.* **2012**, *134*, 244–252. [CrossRef]
16. Xu, Y.; Zhu, W.; Wang, T.; Jin, L.; Liu, T.; Li, X.; Guan, Z.; Jiang, Z.; Meng, X.; Wang, J.; et al. Low molecule weight fucoidan mitigates atherosclerosis in ApoE (-/-) mouse model through activating multiple signal pathway. *Carbohydr. Polym.* **2019**, *206*, 110–120. [CrossRef]
17. Zhao, D.; Xu, J.; Xu, X. Bioactivity of fucoidan extracted from *Laminaria japonica* using a novel procedure with high yield. *Food Chem.* **2018**, *245*, 911–918. [CrossRef]
18. Geng, L.; Hu, W.; Liu, Y.; Wang, J.; Zhang, Q. A heteropolysaccharide from *Saccharina japonica* with immunomodulatory effect on RAW 264.7 cells. *Carbohydr. Polym.* **2018**, *201*, 557–565. [CrossRef]
19. Cao, Y.-G.; Hao, Y.; Li, Z.-H.; Liu, S.-T.; Wang, L.-X. Antiviral activity of polysaccharide extract from *Laminaria japonica* against respiratory syncytial virus. *Biomed. Pharmacother.* **2016**, *84*, 1705–1710. [CrossRef]

20. Jin, W.; Wang, J.; Jiang, H.; Song, N.; Zhang, W.; Zhang, Q. The neuroprotective activities of heteropolysaccharides extracted from *Saccharina japonica*. *Carbohydr. Polym.* **2013**, *97*, 116–120. [CrossRef]
21. Yoon, S.-J.; Pyun, Y.-R.; Hwang, J.-K.; Mourao, P.A.S. A sulfated fucan from the brown alga *Laminaria cichorioides* has mainly heparin cofactor II-dependent anticoagulant activity. *Carbohydr. Res.* **2007**, *342*, 2326–2330. [CrossRef] [PubMed]
22. Maruyama, H.; Tamauchi, H.; Kawakami, F.; Yoshinaga, K.; Nakano, T. Suppressive Effect of Dietary Fucoidan on Proinflammatory Immune Response and MMP-1 Expression in UVB-Irradiated Mouse Skin. *Planta Med.* **2015**, *81*, 1370–1374. [PubMed]
23. Ku, M.-J.; Jung, J.-W.; Lee, M.-S.; Cho, B.-K.; Lee, S.-R.; Lee, H.-S.; Vischuk, O.S.; Zvyagintseva, T.N.; Ermakova, S.P.; Lee, Y.-H. Effect of *Fucus evanescens* Fucoidan on Expression of Matrix Metalloproteinase-1 Promoter, mRNA, Protein and Signal Pathway. *J. Life Sci.* **2010**, *20*, 1603–1610. [CrossRef]
24. Moon, H.J.; Park, K.S.; Ku, M.J.; Lee, M.S.; Jeong, S.H.; Imbs, T.I.; Zvyagintseva, T.N.; Ermakova, S.P.; Lee, Y.H. Effect of *Costatia costata* Fucoidan on Expression of Matrix Metalloproteinase-1 Promoter, mRNA, and Protein. *J. Nat. Prod.* **2009**, *72*, 1731–1734. [CrossRef]
25. Ni, L.; Wang, L.; Fu, X.; Duan, D.; Jeon, Y.J.; Xu, J.; Gao, X. In vitro and in vivo anti-inflammatory activities of a fucose-rich fucoidan isolated from *Saccharina japonica*. *Int. J. Biol. Macromol.* **2020**, *156*, 717–729. [CrossRef] [PubMed]
26. Kammeyer, A.; Luiten, R.M. Oxidation events and skin aging. *Ageing Res. Rev.* **2015**, *21*, 16–29. [CrossRef] [PubMed]
27. Masaki, H. Role of antioxidants in the skin: Anti-aging effects. *J. Dermatol. Sci.* **2010**, *58*, 85–90. [CrossRef]
28. Zhou, X. FAO Global Aquaculture Updates, Notes from the Aquaculture Statistician. In *FAO Aquaculture Newsletter*; FAO Fisheries and Aquaculture Department: Rome, Italy, 2018; Volume 58, p. 135.
29. Ziegler, A.; Jonason, A.S.; Leffell, D.J.; Simon, J.A.; Sharma, H.W.; Kimmelman, J.; Remington, L.; Jacks, T.; Brash, D.E. Sunburn and P53 in the onset of skin-cancer. *Nature* **1994**, *372*, 773–776. [CrossRef]
30. Hamdoun, S.; Efferth, T. Ginkgolic acids inhibit migration in breast cancer cells by inhibition of NEMO sumoylation and NF-kappa B activity. *Oncotarget* **2017**, *8*, 35103–35115. [CrossRef]
31. Baek, S.H.; Ko, J.-H.; Lee, J.H.; Kim, C.; Lee, H.; Nam, D.; Lee, J.; Lee, S.-G.; Yang, W.M.; Um, J.-Y.; et al. Ginkgolic acid inhibits invasion and migration and TGF-β-induced EMT of lung cancer cells through PI3K/Akt/mTOR inactivation. *J. Cell. Physiol.* **2017**, *232*, 346–354. [CrossRef]
32. Kanematsu, S.; Uehara, N.; Miki, H.; Yoshizawa, K.; Kawanaka, A.; Yuri, T.; Tsubura, A. Autophagy inhibition enhances sulforaphane-induced apoptosis in human breast cancer cells. *Anticancer Res.* **2010**, *30*, 3381–3390. [PubMed]
33. Kim, M.Y.; Trudel, L.J.; Wogan, G.N. Apoptosis induced by capsaicin and resveratrol in colon carcinoma cells requires nitric oxide production and caspase activation. *Anticancer Res.* **2009**, *29*, 3733–3740. [PubMed]
34. Danial, N.N. BCL-2 family proteins: Critical checkpoints of apoptotic cell death. *Clin. Cancer Res.* **2007**, *13*, 7254–7263. [CrossRef] [PubMed]
35. Zhuang, L.H.; Wang, B.H.; Sauder, D.N. Molecular mechanism of ultraviolet-induced keratinocyte apoptosis. *J. Interferon Cytokine Res.* **2000**, *20*, 445–454. [CrossRef] [PubMed]
36. Riedl, S.J.; Salvesen, G.S. The apoptosome: Signalling platform of cell death. *Nat. Rev. Mol. Cell Biol.* **2007**, *8*, 405–413. [CrossRef] [PubMed]
37. Xiao, D.; Powolny, A.A.; Singh, S.V. Benzyl isothiocyanate targets mitochondrial respiratory chain to trigger reactive oxygen species-dependent apoptosis in human breast cancer cells. *J. Biol. Chem.* **2008**, *283*, 30151–30163. [CrossRef] [PubMed]
38. Fernando, P.M.D.J.; Piao, M.J.; Hewage, S.R.K.M.; Kang, H.K.; Yoo, E.S.; Koh, Y.S.; Ko, M.H.; Ko, C.S.; Byeon, S.H.; Mun, S.R.; et al. Photo-protective effect of sargachromenol against UVB radiation-induced damage through modulating cellular antioxidant systems and apoptosis in human keratinocytes. *Environ. Toxicol. Pharmacol.* **2016**, *43*, 112–119. [CrossRef]
39. Kim, Y.I.; Oh, W.S.; Song, P.H.; Yun, S.; Kwon, Y.S.; Lee, Y.J.; Ku, S.K.; Song, C.H.; Oh, T.H. Anti-photoaging effects of low molecular-weight fucoidan on ultraviolet B-irradiated mice. *Mar. Drugs* **2018**, *16*, 286. [CrossRef]
40. Yang, H.-M.; Ham, Y.-M.; Yoon, W.-J.; Roh, S.W.; Jeon, Y.-J.; Oda, T.; Kang, S.-M.; Kang, M.-C.; Kim, E.-A.; Kim, D.; et al. Quercitrin protects against ultraviolet B-induced cell death in vitro and in an in vivo zebrafish model. *J. Photochem. Photobiol. B Biol.* **2012**, *114*, 126–131. [CrossRef]

41. Wang, L.; Kim, H.S.; Oh, J.Y.; Je, J.G.; Jeon, Y.J.; Ryu, B. Protective effect of diphlorethohydroxycarmalol isolated from *Ishige okamurae* against UVB-induced damage in vitro in human dermal fibroblasts and *in vivo* in zebrafish. *Food Chem. Toxicol.* **2020**, *136*, 110963. [CrossRef]
42. Wang, L.; Ryu, B.; Kim, W.-S.; Kim, G.H.; Jeon, Y.-J. Protective effect of gallic acid derivatives from the freshwater green alga *Spirogyra* sp. against ultraviolet B-induced apoptosis through reactive oxygen species clearance in human keratinocytes and zebrafish. *Algae* **2017**, *32*, 379–388. [CrossRef]
43. Zha, X.-Q.; Lu, C.-Q.; Cui, S.-H.; Pan, L.-H.; Zhang, H.-L.; Wang, J.-H.; Luo, J.-P. Structural identification and immunostimulating activity of a *Laminaria japonica* polysaccharide. *Int. J. Biol. Macromol.* **2015**, *78*, 429–438. [CrossRef] [PubMed]
44. Rosenkranz, A.R.; Schmaldienst, S.; Stuhlmeier, K.M.; Chen, W.J.; Knapp, W.; Zlabinger, G.J. A microplate assay for the detection of oxidative products using 2′,7′-dichlorofluorescin-diacetate. *J. Immunol. Methods* **1992**, *156*, 39–45. [CrossRef]
45. Kang, M.-C.; Kim, S.Y.; Min, Y.T.; Kim, E.-A.; Lee, S.-H.; Ko, S.-C.; Wijesinghe, W.A.J.P.; Samarakoon, K.W.; Kim, Y.-S.; Cho, J.H.; et al. In vitro and in vivo antioxidant activities of polysaccharide purified from aloe vera (*Aloe barbadensis*) gel. *Carbohydr. Polym.* **2014**, *99*, 365–371. [CrossRef] [PubMed]
46. Naito, Y.; Yoshikawa, T. Neutrophil-dependent oxidative stress in gastrointestinal inflammation. In *Oxidative Stress and Digestive Diseases*; Karger: Basel, Switzerland, 2001; pp. 24–40.
47. Wijesinghe, W.A.J.P.; Jeon, Y.J.; Ramasamy, P.; Wahid, M.E.A.; Vairappan, C.S. Anticancer activity and mediation of apoptosis in human HL-60 leukaemia cells by edible sea cucumber (*Holothuria edulis*) extract. *Food Chem.* **2013**, *139*, 326–331. [CrossRef]
48. Zou, Y.; Fu, X.; Liu, N.; Duan, D.; Wang, X.; Xu, J.; Gao, X. The synergistic anti-inflammatory activities of agaro-oligosaccharides with different degrees of polymerization. *J. Appl. Phycol.* **2019**, *31*, 2547–2558. [CrossRef]

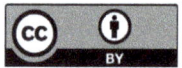

© 2020 by the authors. Licensee MDPI, Basel, Switzerland. This article is an open access article distributed under the terms and conditions of the Creative Commons Attribution (CC BY) license (http://creativecommons.org/licenses/by/4.0/).

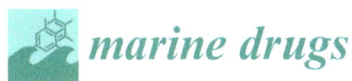

Article

Protective Effect of Fucoidan against MPP+-Induced SH-SY5Y Cells Apoptosis by Affecting the PI3K/Akt Pathway

Huaide Liu [1], Jing Wang [2,3,*], Quanbin Zhang [2,3], Lihua Geng [2,3], Yue Yang [2,3] and Ning Wu [2,3]

1. School of Life Sciences, Nantong University, Seyuan Road 9, Nantong 226019, China; hold126@126.com
2. Key Laboratory of Experimental Marine Biology, Center for Ocean Mega-Science, Institute of Oceanology, Chinese Academy of Sciences, Qingdao 266071, China; qbzhang@qdio.ac.cn (Q.Z.); lhgeng@qdio.ac.cn (L.G.); yueyang@qdio.ac.cn (Y.Y.); wuning@qdio.ac.cn (N.W.)
3. Laboratory for Marine Biology and Biotechnology, Qingdao National Laboratory for Marine Science and Technology, Wenhai Road, Aoshanwei, Jimo, Qingdao 266237, China
* Correspondence: jingwang@qdio.ac.cn; Tel.: +86-532-82898703

Received: 9 May 2020; Accepted: 23 June 2020; Published: 25 June 2020

Abstract: The main pathologic changes of the Parkinson's disease (PD) is dopaminergic (DA) neurons lost. Apoptosis was one of the important reasons involved in the DA lost. Our previous study found a fucoidan fraction sulfated heterosaccharide (UF) had neuroprotective activity. The aim of this study was to clarify the mechanism of UF on DA neurons using human dopaminergic neuroblastoma (SH-SY5Y) cells a typical as a PD cellular model. Results showed that UF prevented MPP+-induced SH-SY5Y cells apoptosis and cell death. Additionally, UF pretreated cells increased phosphorylation of Akt, PI3K and NGF, which means UF-treated active PI3K–Akt pathway. Moreover, UF treated cells decreased the expression of apoptosis-associated protein, such as the ratio of Bax/Bcl-2, GSK3β, caspase-3 and p53 nuclear induced by MPP+. This effect was partially blocked by PI3K inhibitor LY294002. Our data suggested that protective effect of UF against MPP+-induced SH-SY5Y cells death by affecting the PI3K–Akt pathway. These findings contribute to a better understanding of the critical roles of UF in treating PD and may elucidate the molecular mechanisms of UF effects in PD.

Keywords: fucoidan; sulfated heterosaccharide; dopamine neurons apoptosis; PI3K–Akt

1. Introduction

Parkinson's disease (PD) is a neurodegenerative disease characterized by the selective loss of dopaminergic (DA) neurons and the formation of Lewy bodies in the brain. The mainly symptoms was movement disorders such as bradykinesia, myotonia, tremors and abnormal gait [1]. Many reasons such as apoptosis, oxidative stress, genetic factors, environmental factors, mitochondrial dysfunction, ubiquitin-proteasome system dysfunction, immune abnormalities, excitotoxicity and cytotoxicity of calcium may be related to the occurrence of PD [2,3]. Many studies have shown that DA neuron apoptosis has an important effect on the pathogenesis of PD, the number of apoptotic cells in PD patients is nearly 10 times more than normal aged person [4]. However, the exact cause of DA neuron apoptosis is unknown [5]. Oxidative stress, loss of antioxidant function and mitochondrial function damage, can induce DA neuron apoptosis at different levels [6]. The inhibition of pro-apoptotic protein Bax and anti-apoptotic protein Bcl-2 can regulate the apoptosis of DA neurons [7]. Therefore, regulation the expression of apoptosis-associated genes and proteins has become another strategy for the treatment of PD.

The PI3K–Akt pathway plays an important role in neuronal survival and death. Activation the PI3K–Akt pathway can inhibit the activity of downstream caspase-3 and thus inhibit the apoptosis of DA neurons, which can be weakened by the PI3K-specific inhibitor LY294002 [8]. Studies found pretreatment with simvastatin, sulforaphane, erythropoietin, β-interferon and catechins on 6-OHDA-damaged SH-SY5Y cells can increase the PI3K phosphorylation and directly activates the PI3K signaling pathway. Activated Akt can inhibit the activity of downstream caspase-3 and thus inhibit the apoptosis of DA neurons, which can be weakened by the PI3K-specific inhibitor LY294002 [9]. The brain tissues of PD patients and normal people were analyzed by immunofluorescence and western blotting after death. It was found that Akt and activated phosphoSer473-Akt were significantly reduced in the brains of PD patients. Nerve growth factor (NGF) plays an important role in the stages of neuron growth and development, axon growth, transmitter synthesis and cell apoptosis. Studies have shown that the application of corresponding treatments after spinal cord ischemia can induce NGF to activate the PI3K–Akt pathway to inhibit neuronal apoptosis. It can be seen that increase NGF to activate the PI3K–Akt pathway to inhibit DA neuronal apoptosis is a new strategy for the prevention and treatment of PD.

Marine seaweeds produce and accumulate a large number of substances with special chemical structures, physiological activities and functions during their growth and metabolism. The development and utilization of marine biologic resources is an important area and direction for drug candidates. The main feature of the polysaccharides extracted from seaweeds is that it contained sulfated groups. The structures were more complex and the activities were more excellent compared with the polysaccharides extracted from the land plants [10]. Fucoidan is a kind of sulfated polysaccharide extracted from brown algae. It has various biologic activities such as antivirus, antitumor, antimutation, antiradiation and immunity enhancement [11]. The bioactivity such as antioxidant, anticoagulation, neuro-protective activity of fucoidan depends on several structural parameters such as the degree of sulfation (DS), the molecular weight, other substitution groups and position, type of sugar and glycosidic branching. Our preliminary study had shown that the fucoidan with highest sulfated group exhibited stronger activity in scavenging superoxide radical and also hydroxyl radical [12]. The sulfated and benzoylated derivatives of fucoidan could enhance the neuroprotective activity by increasing mitochondrial activity and decreasing LDH and ROS release induced by 6-OHDA ($p < 0.01$ or $p < 0.001$) [13]. Our previous studies found that fucoidan (FPS) can reduce DA neurons damage in phenyl-1,2,3,6-tetrahydropyridine (MPTP)-induced PD mouse model [14,15]. FPS has a protective effects on oxidative damage and inflammatory lesion on DA neurons caused by MPTP in PD mouse, [16]. FPS is a crude polysaccharide prepared from *Saccharina japonica*. After degradation and purification, we got three fractions with different sulfated groups and monosaccharides compositions. Among the samples, UF with highest uronic acid and lowest sulfated groups has the strongest neuroprotective effect both in vitro and in vivo [17]. UF can increase the level of antioxidant enzymes and reduce the level of lipid peroxidation in PD mice [18]. We further found that UF can upregulate the expression of the anti-apoptotic protein Bcl-2, reduce the expression of the pro-apoptotic protein Bax, and significantly inhibit the apoptosis of DA neurons in H_2O_2–induced SH-SY5Y cell model [13]. Therefore, we speculate that UF has effect on the DA neurons apoptosis. However, it is not yet established whether UF exhibited apoptosis activity through PI3K–Akt pathway in a MPP^+ induced neuronal cell line. Can UF activate PI3K by acting on the NGF to cause progressive activation of the PI3K–Akt pathway? How does UF regulate downstream signaling molecules and proteins in the PI3K–Akt pathway?

The aim of this study is to clarify whether UF can activate the PI3K–Akt pathway by acting on NGF protein and illuminate the anti-apoptosis mechanism of UF through the PI3K–Akt pathway. This study will provide experimental foundation and theoretical basis for the application of UF in PD therapy and provide a scientific basis for the development of new and effective anti-PD marine drugs.

2. Result

2.1. Chemical Analysis

The chemical composition of FPS, DF (low molecular weight fucoidan) and UF are shown in Table 1. All these three samples were sulfated heteropolysaccharides; they were mainly made of fucose, uronic acid and sulfated groups. However, the exactly chemical composition were different. The chemical composition of FPS and DF were nearly the same, however. The molecular weight of FPS was 10 times higher than DF. Among the three samples, UF had the highest uronic acid and lowest sulfated groups. The monosaccharides of three samples all contained fucose, galactose, glucose, rhamnose, mannose and xylose. Fucose was the mainly monosaccharide in all three samples, followed with galactose The structure of FPS, DF and UF were published by our group. The backbone of FPS and DF was similar: they were primarily made by (1→3)-linked α-L-fucopyranose residues and a few (1→4)-α-L-fucopyranose linkages. β-D-galactose and fucose were linked at the branch points at C-4 or C-2 of α-L-fucopyranose residues. Sulfate groups occupied at C-4 or C-2, sometimes C-2, 4 to fucose residues and C-3 and/or C-4 to galactose residues. The structure of UF was more complex. The backbone was made by 4-linked uronic acid and 2-linked mannose. The branch chain was composed of 1–3-linked fucose, 1–6-linked galactose and 1–4-linked glucuronic acid. The sulfate group was connected to the C-6 position of mannose. and C-4 or C-2 position of fucose [19].

Table 1. The yield (% compared with the dry *S. japonica*), chemical composition (% dry weight) and molecular weight of fucoidan (FPS), DF and its fraction (UF) isolated from *S. japonica*.

Sample	Yield%	Fucose	Uronic Acid	Sulfate	Molecular Weight (Da)	Neutral Sugar (Mole Ratio) [a]					
						Fuc	Gal	Man	Glc	Rha	Xyl
FPS	2.2	26.12	4.93	28.01	174,000	1.00	0.39	0.098	0.031	0.091	0.022
DF	1.3	28.7	3.65	30.1	9500	1.00	0.58	0.038	0.16	0.054	0.033
UF	0.3	19.12	14.25	21.21	6544	1.00	0.71	0.11	0.26	0.11	0.087

[a] Fuc: fucose; Gal: galactose; Man: mannose; Glc: glucose; Rha: rhamnose; Xyl: xylose.

2.2. Protective Effect of UF on MPP^+-Induced Neurotoxicity in SH-SY5Y Cells

The results of protective effect of UF on MPP^+-induced neurotoxicity in SH-SY5Y cells are shown in Figure 1. The exposure of the SH-SY5Y cells to 100-μM MPP^+ significantly reduced cell viability to 60% compared with that of the normal cells. In contrast, pretreatment with different concentrations of UF reversed the decreased cell viability induced by MPP^+. Co-incubation of UF at the dose of 500 μg/mL and 800 μg/mL increased the cell viability more than 30% compared with the MPP group. When exposed with PI3K inhibitor LY294002, the cell viability decreased in all groups compared with the NC group. The cell viability of NCLY and MPPLY group was nearly 80% and 32% compared with the NC group. Pretreatment with UF increased the cell viability to 55%—especially at the dose of 800 μg/mL.

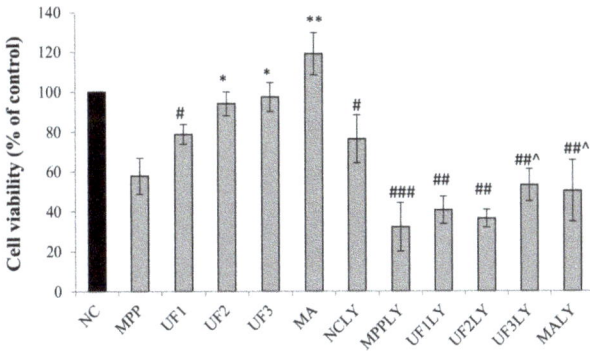

Figure 1. Effect of the samples on the neuronal cell viability induced by MPP^+. # Vs NC $p < 0.05$; ## Vs NC $p < 0.01$; ### Vs NC $p < 0.001$; * Vs MPP $p < 0.05$; ** Vs MPP $p < 0.01$; *** Vs MPP $p < 0.001$; ^ Vs MPPLY $p < 0.05$; ^^ Vs MPPLY $p < 0.01$; ^^^ Vs MPPLY $p < 0.001$.

To determine whether the survival rate of SH-SY5Y neurons increased by UF treatment was related to cell apoptosis, cells were stained with the DNA dye Hoechst 33342/PI to visualize nuclear morphology (Figure 2). The results showed that incubation with MPP$^+$ could cause SH-SY5Y cells apoptosis—including the degeneration of neuritis and shrinkage of cell bodies—as well as fragmentation and condensation of nuclei. Without exposure to MPP$^+$, SH-SY5Y cells exhibited normal cellular morphology. Different doses of UF administration groups could reduce the apoptosis and death rate of SH-SY5Y cells (500 μg/mL and 800 μg/mL, respectively, $p < 0.01$), which indicated that the protective effect of UF on SH-SY5Y cells was related to reducing the apoptosis of SH-SY5Y cells. To determine whether the apoptosis of SH-SY5Y cells caused by MPP$^+$ was related to the PI3K/AKT pathway, we added PI3K/AKT pathway inhibitor LY294002 during cell culture [7,8]. The degree of apoptosis and death rate of SH-SY5Y cells in MPPLY group increased significantly compared with NC group. Different concentrations of UF administration groups could reduce the apoptosis and death rate. The MPP$^+$-induced apoptosis rate was 37.6%; the addition of LY294002 increased the frequency of apoptosis rate to 51.5%. UF at 800 μg/mL greatly reduced MPP$^+$-induced apoptosis to 11.1%. With the addition of LY294002, the effect of UF at 800 μg/mL on MPP$^+$-induced apoptosis was 28.7%. The apoptosis rate was different when cells were pretreatment with UF alone or together with LY294002 (11.1% versus 28.7%, $p < 0.001$). These data suggest that the protective effect of UF on SH-SY5Y cells was partly related to the PI3K/AKT pathway.

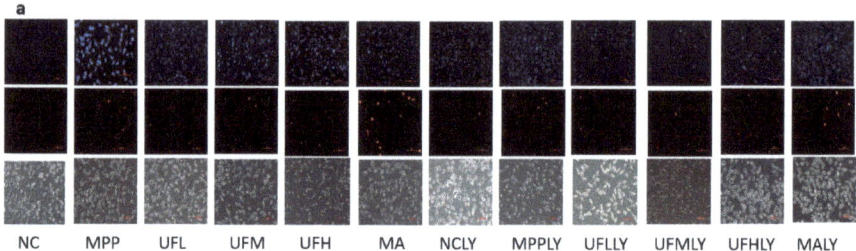

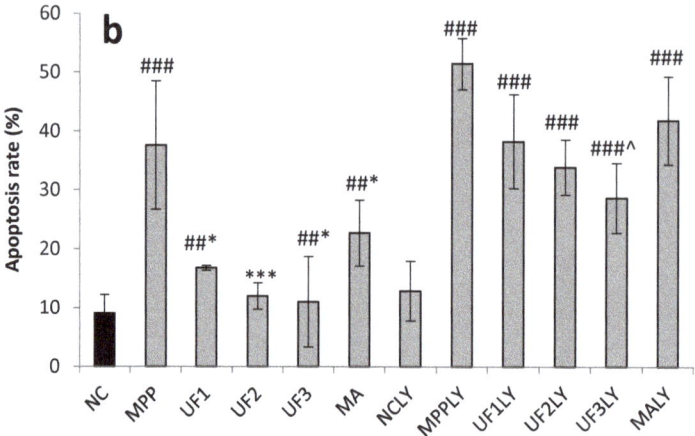

Figure 2. *Cont.*

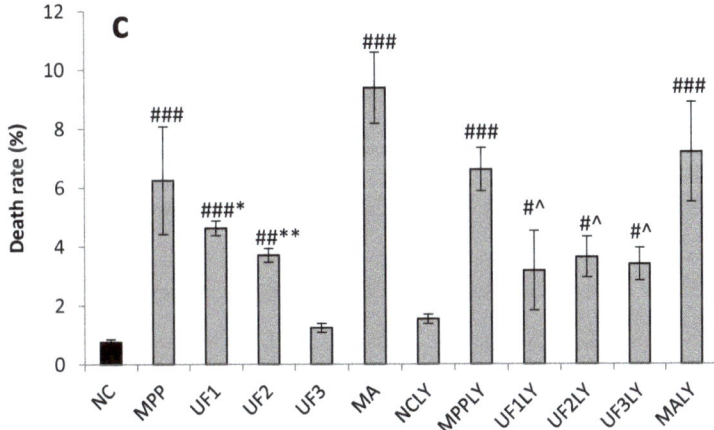

Figure 2. Nuclear morphology of MPP$^+$ and UF treated SH-SY5Y cells for 48 h. (**a**) Protective effects of UF on MPP$^+$-induced cell apoptosis rate %; (**b**) protective effects of UF on MPP$^+$-induced cell Death rate % (**c**) Data are expressed as percentages and represent the mean ± SD of three separate experiments in which at least 200 cells were counted per one treatment group. $^\#$ Vs NC $p < 0.05$; $^{\#\#}$ Vs NC $p < 0.01$; $^{\#\#\#}$ Vs NC $p < 0.001$; * Vs MPP $p < 0.05$; ** Vs MPP $p < 0.01$; *** Vs MPP $p < 0.001$; $^\wedge$ Vs MPPLY $p < 0.05$; $^{\wedge\wedge}$ Vs MPPLY $p < 0.01$; $^{\wedge\wedge\wedge}$ Vs MPPLY $p < 0.001$; Scale bar in the picture is 50 in length.

2.3. UF Effect on the Expression of PI3K, Akt and Its Phosphorylation

Figure 3 summarizes the effect of the samples on the phosphorylation of PI3K and Akt proteins (). The immunochemistry results showed that MPP$^+$ treatment decreased the phosphorylation of PI3K and Akt and inhibited the activation of PI3K/AKT pathway. Different concentrations of UF administration groups promoted the phosphorylation of PI3K and Akt, thereby activating the PI3K/AKT pathway (Figure 3b,c). The ratio of pAkt/tAkt and pPI3K/tPI3K were analyzed; the two ratios were lower in MPP group than in NC group. Different doses of UF treated increased the two ratios, respectively. We also examined whether the PI3K inhibitor LY294002 could inhibit the cytoprotective effect of UF. After incubation with LY294002, the degree of phosphorylated PI3K and Akt decreased significantly compared with NC group. Different concentrations of UF administration groups increased the phosphorylated PI3K and Akt level. Comparing the groups UF1 and UF1LY, UF2 and UF2LY, UF3 and UF3LY, the phosphorylated PI3K and Akt increased rates in UF1LY, UF2LY and UF3LY groups were lower than in the UF1, UF2 and UF3 groups, respectively. The results suggest that UF activated the PI3K/AKT pathway to inhibit the apoptosis of neuron cells and additional LY294002 alleviated UF neuron protective, but not completely. We tested the pAkt and pPI3K protein expression using western blotting to confirm. As we expected, results showed that the expression of pAkt and pPI3K was decreased in MPP group compared with the NC group. UF treatment groups reversed the MPP$^+$ induced pAkt and pPI3K decrease markedly. After incubation with LY294002, the expression of pAkt and pPI3K were lower than the groups without treated with LY294002, respectively. Treatment with UF and positive drug MA increased the expression of pAkt and pPI3K at some extent. Therefore, it is plausible that the degradation pAkt and pPI3K may be regulated by UF and the UF treatment could activate PI3K–Akt pathway.

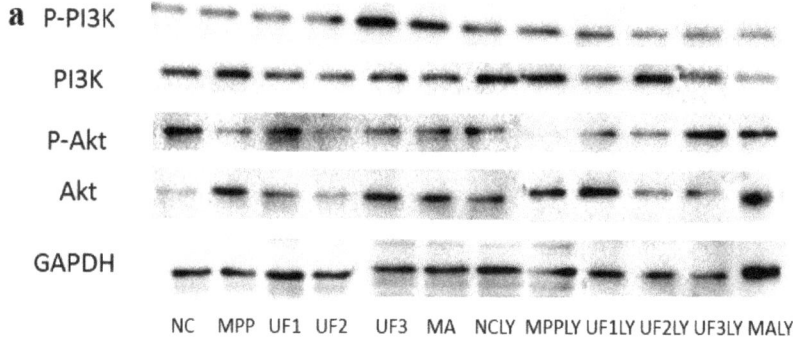

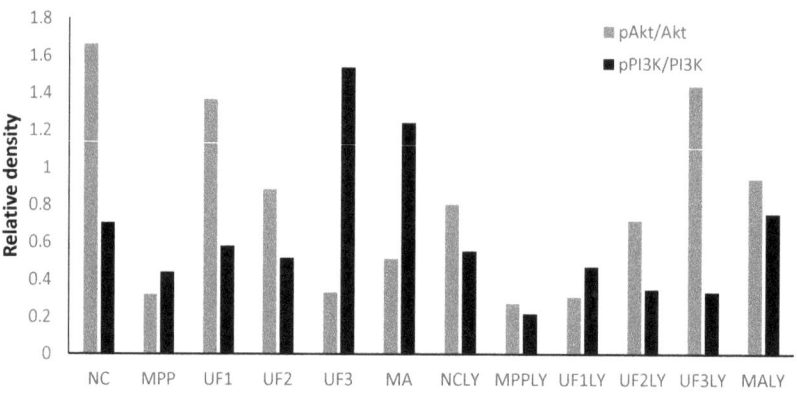

Figure 3. *Cont.*

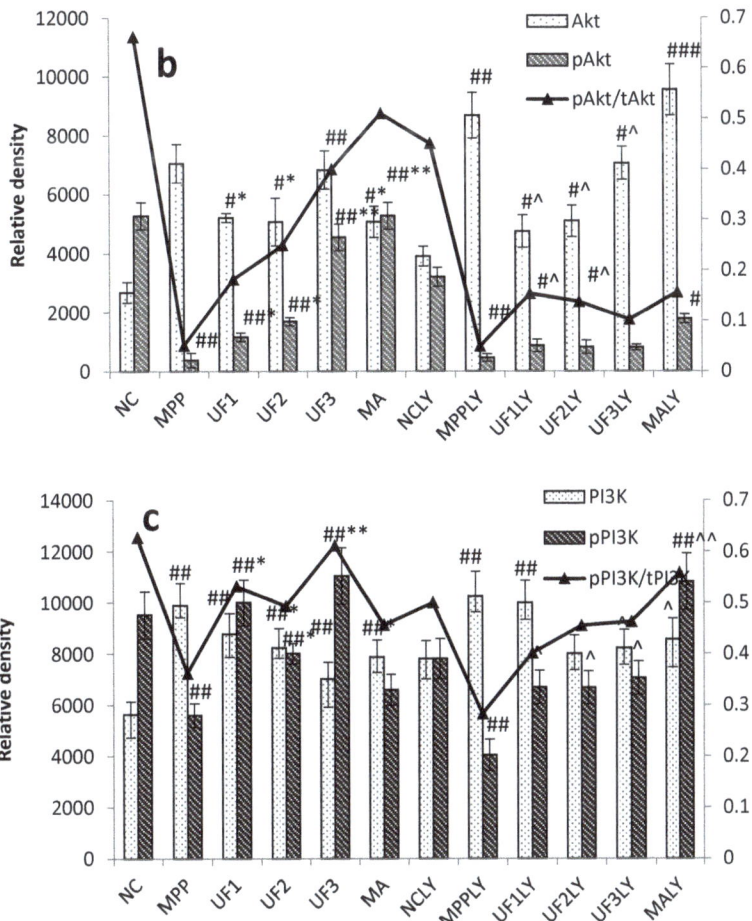

Figure 3. UF effect on the expression of PI3K, Akt and its phosphorylation. (**a**) PI3K, Akt and its phosphorylation results by western blot; (**b**) Akt and its phosphorylation results by immunochemistry method; (**c**) PI3K and its phosphorylation results by immunochemistry method; # Vs NC $p < 0.05$; ## Vs NC $p < 0.01$; * Vs MPP $p < 0.05$; ** Vs MPP $p < 0.01$; ˆ Vs MPPLY $p < 0.05$; ˜ Vs MPPLY $p < 0.01$.

2.4. UF Effect on the Expression of NGF

To determine whether UF treatment could promote the survival of CNS neurons and activation PI3K/AKT pathway, we tested the effectiveness of UF on NGF. The protein expression level of the NGF decreased significantly in the MPP group, however, NGF expression elevated in different doses of the UF treatment groups, especially in the dose of 100-μg/mL UF group (Figure 4a). Moreover, the treatment of cells with 100-μM MPP$^+$ and 20-μM LY294002 significantly decreased the mRNA level of NGF to 0.28 ± 0.03 of the NC group and the UF (800 μg/mL) combined with LY294002 treatment group increased that to 0.75 ± 0.06 of the NC group, respectively (Figure 4b).

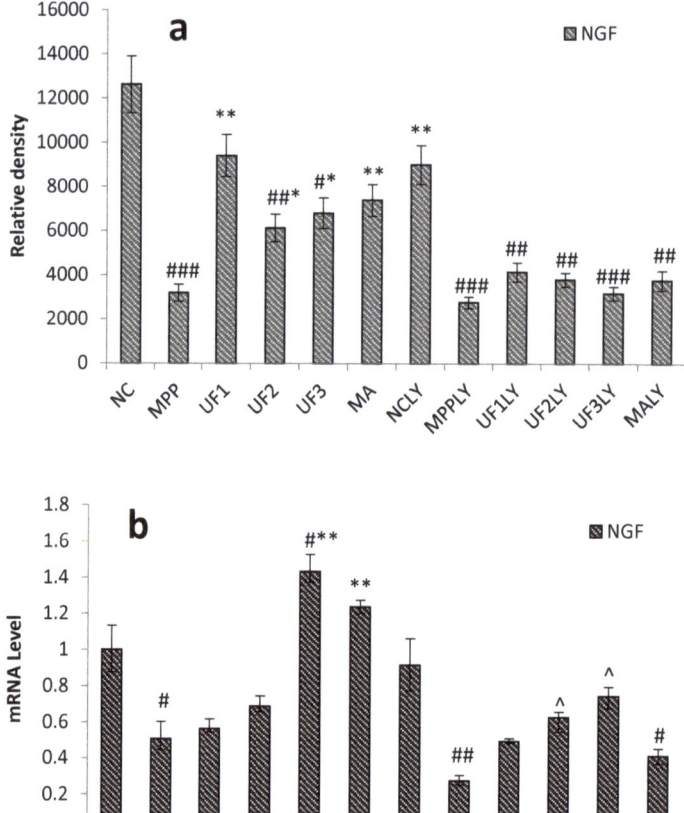

Figure 4. Protective effects of UF on MPP$^+$-induced SH-SY5Y cell of NGF. (**a**) NGF results by immunochemistry method; (**b**) NGF results by RT-PCR method; # Vs NC $p < 0.05$; ## Vs NC $p < 0.01$; ### Vs NC $p < 0.001$; * Vs MPP $p < 0.05$; ** Vs MPP $p < 0.01$; ^ Vs MPPLY $p < 0.05$; ^^ Vs MPPLY $p < 0.01$.

2.5. UF Effect on the Expression of Apoptosis Related Proteins

Figure 5 summarizes apoptosis-related proteins in the PI3K/AKT pathway. From our data we concluded that UF has a certain inhibitory effect on the expression of pro-apoptotic proteins Bax, P53 and GSK3β, and also has a certain promotion effect on the anti-apoptotic protein Bcl-2 (Figure 5a,b). The ratio of Bax/Bcl-2 was increased to 4.2 and 4.7-fold in MPP and MPPLY groups compared with NC group, respectively. UF treatment group decreased the ratio of Bax/Bcl-2 at a dose dependent manner. The ratio of Bax/Bcl-2 in UF3 group was lower than in the NC group. The ratio of Bax/Bcl-2 in UF3LY group was nearly the same as in the NC group. The level of mRNA expression following MPP$^+$ and UF treatment were examined by RT-PCR in order to confirm the protein changes in process of the cell apoptosis (Figure 5c,d). The PD model induced by MPP$^+$ increased the mRNA expression level of pro-apoptosis protein such as Bax, p53 and GSK3β, and decreased the mRNA expression level of anti-apoptosis protein Bcl-2. However, there was a marked decrease in the mRNA expression level of pro-apoptosis protein levels and increase in the mRNA expression level of anti-apoptosis protein levels in the UF-treated groups. We also found that the mRNA expression of the key apoptosis-related proteins Bax, P53 and GSK3β was consistently upregulated to 5.97 ± 0.15, 6.24 ± 0.44 and 7.63 ± 0.52, respectively, in cells treated with 100-μM MPP$^+$ and LY294002, whereas that of Bcl-2 was downregulated to 0.44 ± 0.07 of the control values. However, UF together with LY294002 treatment inhibited the up- or downregulation of Bax, P53, GSK3β and Bcl-2. Compared to the UF treated group, the up- or downregulation ability was weaker.

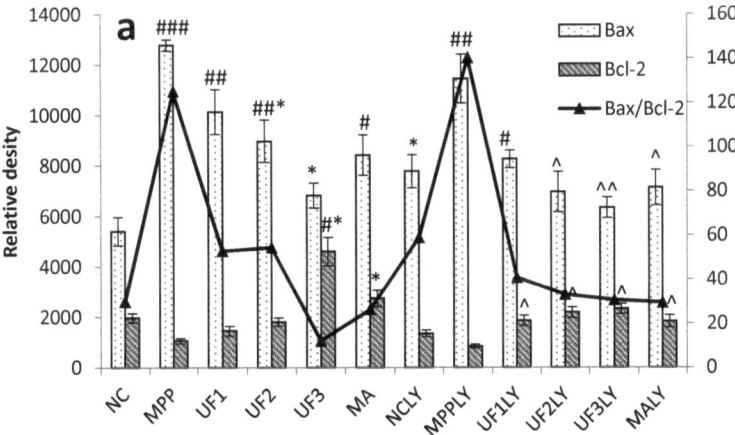

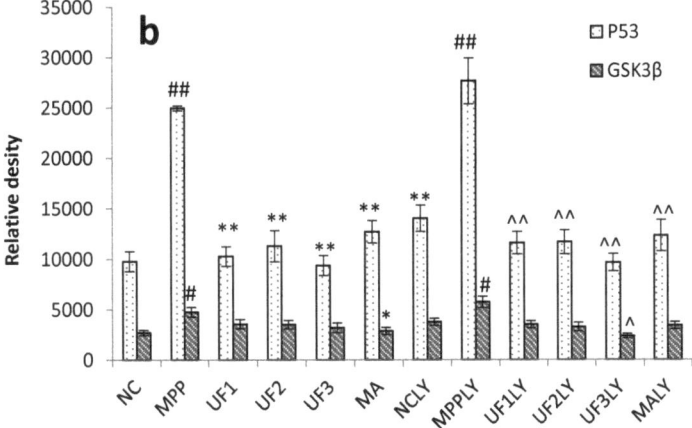

Figure 5. Cont.

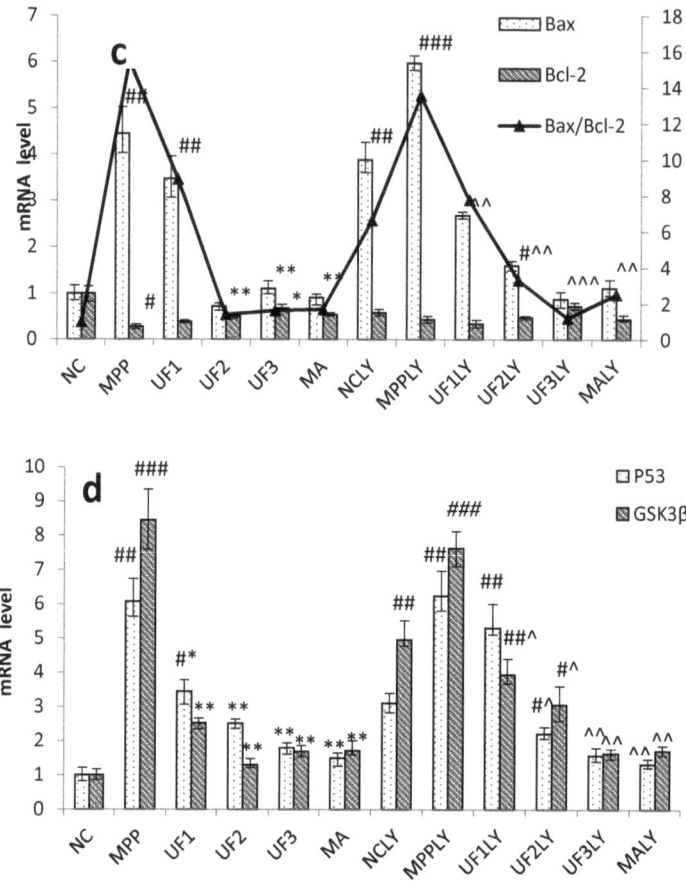

Figure 5. Protective effects of UF on MPP$^+$-induced SH-SY5Y cell of apoptosis relative protein. (**a**) protein expression of Bcl-2 and Bax by immunochemistry method; (**b**) protein expression of p53 and GSK3β by immunochemistry method; (**c**) mRNA expression of Bcl-2 and Bax by RT-PCR method; (**d**) mRNA expression of Bcl-2 and Bax by RT-PCR method $^{\#}$ Vs NC $p < 0.05$; $^{\#\#}$ Vs NC $p < 0.01$; $^{\#\#\#}$ Vs NC $p < 0.001$; * Vs MPP $p < 0.05$; ** Vs MPP $p < 0.01$; ^ Vs MPPLY $p < 0.05$; ^^ Vs MPPLY $p < 0.01$; ^^^ Vs MPPLY $p < 0.001$.

2.6. Caspase-3, -8 and -9 Activity

The treatment of cells with 100-μM MPP$^+$ significantly increased the relative activity of caspase-3 (cas3), caspase-8 (cas8) and caspase-9(cas9) to 0.73 ± 0.2, 2.90 ± 0.43 and 2.06 ± 0.18 of the NC group, respectively (Figure 6); however, this significantly decreased to 0.58 ± 0.13, 1.45 ± 0.32 and 1.16 ± 0.36 of the NC group, respectively, under UF treatment at 100 μg/mL. Moreover, the treatment of cells with 100-μM MPP$^+$ and 20-μM LY294002 significantly increased the relative activity of cas3, cas8 and cas9 to 3.21 ± 0.11 and 4.53 ± 0.56, 3.02 ± 0.27 of the NC group, respectively, which were much higher than MPP group; however, this significantly decreased to 0.94 ± 0.24, 0.84 ± 0.35 and 0.73 ± 0.18 of the control group, respectively, when treated with UF at 800-μg/mL and 20-μM LY294002. These results showed that UF treatment could promote the activity of caspase-3, caspase-8 and caspase-9 did not inhibited by LY294002.

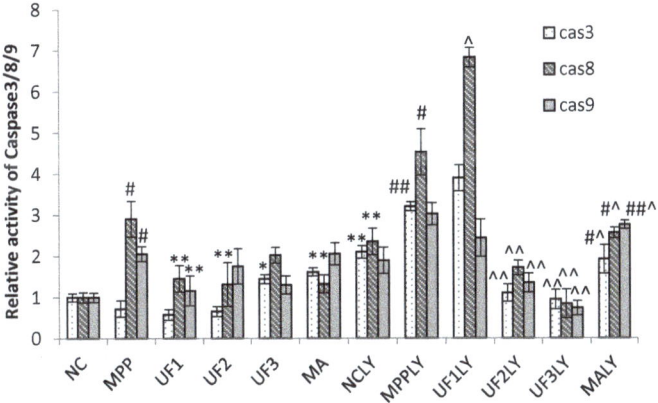

Figure 6. Protective effects of UF on MPP$^+$-induced SH-SY5Y cell of relative activity of caspase-3, caspase-8 and caspase-9. $^\#$ Vs NC $p < 0.1$; $^{\#\#}$ Vs NC $p < 0.01$; * Vs MPP $p < 0.1$; ** Vs MPP $p < 0.01$; $^\wedge$ Vs MPPLY $p < 0.1$; $^{\wedge\wedge}$ Vs MPPLY $p < 0.01$.

3. Discussion

PD is a neurodegenerative disease caused by both genetic and environmental factors. Neuroprotection therapeutic method caused interest in recently. Previous study found fucoidan extracted from brown seaweeds had neuron protective activity which related to its antioxidant activity [15]. Further studies found different fractions of fucoidan exhibited variety neuron protective activities. One fraction UF with higher uronic acid, lower sulfated group content and more complex monosaccharides exhibited the strongest activity. The neuron protective effect of UF may be mediated, in part, through antioxidant activity and the prevention of cell apoptosis [18]. The simplified depiction effect of UF on MPP$^+$-induced cytotoxicity was summarized in Figure 7. UF treatment groups could decrease the cell apoptosis rate and increase the cell vitality. LY294002 could inactivate the PI3K–Akt pathway, thereby inhibiting cell proliferation and inducing apoptosis. The results found that the neuron protective effect of UF was alleviated when treated with LY294002. It is illustrated that the neuron protective effect of UF may relate with the PI3K–Akt pathway.

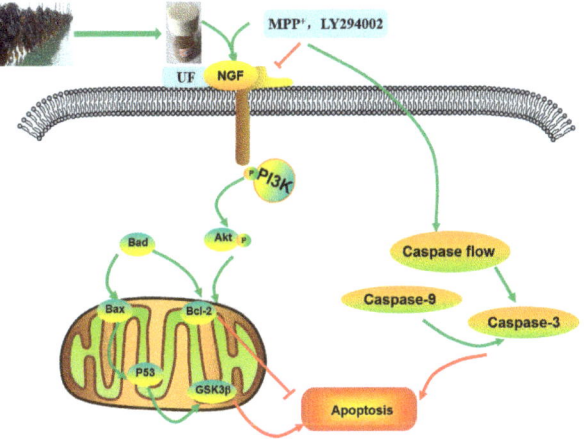

Figure 7. Effect of UF on MPP$^+$-induced SH-SY5Y cells apoptosis.

The PI3K–Akt pathway plays an important role in the survival and maintenance of many neuronal function such as long-term potentiation and memory formation. Inhibition of PI3K activity can offset the ability of nerve growth factors to promote cell survival [8]. Chondroitin sulfate (CS) in the cell matrix can protect SH-SY5Y cells by activating the PI3K–Akt signaling pathway [6]. Nerve growth factor (NGF) is a peptide molecule that plays a nutritional role in nerve cells. In the nervous system, NGF can increase the tolerance of cells under oxidative stress, which is the main mechanism involves NGF-induced activation of the PI3K–Akt pathway. Studies have shown that the application of corresponding treatments after spinal cord ischemia can induce NGF to activate the PI3K–Akt pathway to inhibit neuronal apoptosis [20]. Seow et al. found crude polysaccharides extracted from *Lignosus rhinocerotis* could stimulate neurogenesis without stimulating the production of NGF in PC-12 cells [21]. We found UF had a backbone of alternating 4-linked GlcA and 2-linked Man with the first Man residue from the nonreducing end accidentally sulfated at C6. UF and CS both have GluA and sulfate group, so we suppose UF could combine with NGF and increase the expression of the NGF, then activation the PI3K–Akt pathway. Our study confirmed that UF treatment could increase the expression of NGF, the effect was alleviated when added LY294002, but not disappeared completely. From our data, we suppose UF exhibited protective effect against MPP^+-induced SH-SY5Y cell apoptosis by activating PI3K–Akt pathway through reacting with NGF. The chemical composition and structure of the polysaccharide had relationship with the effect on the NGF, chondroitin sulfate and fucoidan could increase the expression of the NGF protein, however, polysaccharide extracted from *Lignosus rhinocerotis* mimics the neurogenic activity of NGF.

PI3K is one of the signal molecules involved in intracellular signal transduction. When cells are stimulated by stimulating factors such as NGF, the phosphorylation of PI3K is activated. The present results demonstrated that UF treatment could enhance the phosphorylation of PI3K first, and then promoted the phosphorylation of Akt. This effect was alleviated when combined with LY294002.

When phosphorylating the PI3K and Akt, it activates or inhibits its downstream target proteins Bad, Bcl-2, Bax, caspase-9, GSK-3, mTOR, nuclear transcription factors, etc., in turn regulate cell proliferation, differentiation, apoptosis and invasion [22]. The influence of UF on these anti-apoptotic and pro-apoptotic protein were analyzed. Our study showed that UF could partially inhibit MPP^+-induced dysfunction of the Bax/Bcl-2 system and decrease the expression of P53 and GSK3β protein, then inhibited cell apoptosis. This impact was alleviated when adding LY294002 in UF treated groups. As an anti-apoptotic member of the Bcl-2 family, Bcl-2 can bind Bax to form Bax/Bcl-2 heterodimers, thereby, attenuating the pro-apoptotic effect of Bax. Habaike et al. found polysaccharides extracted from *Laricifomes officinalis* Ames could attenuating cell apoptosis, increasing the ratio of Bcl-2/Bax and inhibiting cytochrome C release from mitochondria to cytosol in PC12 cells [23]. An acid-soluble polysaccharide (GFAP) prepared from *Grifola frondosa* could upregulate the expressions of Bax in HCC cells and induced the cell apoptosis [24]. The UF is a heteropolysaccharide with uronic acid and sulfate group, we suppose it can react with Bax and effect the formation of Bax/Bcl-2 heterodimers. P53 and GSK3β are thought to be a key factor in the subsequent apoptotic processes among the pro-apoptotic proteins. UF can react with these two proteins directly and reduce the cell apoptosis in the H_2O_2-reduced cell model [25].

Caspase family such as caspase-3 (cas3), caspase-8 (cas8) and caspase-9 (cas9) are crucial checkpoint in cell commitment to apoptosis. Cas3 is a critical executor of apoptosis being responsible for the proteolytic cleavage of many key proteins, which damage initiates the cell death program. Yu et al. found an acid-soluble polysaccharide could trigger apoptosis of HCC cells through mitochondria apoptotic pathway in a caspases-dependent pattern [24]. It means the acid polysaccharide could react with caspases-dependent pattern, it could decrease or increase the expression of caspase protein, which confirmed by our results. The addition of UF significantly attenuated the expression of cas3 in MPP^+-induced SH-SY5Y cells, confirming UF had effect in terms of apoptosis process. LY294002 used did not lead to a complete inhibition of initiation-programmed cell death by UF treated groups, suggesting that other pathways are also involved. Cas8 and cas9 have shown increase in MPP^+

and MPP$^+$+LY294002 groups simultaneously, UF treated groups could decrease this rising tendency. The observed changes may suggest that UF could significantly decrease cas3, cas8 and casp9 activation, the consequence of which is apoptosis.

Our study showed that UF treatment could reversed the toxic effect of MPP$^+$ on SH-SY5Y cells by activation the PI3K–Akt pathway. Addition of LY294002 significantly inhibited the PI3K–Akt pathway active and enhanced DNA fragmentation in SH-SY5Y cells, UF treated groups could still alleviate the cell apoptosis. In the present study, we demonstrated for the first time that UF attenuated the MPP$^+$ induced apoptosis via reacting with NGF, Bax and cas3. Our data indicated that UF inhibited cell apoptosis by participating in PI3K–Akt pathway partially.

4. Materials and Methods

4.1. Preparation of Sulfated Polysaccharides

Saccharina japonica (Laminariaceae), cultured along the coast of Dandong, China, was collected in August 2015, authenticated by Prof. Lanping Ding and stored as a voucher specimen (No. 83) in the Institute of Oceanology, CAS. The fresh algae were promptly washed, sun dried and kept in plastic bags at room temperature until use. FPS and UF were prepared according to our previous methods with minor modifications (Figure 8) [12,26]. Briefly, FPS was extracted in water solution at 120 °CC using autoclave from *Saccharina japonica*. DF was prepared using ascorbate and hydrogen peroxide (30 mmol/L, 1:1) degradation method. UF were obtained using DEAE-Sepharose FF exchange chromatography previously described.

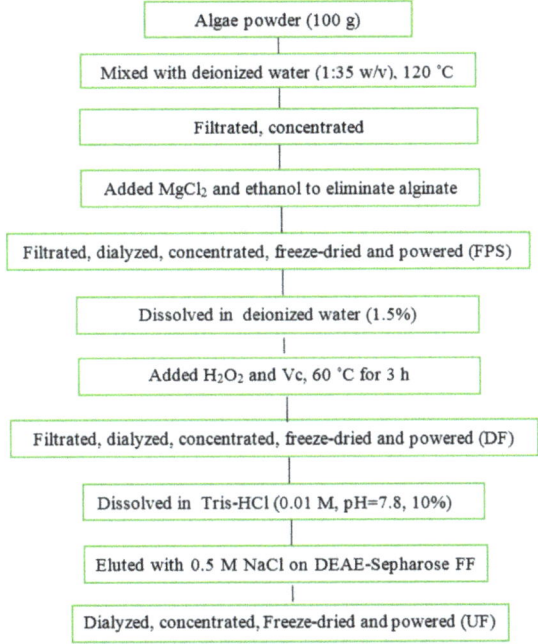

Figure 8. Flowchart of the extraction for UF.

4.2. Analytical Methods

The total sugar content of samples were determined according to the method of Dubois et al. using L-fucose as the standard [27]. The sulfate content was analyzed by ion chromatography using K_2SO_4 as the standard. Uronic acid was estimated via a modified carbazole method using D-glucuronic acid as the standard [28]. The neutral sugar composition was determined by PMP-HPLC precolumn derivatization chromatography using ribose as interior label [29]. The molecular weight was assayed by an HP-GPC chromatography using a series of dextrans with different molecular weights as standards. A series of dextrans were purchased from the National Institute for the Control of Pharmaceutical and Biologic Products (China). Other standard reagents were purchased from Sigma-Aldrich (Milwaukee, WI, USA).

4.3. Cell Culture and Treatments

A dopaminergic cell line SH-SY5Y was used to establish an in vitro PD model. SH-SY5Ycells were kindly provided by Professor Ning Song (QingDao University) and maintained in Dulbecco's modified Eagle medium/F12 supplemented with 10% newborn calf serum (Gibco) in an incubator with an atmosphere of 5% CO_2 at 37 °C. For all experiments, the cells were seeded on 96-well plates, 24-well plates or 6-well plates at a density of 1×10^4 cells–1×10^5 cells/mL for 24 h. Then the cells were incubated with MPP^+ for 30 min, then treated with different reagents for 24 h. The cells were divided into 12 groups. 1. NC group: treated with DMEM; 2: MPP group: treated with 100-μM MPP^+; 3. UF1 group: treated with 100-μM MPP^+ and 100-μg/mL UF; 4. UF2 group: treated with 100-μM MPP^+ and 500-μg/mL UF; 5. UF3 group: treated with 100-μM MPP^+ and 800-μg/mL UF; 6. MA group: treated with 100-μM MPP^+ and 100-mM positive drugs Modopar; 7. NCLY group: treated with DMEM and 20-μM LY294002; 8: MPPLY group: treated with 100-μM MPP^+ and 20-μM LY294002; 9. UF1LY group: treated with 100-μM MPP^+, 100-μg/mL UF and 20-μM LY294002; 10. UF2LY group: treated with 100-μM MPP^+, 500-μg/mL UF and 20-μM LY294002; 11. UF3LY group: treated with 100-μM MPP^+, 800-μg/mL UF and 20-μM LY294002; 12. MALY group: treated with 100-μM MPP^+, 100-mM positive drugs Modopar and 20-μM LY294002. All the group had six wells and all the experiments were repeated three times in different batches of cells.

4.4. Measurement of Cell Viability by MTT

SH-SY5Y cells were plated at a density of 1×10^4 cells/100 μL in 96-well plates. Cell viability was quantitatively assessed using the MTT ([3-(4,5-dimethyl-2-thiazolyl)-2,5-diphenyl tetrazolium bromide]) assay [9]. After 24 h treatment, 20 μL MTT (0.5 mg/mL) regent was added to each well and incubated at 37 °C for 4 h. The medium was removed and washed twice with phosphate buffer solution (pH 7.4), then 200 μL DMSO was added to solubilize the formazan crystals. Cell viability was measured at 494 nm by spectrophotometer (Bio-Tec Gen 5, Winooski, VT, USA). Unless stated otherwise, all other chemicals were purchased from Sigma-Aldrich.

4.5. Observation of Morphologic Changes

Cells were seeded in 24-well plates at a density of 1×10^5 for 24 h. After treatment for 24 h, cells were washed with phosphate-buffered saline and stained with 400 μL Hoechst 33,342 (2.5 μg/mL) for 5 min in the dark. After removing the medium and washed twice with phosphate buffer solution (pH 7.4), 400 μL PI (12.5 μg/mL) was added for 5 min in the dark. Cells with typical apoptotic nuclear morphology such as nuclear shrinkage and fragmentation and micronuclei formation were identified under fluorescent microscope and counted using randomly selected fields on numbered slides. The percentage of apoptotic cells was scored by counting at least 200 cells per treatment group and the average percentage of apoptotic cells was determined for each UF treatment and expressed as the mean ± SD.

4.6. Immunocytochemistry

Immunocytochemistry was performed and modified according to Iida's study. Briefly, SH-SY5Y cells were seeded in 12-wells plates and incubation with MPP^+ and different reagent for 24 h. After washing with PBS for three times and fixing with PBS containing 4% (wt/vol) paraformaldehyde for 15 min and then permeabilized with 0.5% (wt/vol) Triton X-100 and blocked with 5% goat serum for

1 h at room temperature. Subsequently, the cells were incubated with rabbit monoclonal anti-Akt (1:200), anti-PI3K (1:200), anti-Bax (1:100), anti-Bcl-2 (1:100), anti-GSK3β (1:200), anti-pPI3K (1:200), anti-p53 (1:100), anti-NGF (1:200), anti-pAkt (1:200) antibodies at 4 °C overnight. After washing with PBST and incubated with the second antibody (1:200) in PBST for 1 h. After the samples were washed with PBS three times, they were embedded in DAPI for 5 min and then washed with PBST 4 times. The images were obtained using an Olyba microscope. The mean fluorescence intensity was calculated by Image-Pro (Rockville, MD, USA).

4.7. Western Blot Analysis

Cells were lysed in lysis solution (Ambion, Grand Island, NY, USA) and incubated at 95 °C for 10 min. Protein concentration was determined by the Bradford assay kit (Takara Biotechnology, Dalian, China). Twenty micrograms of total proteins was separated by 10%–12% sodium dodecyl sulfate polyacrylamide gels and then transferred to polyvinylidene difluoride membranes. Blots were probed with rabbit monoclonal anti-Akt (1:1000), anti-pAkt (1:1000), anti-PI3K (1:1000), anti-pPI3K (1:1000). Blots were also probed with rabbit monoclonal anti-GAPDH antibody (Milwaukee, WI, USA, Sigma, 1:10,000) as a loading control. Anti-rabbit secondary antibodies conjugated to horseradish peroxidase were used at 1:10,000 (Santa Cruz Biotechnology, Santa Cruz, CA, USA). UVP BioSpectrum®CCD imaging system (Davis, CA, USA) was used for imaging and analysis. Camera settings were manipulated in preview mode to optimize the exposure and determine the appropriate final exposure settings. Exposures of 30 s up to 5 min were used for data collection. Results were analyzed through scanning densitometry by UVP Vision Works LS Software (UVP, Cambridge, UK).

4.8. Total RNA Extraction and Real Time PCR

SH-SY5Y Cells were seeded in 6-wells plates and incubation with MPP$^+$ and different reagent for 24 h. Total RNA was isolated by Trizol Reagent (Takara Biotechnology, Dalian, China) ccording to the manufacturer's instructions. From each sample, 1 μg of total RNA was retrotranscripted into cDNA (Takara RR047A, Dalian, China). Then, 2 μL of each sample was used as a template for amplification reactions conducted with the SYBR Premix Ex TaqTMII (Takara Biotechnology, Dalian, China) following the manufacturer's instructions. The PCR amplifications were conducted using a life Technology 7500 fast Real-time PCR system. The expression of house-keeping gene, GAPDH mRNA, was served as the standardized control. Primer (showed in Table 2) selection was performed using the Primer Premier Design Software, version 1.0 (Idaho Technology, Inc., Alameda, CA, USA). The mRNA level for the control group was set as 100%.

Table 2. Primers used for real-time RT-PCR.

Target Gene		Primer Sequences	Amplicon (bp)
Bax	FP	GGCGAATTGGACATGAAC	182
	RP	CCGAAGTAGGAGAGGAGG	
Bcl-2	FP	CCCCAGAAGAAACTGAACC	195
	RP	GCATCTCCTTGTCTACGC	
GSK3β	FP	ATTCCCTCAAATTAAGGCACCTCC	142
	RP	ATACTCCAGCAGACGGCTACACAG	
p53	FP	GGCGAATTGGAGATGAAC	156
	RP	CCGAAGTAGGAGAGGAGG	
GAPDH	FP	TTCACCACCATGGAGAAGGC	247
	RP	GGCATGGACTGTGGTCATGA	
NGF	FP	TCCAGGTGCATAGCGTAATG	195
	RP	CTCCGGTGAGTCCTGTTGAA	

4.9. Caspase-3, -8 and -9 Activity

After treatment of cells with UF for 24 h, the cells were harvested using cell scrapers and washed in ice-cold PBS. Then, the cells were lysed for 30 min on the ice in 100 µL of Cell Lysis Reagent supplemented with complete protease inhibitor cocktail. The protein concentration of cell lysates was determined by Bicinchoninic acid (BCA) assay (Takara Biotechnology, Dalian, China).

4.10. Statistical Analysis of Data

The data are presented as the mean values ± 1 SD (n = 8–10). The data were analyzed by a one-way ANOVA, a Duncan's multiple-range test and an LSD test at a significance level of $p < 0.05$. SPSS 22.0 software (New York, NY, USA) was used for the analysis.

5. Conclusions

Fucoidan is a kind of sulfated polysaccharide extracted from brown algae. UF is a heteropolysaccharide purified from fucoidan. In our previous study, we found UF had excellent neuron protective activity. However, the mechanism is still unknown. In our present study, we demonstrated that UF could act on the extracellular growth factor NGF and cause progressive activation of the PI3K–Akt pathway. Furthermore, this study provides further insight into the mechanisms of UF, including regulating downstream signaling molecules and proteins of the PI3K–Akt pathway and the a alleviate effect by adding LY294002, which means the neuron protective activity of UF was partly through PI3K–Akt pathway. These findings contribute to a better understanding of the critical roles of UF in treating PD and may elucidate the molecular mechanisms of UF effects in PD.

Author Contributions: Conceptualization, H.L.; formal analysis, N.W.; funding acquisition, J.W.; investigation, Jing Wang; methodology, H.L., L.G. and Y.Y.; project administration, Q.Z.; supervision, N.W. All authors have read and agreed to the published version of the manuscript.

Funding: This research was funded by the National Key research and Development Program of China (Grant No. 2018YFD0901104, 2019YFD0900705), Major Scientific & Engineering Projects of Innovation in Shandong Province (Grant No.2019JZZY010818), Shandong Provincial Natural Science Foundation (Grant No.ZR2019BD053), the Youth Innovation Promotion Association of CAS under Grant (No. 2016190), the Science and Technology project of Fujian Province (No. 2017T3015).

Acknowledgments: We thank the students Zhenzhen Deng and Yue Jin for their help with the experiment.

Conflicts of Interest: The authors declare no conflict of interest.

References

1. Mariani, S.; Ventriglia, M.; Simonelli, I.; Bucossi, S.; Siotto, M.; Donno, S.; Vernieri, F.; Squitti, R. Association between sex, systemic iron variation and probability of Parkinson's disease. *Int. J. Neurosci.* **2016**, *126*, 354–360. [CrossRef]
2. Sarrafchi, A.; Bahmani, M.; Shirzad, H.; Rafieian-Kopaei, M. Oxidative stress and Parkinson's disease: New hopes in treatment with herbal antioxidants. *Curr. Pharm. Des.* **2015**, *22*, 238–246. [CrossRef] [PubMed]
3. Naughton, C.; Moriarty, N.; Feehan, J.; O'Toole, D.; Dowd, E. Differential pattern of motor impairments in neurotoxic, environmental and inflammation-driven rat models of Parkinson's disease. *Behav. Brain Res.* **2016**, *296*, 451–458. [CrossRef] [PubMed]
4. Tatton, N.A.; Maclean-Fraser, A.; Tatton, W.G.; Perl, D.P.; Olanow, C.W. A fluorescent double-labeling method to detect and confirm apoptotic nuclei in Parkinson's disease. *Ann. Neurol.* **1998**, *44*, S142–S148. [CrossRef] [PubMed]
5. Tatton, W.G.; Chalmers-Redman, R.; Brown, D.; Tatton, N. Apoptosis in Parkinson's disease: Signals for neuronal degradation. *Ann. Neurol.* **2003**, *53*, S61–S70. [CrossRef] [PubMed]
6. Perier, C.; Bove, J.; Vila, M. Mitochondria and Programmed Cell Death in Parkinson's Disease: Apoptosis and Beyond. *Antioxid. Redox Signal.* **2012**, *16*, 883–895. [CrossRef]

7. Cheung, E.C.C.; Melanson-Drapeau, L.; Cregan, S.P.; Vanderluit, J.L.; Ferguson, K.L.; McIntosh, W.C.; Park, D.S.; Bennett, S.A.L.; Slack, R.S. Apoptosis-inducing factor is a key factor in neuronal cell death propagated by BAX-dependent and BAX-independent mechanisms. *J. Neurosci.* **2005**, *25*, 1324–1334. [CrossRef]
8. Yao, R.; Cooper, G.M. Requirement for phosphatidylinositol-3 kinase in the prevention of apoptosis by nerve growth factor. *Science* **1995**, *267*, 2003–2006. [CrossRef]
9. Abarikwu, S.O.; Farombi, E.O.; Pant, A.B. Biflavanone-kolaviron protects human dopaminergic SH-SY5Y cells against atrazine induced toxic insult. *Toxicol. In Vitro* **2011**, *25*, 848–858. [CrossRef]
10. Ale, M.T.; Mikkelsen, J.D.; Meyer, A.S. Important Determinants for Fucoidan Bioactivity: A Critical Review of Structure-Function Relations and Extraction Methods for Fucose-Containing Sulfated Polysaccharides from Brown Seaweeds. *Mar. Drugs* **2011**, *9*, 2106–2130. [CrossRef]
11. Wijesinghe, W.A.; Jeon, Y.-J. Biological activities and potential industrial applications of fucose rich sulfated polysaccharides and fucoidans isolated from brown seaweeds: A review. *Carbohydr. Polym.* **2012**, *88*, 13–20. [CrossRef]
12. Wang, J.; Zhang, Q.; Zhang, Z.; Li, Z. Antioxidant activityof sulfated polysaccharide fractions extracted from Laminaria japonica. *Int. Biol. Macromol.* **2008**, *42*, 127–132. [CrossRef] [PubMed]
13. Liu, H.D.; Wang, J.; Zhang, Q.B.; Zhang, H. The effect of different substitute groups and molecular weights of fucoidan on neuroprotective and anticomplement activity. *Int. J. Biol. Macromol.* **2018**, *113*, 82–89. [CrossRef] [PubMed]
14. Cui, Y.Q.; Zhang, L.J.; Zhang, T.; Luo, D.Z.; Jia, Y.J.; Guo, Z.X.; Zhang, Q.B.; Wang, X.; Wang, X.M. Inhibitory effect of fucoidan on nitric oxide production in lipopolysaccharide-activated primary microglia. *Clin. Exp. Pharmacol. Physiol.* **2010**, *37*, 422–428. [CrossRef]
15. Luo, D.; Zhang, Q.; Wang, H.; Cui, Y.; Sun, Z.; Yang, J.; Zheng, Y.; Jia, J.; Yu, F.; Wang, X. Fucoidan protects against dopaminergic neuron death in vivo and in vitro. *Eur. J. Pharmacol.* **2009**, *617*, 33–40. [CrossRef]
16. Cui, Y.Q.; Jia, Y.J.; Zhang, T.; Zhang, Q.B.; Wang, X.M. Fucoidan Protects against Lipopolysaccharide-Induced Rat Neuronal Damage and Inhibits the Production of Proinflammatory Mediators in Primary Microglia. *Cns Neurosci. Ther.* **2012**, *18*, 827–833. [CrossRef]
17. Jin, W.; Wang, J.; Jiang, H.; Song, N.; Zhang, W.; Zhang, Q. The neuroprotective activities of heteropolysaccharides extracted from Saccharina japonica. *Carbohydr. Polym.* **2013**, *97*, 116–120. [CrossRef]
18. Wang, J.; Liu, H.; Jin, W.; Zhang, H.; Zhang, Q. Structure-activity relationship of sulfated hetero/galactofucan polysaccharides on dopaminergic neuron. *Int. J. Biol. Macromol.* **2016**, *82*, 878–883. [CrossRef]
19. Jin, W.; Wang, J.; Ren, S.; Song, N.; Zhang, Q. Structural Analysis of a Heteropolysaccharide from Saccharina japonica by Electrospray Mass Spectrometry in Tandem with Collision-Induced Dissociation Tandem Mass Spectrometry (ESI-CID-MS/MS). *Mar. Drugs* **2012**, *10*, 2138–2152. [CrossRef]
20. Patapoutian, A.; Reichardt, L.F. Trk receptors: Mediators of neurotrophin action. *Curr. Opin. Neurobiol.* **2001**, *11*, 272–280. [CrossRef]
21. Seow, S.L.S.; Eik, L.F.; Naidu, M.; David, P.; Wong, K.H.; Sabaratnam, V. Lignosus rhinocerotis (Cooke) Ryvarden mimics the neuritogenic activity of nerve growth factor via MEK/ERK1/2 signaling pathway in PC-12 cells. *Sci. Rep.* **2015**, *5*, 13. [CrossRef] [PubMed]
22. Manning, B.D.; Cantley, L.C. AKT/PKB Signaling: Navigating Downstream. *Cell* **2007**, *129*, 1261–1274. [CrossRef] [PubMed]
23. Habaike, A.; Yakufu, M.; Cong, Y.; Gahafu, Y.; Li, Z.; Abulizi, P. Neuroprotective effects of Fomes officinalis Ames polysaccharides on A beta(25-35)-induced cytotoxicity in PC12 cells through suppression of mitochondria-mediated apoptotic pathway. *Cytotechnology* **2020**. [CrossRef] [PubMed]
24. Yu, J.; Liu, C.; Ji, H.-Y.; Liu, A.-J. The caspases-dependent apoptosis of hepatoma cells induced by an acid-soluble polysaccharide from Grifola frondosa. *Int. J. Biol. Macromol.* **2020**, *159*, 364–372. [CrossRef]
25. Wang, J.; Liu, H.D.; Zhang, X.; Li, X.P.; Geng, L.H.; Zhang, H.; Zhang, Q.B. Sulfated Hetero-Polysaccharides Protect SH-SY5Y Cells from H2O2-Induced Apoptosis by Affecting the PI3K/Akt Signaling Pathway. *Mar. Drugs* **2017**, *15*, 110. [CrossRef]
26. Wang, J.; Wang, F.; Zhang, Q.; Zhang, Z.; Shi, X.; Li, P. Synsesized different derivatives of low molecular fucoidan extracted from Laminaria japonica and their potential antioxidant activity in vitro. *Int. J. Biol. Macromol.* **2009**, *44*, 379–384. [CrossRef]

27. Dubois, M.; Gilles, K.A.; Hamilton, J.K.; Rebers, P.T.; Smith, F. Colorimetric Method for Determination of Sugars and Related Substabces. *Anal. Chem.* **1956**, *28*, 350–357. [CrossRef]
28. Bitter, T.; Muir, H.M. A modified uronic acid carbazole reaction. *Anal. Biochem.* **1962**, *4*, 330–334. [CrossRef]
29. Honda, S.; Akao, E.; Suzuki, S.; Okuda, M.; Kakehi, K.; Nakamura, J. High-performance liquid chromatography of reducing carbohydrates as strongly ultraviolet-absorbing and electrochemically sensitive 1-phenyl-3-methyl5-pyrazolone derivatives. *Anal. Biochem.* **1989**, *180*, 351–357. [CrossRef]

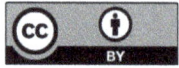

© 2020 by the authors. Licensee MDPI, Basel, Switzerland. This article is an open access article distributed under the terms and conditions of the Creative Commons Attribution (CC BY) license (http://creativecommons.org/licenses/by/4.0/).

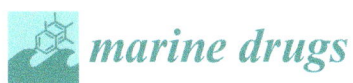

Article

Degradation of *Sargassum crassifolium* Fucoidan by Ascorbic Acid and Hydrogen Peroxide, and Compositional, Structural, and In Vitro Anti-Lung Cancer Analyses of the Degradation Products

Tien-Chiu Wu [1,†], Yong-Han Hong [2,†], Yung-Hsiang Tsai [3], Shu-Ling Hsieh [3], Ren-Han Huang [4], Chia-Hung Kuo [3,*] and Chun-Yung Huang [3,*]

[1] Division of General Internal Medicine, Department of Internal Medicine, Kaohsiung Medical University Hospital, Kaohsiung Medical University, No. 100, Tzyou 1st Rd., Sanmin District, Kaohsiung City 80708, Taiwan; 960552@ms.kmuh.org.tw
[2] Department of Nutrition, I-Shou University (Yanchao Campus), No. 8, Yida Rd., Jiaosu Village, Yanchao District, Kaohsiung City 82445, Taiwan; yonghan@isu.edu.tw
[3] Department of Seafood Science, National Kaohsiung University of Science and Technology, No. 142, Haijhuan Rd., Nanzih District, Kaohsiung City 81157, Taiwan; yht@nkust.edu.tw (Y.-H.T.); slhsieh@nkust.edu.tw (S.-L.H.)
[4] Department of Nursing, Mackay Medical College, No. 46, Sec. 3, Zhongzheng Rd., Sanzhi District, New Taipei City 25245, Taiwan; lisa68850@gmail.com
* Correspondence: kuoch@nkust.edu.tw (C.-H.K.); cyhuang@nkust.edu.tw (C.-Y.H.); Tel.: +886-7-3617141 (ext. 23646) (C.-H.K.); +886-7-3617141 (ext. 23606) (C.-Y.H.)
† These authors contributed equally to this work.

Received: 9 May 2020; Accepted: 24 June 2020; Published: 26 June 2020

Abstract: Fucoidans possess multiple biological functions including anti-cancer activity. Moreover, low-molecular-weight fucoidans are reported to possess more bioactivities than native fucoidans. In the present study, a native fucoidan (SC) was extracted from *Sargassum crassifolium* pretreated by single-screw extrusion, and three degraded fucoidans, namely, SCA (degradation of SC by ascorbic acid), SCH (degradation of SC by hydrogen peroxide), and SCAH (degradation of SC by ascorbic acid + hydrogen peroxide), were produced. The extrusion pretreatment can increase the extraction yield of fucoidan by approximately 4.2-fold as compared to the non-extruded sample. Among SC, SCA, SCH, and SCAH, the chemical compositions varied but structural features were similar. SC, SCA, SCH, and SCAH showed apoptotic effects on human lung carcinoma A-549 cells, as illustrated by loss of mitochondrial membrane potential (MMP), decreased B-cell leukemia-2 (Bcl-2) expression, increased cytochrome c release, increased active caspase-9 and -3, and increased late apoptosis of A-549 cells. In general, SCA was found to exhibit high cytotoxicity to A-549 cells and a strong ability to suppress Bcl-2 expression. SCA also showed high efficacy to induce cytochrome c release, activate caspase-9 and -3, and promote late apoptosis of A-549 cells. Therefore, our data suggest that SCA could have an adjuvant therapeutic potential in the treatment of lung cancer. Additionally, we explored that the Akt/mammalian target of rapamycin (mTOR) signaling pathway is involved in SC-, SCA-, SCH-, and SCAH-induced apoptosis of A-549 cells.

Keywords: ascorbic acid; anti-lung cancer; apoptosis; brown algae; fucoidan; human lung carcinoma A-549 cells; hydrogen peroxide; *Sargassum crassifolium*

1. Introduction

Lung cancer is one of the most commonly diagnosed cancers and is also one of the most deadly forms of cancer worldwide [1]. It is reported that 80% of lung cancers belong to the non-small-cell lung cancer (NSCLC) subtype that can be further divided into two classes: (1) lung adenocarcinoma (LUAD; 50%) and (2) lung squamous cell carcinoma (LUSC; 30%) [2,3]. In Taiwan, lung cancer is currently the most prevalent and most frequent cause of cancer-related mortality [4]. As such, it is crucial to develop novel agents and identify novel targets for the therapeutic treatment of lung cancer in order to improve patient outcomes.

Previous investigations reported that many anti-cancer drugs have drawbacks, such as side effects and toxicity [5]. Thus, there is a need for safer anti-cancer agents, particularly ones that can be manufactured using readily available naturally derived ingredients that cause no or minimal side effects. In recent years, researchers increasingly turned their efforts toward natural bioactive compounds due to their possible therapeutic activity in cancer at non-toxic levels [6]. Fucoidan is a water-soluble fucose-containing sulfated polysaccharide that is most commonly isolated from brown algae [7], and its α-L-fucose-enriched backbone also contains other monosaccharides, including glucose, xylose, galactose, and mannose [8]. Fucoidan possesses remarkable biological functions, including antioxidant, antitumor, anti-inflammatory, immunoregulatory, and antithrombotic activities [9]. These biological activities vary according to differences in the degree of sulfation, sulfation pattern, glycosidic branches, and molecular weight (MW) of fucoidan [9]. Low-molecular-weight (LMW) fucoidan is a highly sulfated fragment derived from fucoidan, and it received considerable attention due to its strong bioactivities with respect to anti-inflammatory, anticoagulant, antiangiogenic, antithrombosis, antioxidant, and anti-obesity effects [10,11]. In addition, LMW fucoidan is reported to be capable of modulating cell adhesion factor [12] and growth factor [13].

The process of extrusion comprises a short-duration, high-temperature bioreaction that involves mixing, heating, shearing, pressurizing, and shaping. During extrusion, the raw materials undergo mechanical shearing at high temperature with a very low moisture content and, thus, the properties of the extruded products, such as texture, microstructure, color, and flavor, are extensively modified [14]. Extrusion cooking provides numerous advantages, such as easy operation, continuous production, low manpower, high production yield, minimal waste, and a diversity of products [15]. Extruders are traditionally used to produce a wide variety of commonly consumed snacks, including corn curls, breadsticks, flatbreads, extruded corn ball, extruded puffed rice cereals, croutons, and breakfast cereals. Extrusion technology is also widely employed in the production of non-snack food products and other applications, such as biomass processing, and in the chemical, polymer, and energy industries [16]. Previous investigations indicated that extrusion can be successfully employed for the pretreatment of rice straw, which involves accelerating the saccharification of rice straw by enzymatic hydrolysis [17]. Fish scale is a good source for extraction of gelatin (a denatured form of collagen). However, it is known that fish scale is composed of collagen and hydroxyapatite, which are tightly linked together and difficult to separate. Extrusion was also adopted to pretreat fish scale to facilitate the separation of collagen and hydroxyapatite [15,18]. Soybean dregs can be pretreated by extrusion to decrease the quantity of insoluble dietary fiber (IDF) and increase soluble dietary fiber (SDF) in soybean residues [19]. Similarly, extrusion can be applied in the pretreatment of orange pomace to redistribute the IDF to SDF and to obtain a greater amount of soluble dietary fiber [20]. Moreover, the saccharification effect of lignocellulose can be improved by subjecting lignocellulosic biomass to bioextrusion pretreatment [21]. Therefore, we were interested in determining whether extrusion could be used to pretreat brown seaweeds in order to disrupt the natural anti-degradation barriers of seaweeds and enhance the release of polysaccharide from seaweed by water extraction alone. In the present study, we extracted fucoidan from *Sargassum crassifolium* pretreated by single-screw extrusion. The extracted fucoidan (native fucoidan, namely, SC) was then treated with different combinations of ascorbic acid (AA), hydrogen peroxide (H_2O_2), and AA + H_2O_2 to obtain degraded fucoidans. The composition, structure, and in vitro anti-lung cancer activity of native and degraded fucoidans were evaluated. This paper presents, for the first time to the authors' knowledge, the in vitro anti-lung cancer activity of native and degraded fucoidans prepared from *S. crassifolium* pretreated by single-screw extrusion. In addition, we attempted to elucidate the underlying mechanisms involved in the fucoidan-induced lung cancer cell death. The result of this study may help to inform future research into the possible applications of degraded fucoidans as natural chemopreventive agents for the adjuvant treatment of cancer, especially lung cancer.

2. Results and Discussion

2.1. Preparation of Native and Degraded Fucoidans from S. crassifolium Pretreated by Single-Screw Extrusion

S. crassifolium consists of 0.98% lipid, 2.36% protein, 34.0% ash, and 62.7% carbohydrate (dry basis), according to previous research [22]. The predominant component in S. crassifolium is carbohydrate (more than 50%), which indicates that S. crassifolium is a good source for extraction of fucoidan. A single-screw extrusion process was used for pretreatment of brown algae before isolation of fucoidan. The extrusion parameters employed were raw material moisture content 35%, feed rate 10.4 kg/h, barrel temperature 115 °C, screw speed 360 rpm, and rounded die head with a diameter of 5 mm, and these parameters were developed previously by our laboratory [15] with minor modification. After extrusion, the algal extrudate was extracted using hot water (85 °C) for 1 h with shaking. Following the removal of alginic acid, the fucoidan extracts were precipitated by 50% ethanol and recovered by centrifugation using the method developed previously by our laboratory [23], and then the native fucoidan (namely, SC) was obtained. The extraction yields of fucoidans from non-extruded and single-screw-extruded S. crassifolium were 2.69 ± 0.97 and 11.3 ± 1.3 g/100 g, dry basis, respectively. These data indicate that the extrusion process augments the extraction yield of fucoidan by 4.2-fold (11.3/2.69 = 4.2), as compared to non-extruded sample. The extrusion process would, therefore, certainly provide a higher production rate and lower production cost in the commercial manufacture of fucoidan. The results of a similar experiment conducted by the authors suggested that the extrusion process also increases the extraction yield of gelatin from fish scale by a maximal value of 3.3-fold with 50 °C water extraction [15]. SC was, thus, utilized for further degradation experiments using different degradation reagent combinations including AA, H_2O_2, and AA + H_2O_2. Then, three degraded fucoidans, namely, SCA (degraded by AA), SCH (degraded by H_2O_2), and SCAH (degraded by AA + H_2O_2), were obtained. The native and degraded fucoidans were subsequently subjected to physicochemical, compositional, structural, and in vitro anti-lung cancer analyses.

2.2. Compositional and Physicochemical Analyses of Native and Degraded Fucoidans

Zhang and his coworkers utilized AA, H_2O_2, or a combination of AA + H_2O_2 to degrade raw polysaccharide from *Enteromorpha linza*, and they successfully obtained its lower-molecular-weight fractions [24]. In the present study, we followed the methods of Zhang et al. [24] to degrade SC with minor modification. The SC was degraded by 10 mM AA, 10 mM H_2O_2, or a mixed solution of 10 mM H_2O_2 and 10 mM AA for 16 h, respectively, and three degradation derivatives, namely, SCA, SCH, and SCAH, were obtained. To examine whether the degradation reagents could successfully degrade fucoidan, the intrinsic viscosities and molecular weights of native and degraded fucoidans were analyzed. Previous investigations suggested that the degradation of fucoidan solution resulted in a decline of its intrinsic viscosity [10,24]. As shown in Table 1, the viscosities of SC, SCA, SCH, and SCAH were 113.9% ± 2.4%, 78.6% ± 4.2%, 102.5% ± 0.9%, and 36.9% ± 2.6%, respectively, indicating that all degrading reagents could successfully degrade SC. Moreover, among SCA, SCH, and SCAH, SCAH had the lowest viscosity value, which suggests that the combination of AA and H_2O_2 may degrade SC more efficiently. High-performance liquid chromatography (HPLC) gel filtration is a powerful research tool that is used to accurately characterize the molecular weight distribution of polysaccharides [23]. Here, we applied an HPLC gel filtration method to analyze the molecular weight distributions of SC, SCA, SCH, and SCAH, as shown in Table 1. The results showed that the peak molecular weight (molecular weight of the highest peak) for SC was 427.8 kDa (the peak was in the molecular weight range of 188.7–1064 kDa) (peak area = 100.0%), while that for SCA was 455.1 kDa (the peak was in the molecular weight range of 216.2–898.9 kDa) (peak area = 50.3%) and 3.06 kDa (the peak was in the molecular weight range of 1.65–9.95 kDa) (peak area = 49.7%), that for SCH was 427.8 kDa (the peak was in the molecular weight range of 194.3–998.1 kDa) (peak area = 61.0%) and 3.14 kDa (the peak was in the molecular weight range of 1.90–15.54 kDa) (peak area = 39.0%), and that for SCAH was 487.1 kDa (the peak was in the molecular weight range of 264.5–956.4 kDa) (peak area = 49.2%) and 3.11 kDa (the peak was in the molecular weight range of 1.66–12.55 kDa) (peak area = 50.8%). When examining the molecular weight intervals of peak 2 (Table 1) of the three degraded fucoidans, it was found that SCA (1.65–9.95 kDa) possessed the lowest molecular weight, followed by SCAH (1.66–12.55 kDa), and then SCH (1.90–15.54 kDa). Moreover, it was also found that SCAH had the highest amount of low-molecular-weight fraction (50.8%), followed by SCA (49.7%), and then SCH (39.0%). However, the difference between SCAH and SCA is not obvious. These data show that SCA, SCH, and SCAH were partially degraded, with a high-molecular-weight fraction (peak molecular weight approximately 427.8–487.1 kDa) and a low-molecular-weight fraction (peak molecular weight approximately 3.06–3.14 kDa) coexisting in SCA, SCH, and SCAH. In this case, it was also found that 10 mM AA, 10 mM H_2O_2, or a mixed solution of 10 mM H_2O_2 and 10 mM AA could only partially degrade SC. For SCA, SCH, and SCAH, the separation of high-molecular-weight and low-molecular-weight fractions is feasible. However, the separation process is complicated, time-consuming, and costly, which might be detrimental for future commercialized applications. In addition, previous studies suggested that high-molecular-weight fucoidans (molecular weight approximately 735–750 kDa) exhibited good pharmacokinetic and tissue distribution after in vivo oral and topical applications [25,26]. Therefore, these degraded fucoidans (SCA, SCH, and SCAH) were directly utilized for further experiments. Since the molecular weight compositions of SC, SCA, SCH, and SCAH are varied, the biological functions, such as the anti-cancer activity of these fucoidans, warrant further investigation. Previous studies suggested that polyphenols are usually coextracted with fucoidans [23]. We also found that the coextracted polyphenols in SCA, SAH, and SCAH were diminished as compared to that of SC (Table 1), indicating that the polyphenols were also partially degraded by these degradation reagents. Previous studies revealed that continuous addition of H_2O_2 during the degradation reaction facilitates the generation of lower-molecular-weight products [27]. Thus, further elucidation of degradation reagents and degradation methods which can thoroughly degrade SC is needed. Previous studies revealed that the bioactive properties of fucoidan may vary depending on the molecular weight, sulfate content, sugar type, and monosaccharide composition [28–30]. Here, we analyzed the chemical and monosaccharide compositions of SC, SCA, SCH, and SCAH. The data depicted in Table 1 suggest that the total sugar contents of SCA, SCH, and SCAH ranged from 30.83% ± 0.21% to 41.70% ± 0.91% (w/w, dry basis), which were lower than that of SC (45.58% ± 0.80%). This observation was consistent with data reported by Hou et al. [31], which suggested that the total sugar content of fucoidan decreased with the reduction in molecular weight of fucoidan after degradation by hydrogen peroxide. A possible reason for this phenomenon may be the destruction of the sugar unit under the degradation process [31]. L-Fucose was found to be the predominant sugar unit in fucoidan, and the content of fucose may have a role in biological functions [32,33]. In addition, previous studies suggested that monosaccharides, such as L-fucose, have anticancer potential. It is documented that deficient fucosylation may play an important role in the pathogenesis of cancer. The supplementation of L-fucose could restore fucosylation in both in vitro and in vivo conditions and could alleviate cancer symptoms [34]. The fucose contents of SC, SCA, SCH, and SCAH were 27.31% ± 1.59%, 35.22% ± 2.79%, 20.08% ± 1.68%, and 30.08% ± 3.11%, respectively. Previous studies suggested that the fucose content of fucoidan increased with the reduction in molecular weight of fucoidan after degradation by hydrogen peroxide and ascorbic acid [35]. However, another report revealed that the fucose content of fucoidan decreased with the reduction in molecular weight of fucoidan after degradation by hydrogen peroxide [31]. Therefore, the precise effects of degradation conditions on the fucose content of fucoidan remain to be elucidated. In general, our data suggest that SCA had the highest fucose content. Thus, their anticancer potential, especially that of SCA, warrants further study. The presence of sulfate in fucoidan may be related to its biological functions [36,37]. We, thus, measured the sulfate contents of SC, SCA, SCH, and SCAH, and the percentages were 18.64% ± 1.43%, 13.67% ± 2.19%, 19.23% ± 0.83%, and 20.39% ± 3.28%, respectively. Our data suggest that the sulfate contents seem to be unrelated to the degradation treatments. These data are in line with previous reports suggesting that there is no relationship between the sulfate content of fucoidan and the reduction in molecular weight of fucoidan after degradation by hydrogen peroxide + ascorbic acid or hydrogen peroxide [24,31]. The monosaccharide compositions of the fucoidans were analyzed, and the data are presented in Table 1. For SC, fucose, galactose, glucuronic acid, and galacturonic acid were the major neutral sugar constituents, and the minor sugar units were mannose and xylose. After degradation, the amounts of glucuronic acid and galacturonic acid in degraded fucoidans seemed to have decreased. In summary, intrinsic viscosity and molecular weight analyses showed that all of the tested degradation reagents could degrade SC. The native and degraded fucoidans contained different amounts of total sugar, fucose, and sulfate, and they had dissimilar monosaccharide compositions. Since differences in physicochemical characteristics among SC, SCA, SCH, and SCAH were found, the biological functions of these fucoidan extracts warrant further investigation.

Table 1. Viscosity, molecular weight, and composition analyses of *Sargassum crassifolium* fucoidan (SC) and that degraded by ascorbic acid (SCA), hydrogen peroxide (SCH), and their combination (SCAH).

Viscosity	SC [3]	SCA [3]	SCH [3]	SCAH [3]
Intrinsic viscosity (mL/g)	113.9 ± 2.4 [d]	78.6 ± 4.2 [b]	102.5 ± 0.9 [c]	36.9 ± 2.6 [a]
Molecular Weight (MW)	SC	SCA	SCH	SCAH
Peak 1 (Peak MW [1] (kDa))	427.8	455.1	427.8	487.1
Peak 1 (MW interval (kDa))	188.7–1064	216.2–898.9	194.3–998.1	264.5–956.4
Peak 1 (Peak area (%))	100.0	50.3	61.0	49.2
Peak 2 (Peak MW (kDa))	ND [4]	3.06	3.14	3.11
Peak 2 (MW interval (kDa))	ND	1.65–9.95	1.90–15.54	1.66–12.55
Peak 2 (Peak area (%))	ND	49.7	39.0	50.8
Chemical Composition	SC	SCA	SCH	SCAH
Total sugar (%) [2]	45.58 ± 0.80 [d]	41.70 ± 0.91 [c]	30.83 ± 0.21 [a]	33.83 ± 0.71 [b]
Fucose (%) [2]	27.31 ± 1.59 [b]	35.22 ± 2.79 [c]	20.08 ± 1.68 [a]	30.08 ± 3.11 [b]
Sulfate (%) [2]	18.64 ± 1.43 [b]	13.67 ± 2.19 [a]	19.23 ± 0.83 [b]	20.39 ± 3.28 [b]
Polyphenols (%) [2]	1.85 ± 0.07 [c]	1.29 ± 0.02 [b]	1.17 ± 0.02 [a]	1.12 ± 0.01 [a]
Monosaccharide Composition (Molar Ratio)	SC	SCA	SCH	SCAH
Fucose	1	1	1	1
Galactose	0.24	0.30	0.27	0.28
Glucuronic acid	0.19	0.01	0.07	0.03
Galacturonic acid	0.15	0.11	0.06	0.05
Mannose	0.08	0.05	0.07	0.06
Xylose	0.04	0.05	0.10	0.02

[1] Peak MW: molecular weight of the highest peak. [2] Total sugars (%), fucose (%), sulfate (%), and polyphenols (%) = (g/g, dry basis) × 100. [3] Experiments were performed in triplicate; values in the same row with varying letters (in [a], [b], [c], and [d]) differ ($p < 0.05$). [4] ND: not detected.

2.3. Structural Analyses of Native and Degraded Fucoidans

Fourier-transform infrared (FTIR) and nuclear magnetic resonance (NMR) spectroscopy techniques were utilized to characterize the structures of native and degraded fucoidans. The FTIR spectra of SC, SCA, SCH, and SCAH within the range of 4000–400 cm^{-1} are depicted in Figure 1. IR bands at 3401, 2940, 1230, and 1055 cm^{-1} are due to the presence of OH and H_2O stretching vibration, mainly by C–H stretching of the pyranoid ring or the C-6 group of fucose and galactose units, the S=O stretching of sulfates, and the C–O–C stretching vibrations in rings or C–O–H in the glucosidal bond [38,39]. Strong absorption bands were observed at 1621 and 1421 cm^{-1}, which can be attributed to scissoring vibration of H_2O and in-plane ring CCH, COH, and OCH vibrations, characterized by the absorption of polysaccharide [38–40]. The absorption bands at 900 and 837 cm^{-1} can be attributed to the presence of

C1–H bending in the β-anomeric link (probably galactose) and equatorial C–O–S bending vibration of sulfate substituents at the axial C-4 position [41]. The bands near 620 and 580 cm^{-1} could be assigned to the symmetric and anti-symmetric O=S=O deformations [42]. Due to the resemblance of the FTIR spectra in SC, SCA, SCH, and SCAH, the structural aspects of these sulfated polysaccharides were not obviously altered by the degrading treatments. NMR spectroscopy is usually adopted to analyze polysaccharides with complex structures [43]. In this study, we utilized ^{1}H-NMR and ^{13}C-NMR spectra to examine the structural features of SC, SCA, SCH, and SCAH. The ^{1}H-NMR spectra (Figure S1A, Supplementary Materials) for SC, SCA, SCH, and SCAH revealed that the signals between 5.5 and 5.0 ppm corresponded to L-fucopyranosyl units [44], the signal at 4.46 ppm, which was obvious in SCA and SCAH, indicates H-2 of a 2-sulfated fucopyranose residue [44], and the signal arising from 4.13 ppm at 4[H] represents 3-linked α-L-fucose [40]. The signals with ppm of 4.07/3.95 (6[H]/6'[H]) correspond to a (1-6)-β-D-linked galacton [45]. The signals between 3.9 and 3.6 ppm may be due to the presence of mannitol [46,47], which is often coextracted with fucoidan. The signal at 3.78 ppm (3[H]) (most notably in SC) can be attributed to 4-linked β-D-galactose, whereas the signal at 3.72 ppm can be assigned to (4[H]) 2,3-linked α-β-mannose [40]. The signals between 2.21 and 2.14 ppm may be tentatively assigned to methyl protons in O-acetyls [40,48], which are often present in algal polysaccharides [48]. The signal obtained at 1.92 ppm (1[H]) signifies alkyl at a sulfonyl-attached proton, and 1.23 ppm (6[H]) indicates an alkane proton in two methyl groups [49]. Due to the similar structural features observed among SC, SCA, SCH, and SCAH (Figure S1, Supplementary Materials) by ^{1}H-NMR analysis, it appears that the structural characteristics of fucoidan were not evidently altered by the treatments with degrading reagents. The ^{13}C-NMR spectra (Figure S1B, Supplementary Materials) for SC, SCA, SCH, and SCAH revealed that the prominent signal at 101.6 ppm and peaks between 65 and 80 ppm correspond to (1-6)-β-D-linked galacton [45].The signal at 100.3 ppm can be assigned to (1,3)-linked α-L-fucopyranose residues [47]. The signals at 62.0 ppm 66.7 ppm were attributed to β-D-galactopyranose residues [50]. The signals at 19–20 ppm revealed the presence of O-acetyl groups [51]. Due to the similar structural features observed among SC, SCA, SCH, and SCAH (Figure S1B, Supplementary Materials) by ^{13}C-NMR analysis, it appears that the structural characteristics of fucoidan were not obviously altered by the treatments with degrading reagents. In summary, the FTIR, ^{1}H-NMR, and ^{13}C-NMR data provide evidence that SC, SCA, SCH, and SCAH possess characteristic structural features of fucoidan. As SCA, SCH, and SCAH are partially degraded derivatives of SC, these four compounds exhibited similar structural features. Therefore, in our case, the differences in bioactivities among SC, SCA, SCH, and SCAH may not be predominantly attributed to their structure since they share similar structural features.

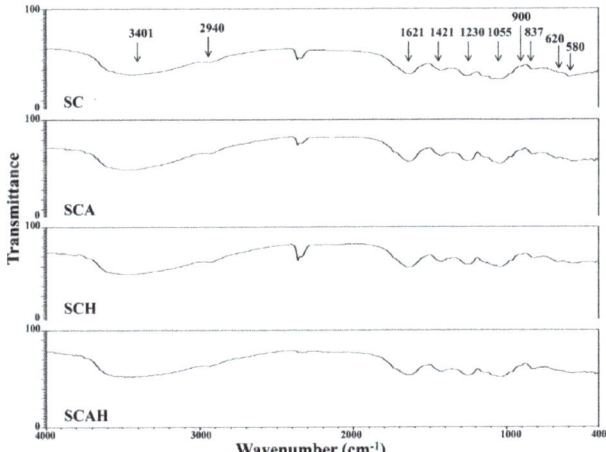

Figure 1. Fourier-transform infrared (FTIR) spectra for SC, SCA, SCH, and SCAH. The characteristic peaks are labeled.

2.4. SC, SCA, SCH, and SCAH Exhibited Cytotoxic Effects on A-549 Cells

The inhibition of cancer cell proliferation can be utilized to evaluate the potential anti-cancer ability of novel substances [33]. Here, we utilized an in vitro model (A-549 cells) to monitor the anti-lung cancer effects of the native and degraded fucoidans. In the preliminary experiments, A-549 cells were treated with 500 µg/mL of native and degraded fucoidans for 24, 48, or 72 h. It was found that a treatment time of 48 h was optimal for the induction of cytotoxicity in A-549 cells. For the purpose of ensuring consistency, the treatment time of cells was, thus, set to 48 h in all cellular experiments. As shown in Figure 2A, all fucoidans (SC, SCA, SCH, and SCAH) decreased the ratios of live A-549 cells, and SCA, SCH, and SCAH exhibited greater cytotoxic effects on A-549 cells than SC. Moreover, as shown in Figure 2B, among SCA, SCH, and SCAH, SCA showed cytotoxicity to A-549 cells with the lowest half maximal inhibitory concentration (IC_{50}) value, indicating that SCA exhibited the greatest cytotoxicity to A-549 cells. These results indicate that degraded fucoidans may have stronger inhibitory effects on A-549 cells as compared to native fucoidan. BEAS-2B is a non-cancerous bronchial epithelial cell line, which can be used to represent normal human lung cells [52]. Additionally, we conducted a similar experiment utilizing BEAS-2B cells in an effort to determine whether or not these fucoidans exerted toxic effects on normal cells. The results suggest that SC and SCH exhibited the greatest cytotoxicities to BEAS-2B cells, followed by SCAH, and the least cytotoxic was SCA (Figure 2C). In addition, it was found that, at the concentration of 200 µg/mL, A-549 cells showed survival rates of approximately 50.4–58.0% and BEAS-2B cells showed survival rates of approximately 73.8–94.1% following exposure to each of the fucoidan extracts. Therefore, a concentration of 200 µg/mL was chosen for all of the tested fucoidans, and a treatment duration of 48 h was used for further in vitro anti-lung cancer experiments. Interestingly, SCA was highly cytotoxic to A-549 cells (survival rate 53.8% ± 3.1%), but only had a weak cytotoxic effect on BEAS-2B cells (survival rate 94.1% ± 2.5%) at a dose of 200 µg/mL and a treatment duration of 48 h (Figure 2A,C), indicating that SCA may be a better anti-lung tumor candidate. Taken together, all of the tested fucoidan extracts exhibited growth suppression of A-549 cells. SCA was shown to be a better choice as an anti-lung cancer agent due to its strong cytotoxic effect on A-549 cells and its low cytotoxic impact on normal lung cells.

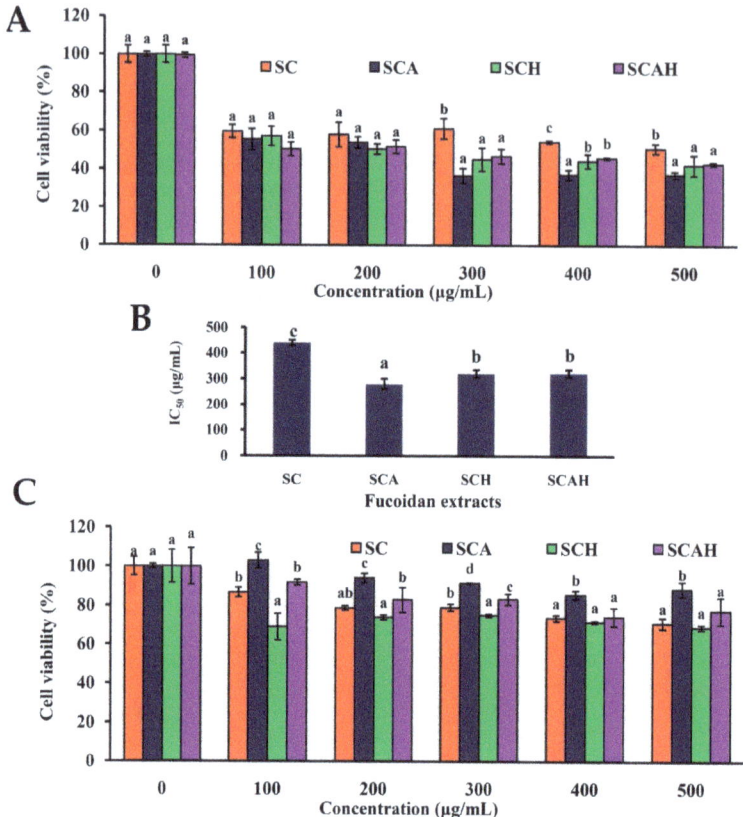

Figure 2. Effects of SC, SCA, SCH, and SCAH on cell viabilities of A-549 and BEAS-2B cells: (**A**) A-549 cells were co-incubated with various concentrations of SC, SCA, SCH, and SCAH for 48 h, and cell viability was assessed. Bars in the same treating concentration bearing different letters (in a, b, and c) significantly differ at the level of 0.05; (**B**) bar graphs show the half maximal inhibitory concentration (IC_{50}) values (the inhibitory concentrations at 50% growth of A-549 cells) of SC, SCA, SCH, and SCAH as determined for (**A**). Bars bearing different letters (in a, b, and c) significantly differ at the level of 0.05; (**C**) BEAS-2B cells were co-incubated with various concentrations of SC, SCA, SCH, and SCAH for 48 h, and the cell survival was evaluated. Bars in the same treating concentration bearing different letters (in a, b, c, and d) significantly differ at the level of 0.05. Experiments were repeated three times.

2.5. SC, SCA, SCH, and SCAH Decreased Mitochondrial Membrane Potential (MMP) in A-549 Cells

Two fundamental pathways, namely, the intrinsic pathway (the mitochondria pathway) and the extrinsic pathway (death receptor pathway), are involved in cellular apoptosis [53]. The intrinsic pathway operates several processes involving the loss of mitochondrial membrane potential (MMP), release of cytochrome c, and formation of an apoptotic complex in which caspase-9 and caspase-3 are activated [54]. Mitochondrial dysfunction is suggested to play a central role in the mitochondria-dependent apoptotic pathway. Generally, loss of MMP can be regarded as an early event in the apoptotic process [55]. Thus, we evaluated the effects of SC, SCA, SCH, and SCAH on the MMP of A-549 cells. A potentiometric fluorescent tetramethylrhodamine ethyl ester (TMRE) dye, which is a cell-permeable, positively charged dye, can stably accumulate in active mitochondria due to their relatively negative charge. The loss of MMP may result in a decline of TMRE accumulation in mitochondria [22]. A statistically significant reduction in MMP was observed in A-549 cells following exposure to SCA, SCH, and SCAH at a dose of 200 µg/mL for 48 h, as compared to that of the untreated control (Figure 3). The greatest loss of MMP was induced by SCAH, followed by SCA and SCH, and SC had a similar effect on MMP as compared to the untreated control. These data indicate that degraded fucoidans (SCA, SCH, and SCAH) have a strong capability to induce loss of MMP in A-549 cells.

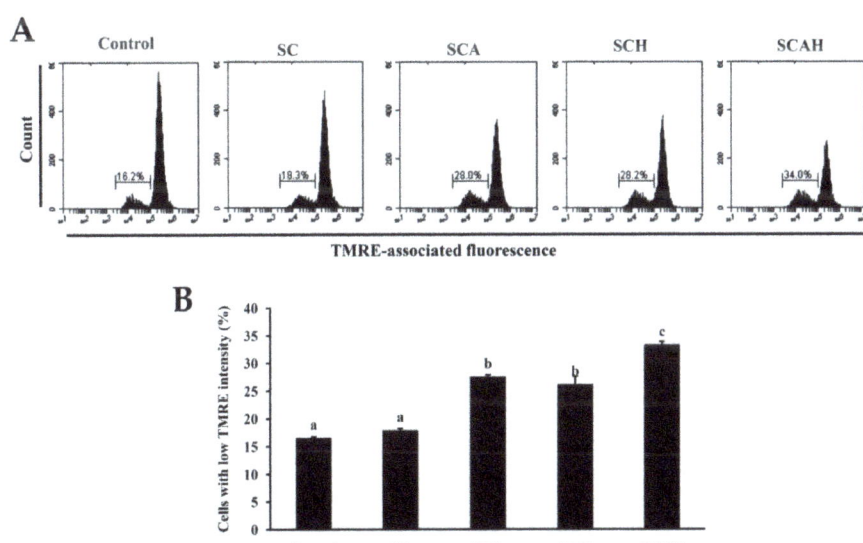

Figure 3. Effects of SC, SCA, SCH, and SCAH treatments on mitochondrial membrane potential (MMP) of A-549 cells. A-549 cells were treated without and with 200 µg/mL SC, SCA, SCH, and SCAH for 48 h, and MMP was determined by tetramethylrhodamine ethyl ester (TMRE) staining and flow cytometry: (**A**) histograms; (**B**) bar chart. Experiments were repeated three times. Bars bearing different letters (in a, b, and c) significantly differ at the level of 0.05.

2.6. SC, SCA, SCH, and SCAH Decreased B-cell leukemia-2 (Bcl-2) Expression of A-549 Cells

Bcl-2 belongs to the anti-apoptotic class of B-cell leukemia-2 (Bcl-2) gene product family proteins, and it is proposed to block MMP depolarization, which then retards the activation of various death effectors, such as release of cytochrome c, apoptosis-inducing factor (AIF), and Smac/Diablo [56]. In contrast, the suppression of Bcl-2 expression brings about cellular apoptosis. The effects of SC, SCA, SCH, and SCAH on Bcl-2 expression in A-549 cells were examined, and the data are shown in Figure 4. A statistically significant decrease in the level of Bcl-2 was observed in A-549 cells following exposure to SC, SCA, SCH, and SCAH at a dose of 200 µg/mL for 48 h as compared to the untreated control. Among the fucoidans tested, SCA and SCAH exhibited the greatest suppression of Bcl-2. In addition, the degraded fucoidans (SCA, SCH, and SCAH) appeared to have stronger activity in suppressing Bcl-2 expression in A-549 cells compared with SC.

2.7. SC, SCA, SCH, and SCAH Increase Cytochrome C Release of A-549 Cells

Previous investigations suggested that a decline in MMP results in matrix condensation and exposure of cytochrome c to the intermembrane space, which then facilitates cytochrome c release, resulting in apoptotic death [57]. Here, the effects of SC, SCA, SCH, and SCAH exposure on cytochrome c release in A-549 cells were examined, and the data are shown in Figure 5. A statistically significant decrease in the high fluorescence level of cytochrome c was observed in A-549 cells after exposure to SC, SCA, SCH, and SCAH at a dose of 200 µg/mL for 48 h as compared to the untreated control. Among the fucoidans tested, SCA and SCAH diminished cytochrome c to the greatest extent.

In addition, the degraded fucoidans (SCA, SCH, and SCAH) appeared to exhibit stronger activity in the augmentation of cytochrome c release in A-549 cells compared with SC.

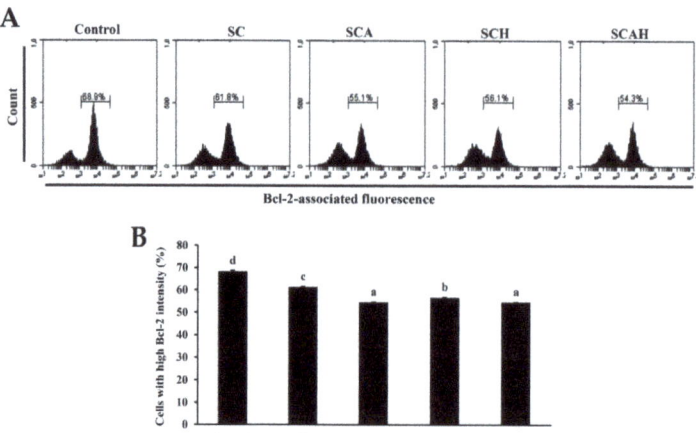

Figure 4. Effects of SC, SCA, SCH, and SCAH treatments on B-cell leukemia-2 (Bcl-2) expression in A-549 cells. A-549 cells were treated without and with 200 µg/mL SC, SCA, SCH, and SCAH for 48 h, and fluorescence histograms of immunolabeled Bcl-2 were determined by flow cytometry: (**A**) histograms; (**B**) bar chart. Experiments were repeated three times. Bars bearing different letters (in a, b, c, and d) significantly differ at the level of 0.05.

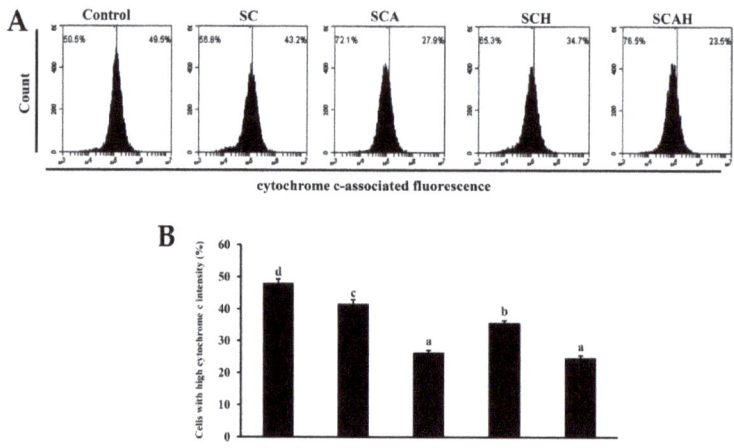

Figure 5. Effects of SC, SCA, SCH, and SCAH treatments on the amount of cytochrome c release in A-549 cells. A-549 cells were treated without and with 200 µg/mL SC, SCA, SCH, and SCAH for 48 h, and flow-cytometric profiles of immunolabeled cytochrome c were determined: (**A**) histograms; (**B**) bar chart. Experiments were repeated three times. Bars bearing different letters (in a, b, c, and d) significantly differ at the level of 0.05.

2.8. SC, SCA, SCH, and SCAH Increase Active Caspase-9 and -3 of A-549 Cells

In the mitochondrion-dependent pathway, the release of cytochrome c from the mitochondrial intermembrane space triggers the formation of an apoptosome, which induces the activation of caspase-9 and caspase-3 [58]. In the present study, the effects of SC, SCA, SCH, and SCAH on the activation of caspase-9 and -3 in A-549 cells were evaluated. The results shown in Figure 6 suggest that a statistically significant increase in the levels of active caspase-9 and -3 occurred in A-549 cells after exposure to SC, SCA, SCH, and SCAH at a dose of 200 µg/mL for 48 h as compared to the untreated control. Among the fucoidans tested, SCA exhibited the greatest effect on the upregulation of caspase-9, whereas SCAH induced the largest upregulation of caspase-3. In addition, the degraded fucoidans (SCA, SCH, and SCAH) showed stronger activity in terms of activation of caspase-9 and -3 in A-549 cells compared with SC.

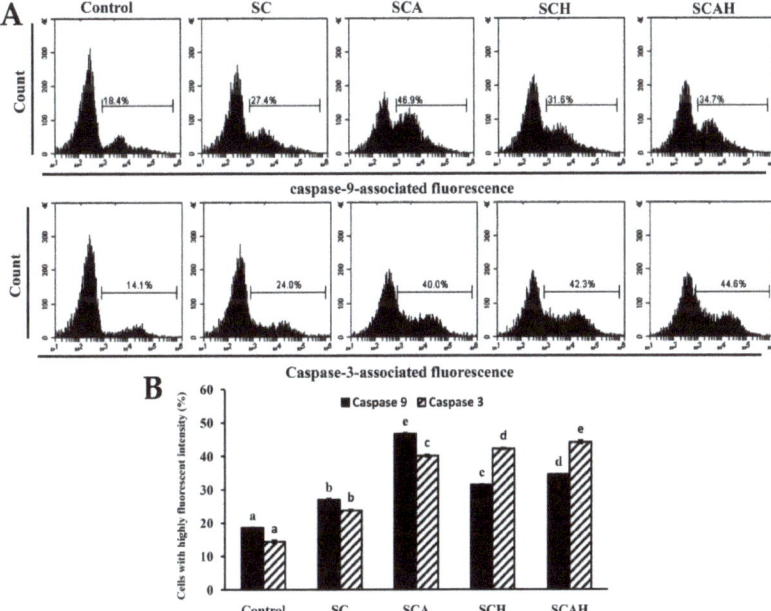

Figure 6. Effects of SC, SCA, SCH, and SCAH treatments on the activation of caspase-9 and -3 in A-549 cells. A-549 cells were treated without and with 200 µg/mL SC, SCA, SCH, and SCAH for 48 h, and the flow-cytometric profiles of immunolabeled caspase-9 and -3 were determined: (**A**) histograms; (**B**) bar chart. Bars in the same caspase-9 or caspase-3 group bearing different letters (in a, b, c, d, and e) significantly differ at the level of 0.05. Experiments were repeated three times.

2.9. SC, SCA, SCH, and SCAH Induce Apoptosis of A-549 Cells

Once caspase-3 is activated, the cells undergo late-stage apoptosis, and apoptotic cell death is inevitable [55]. To discriminate between early and late apoptosis of cells, a flow-cytometric based Annexin V/propidium iodide (PI) Cell Apoptosis kit was used to detect the apoptotic rate of cells after SC, SCA, SCH, and SCAH treatments. According to the data shown in Figure 7, late apoptosis of cells predominated in SC-, SCA-, SCH-, and SCAH-induced cell death. There were statistically significant increases from 14.0% ± 0.3% (control) to 40.0% ± 0.1% (SC), 45.9% ± 1.1% (SCA), 39.7% ± 1.2% (SCH), and 27.7% ± 0.8% (SCAH), in the percentages of late apoptotic cells, and significant reductions from 71.4% ± 0.6% (control) to 44.3% ± 0.9% (SC), 37.9% ± 0.5% (SCA), 39.1% ± 0.4% (SCH), and 55.2% ± 2.7% (SCAH), in the percentages of live cells. Among the degraded fucoidans, SCA induced the largest number of late apoptotic cells. In addition, the percentage of live cells in the non-treated control was 71.4% ± 0.6%, suggesting that A-549 cells alone also showed ongoing apoptotic and necrotic effects after 48 h of starvation. Further investigations regarding the optimal treatment conditions satisfying both the control and the experimental group are needed. The in vitro anti-lung cancer potential of fucoidan was examined previously by other investigators. A-549 cells were exposed to fucoidan extracted from *Padina distromatica* at 1000 µg/mL for 48 h and showed a survival rate of approximately 65.44% ± 1.35% [59]. Compared with *P. distromatica* fucoidan, the cytotoxic effect of SCA to A-549 cells was higher (treatment of A-549 cells at 300 µg/mL for 48 h resulted in a survival rate of 36.5% ± 3.9%, Figure 2A). In addition, the fucoidan extracted from *Turbinaria conoides* exhibited a survival rate of approximately 35% when used to treat A-549 cells at 250 µg/mL for 72 h [60]; therefore, in general, it also showed that the cytotoxic effect of SCA to A-549 cells was higher than *T. conoides* fucoidan, since the treating concentration was similar but the treatment duration of SCA was shorter (48 h) (Figure 2A). These data suggest that SCA may serve as a good anti-lung cancer candidate as compared to other reported data. Moreover, Boo et al. utilized commercialized *Undaria pinnatifida* fucoidan (obtained from Sigma) and determined that fucoidan induces apoptosis in A-549 cells via caspase-9 activation, cleavage of poly-ADP-ribose polymerase (PARP), and activation of extracellular signal-regulated kinases (ERK) 1/2, as well as downregulation of phospho-p38 and phospho- phosphatidylinositol 3-kinase (PI3K)/Akt expression [61]. In the present study, we utilized fucoidan from *S. crassifolium* and its degraded products, and we revealed that these fucoidan extracts showed apoptotic effects on A-549 cells via loss of MMP, decreased Bcl-2 expression, increased cytochrome c release, increased active caspase-9 and -3, and augmented late apoptosis of A-549 cells. These data provide evidence that fucoidan and its degraded products induced apoptosis of A-549 cells. Taken together, SC-, SCA-, SCH-, and SCAH-induced cell death was found to involve mitochondrial-dependent apoptosis as elucidated by the loss of MMP, decreased Bcl-2 expression, increased release of cytochrome c, increased activation of caspase-9 and -3, and increased late apoptosis of cells. Generally, degraded fucoidans had a more potent effect in terms of inducing apoptosis of A-549 cells compared with SC. Since SCA has a high amount of low-molecular-weight fraction, the highest fucose content, is highly cytotoxic to A-549 cells, has a low cytotoxic effect on BEAS-2B cells, and exhibits the highest ability to suppress Bcl-2 expression, induce cytochrome c release, activate caspase-9, and promote late apoptosis of A-549 cells; thus, it can be recommended as a potential therapeutic agent for preventive or auxiliary treatment of lung cancer.

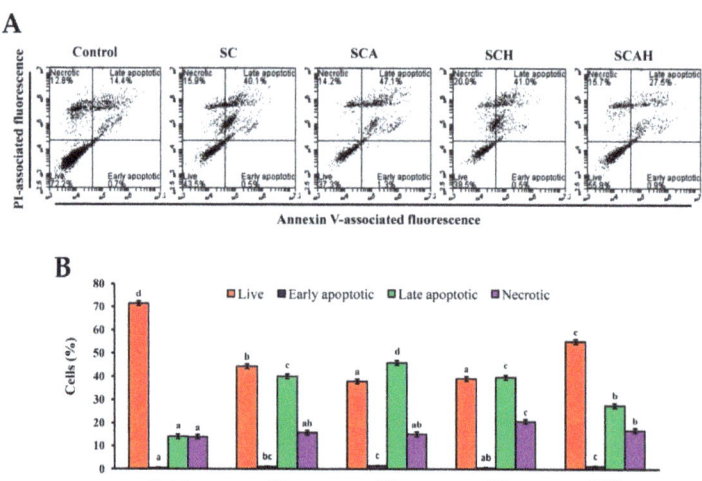

Figure 7. SC, SCA, SCH, and SCAH induce apoptosis in A-549 cells. Flow-cytometric analysis of Annexin V-fluorescein isothiocyanate (FITC)/propidium iodide (PI)-stained A-549 cells treated without and with 200 µg/mL SC, SCA, SCH, and SCAH for 48 h: (**A**) histograms; (**B**) bar chart. Bars in the same cell population bearing different letters (in a, b, c, and d) significantly differ at the level of 0.05. Experiments were repeated three times.

2.10. The Akt/mTOR Pathway Is Involved in SC-, SCA-, SCH-, and SCAH-Induced Apoptosis of A-549 Cells

Previous studies indicated that the Akt/mammalian target of rapamycin (mTOR) pathway is closely related to a variety of cellular functions including adhesion, invasion, proliferation, angiogenesis, migration, and survival [62]. In addition, the Akt/mTOR signaling cascade is frequently activated in diverse cancers [63–65]. As the Akt/mTOR pathway is frequently activated in cancer, numerous research efforts sought to target this pathway with a view to developing pharmacologic interventions for various cancers, such as colon cancer [66], endometrial cancer [67], breast cancer [68], prostate cancer [69], human small-cell lung cancer cells [70], non-small-cell lung cancer [71], and ovarian cancer [72]. In the present study, a flow-cytometric approach was conducted to evaluate the expression levels of p-Akt, Akt serine/threonine kinase 1 (Akt1), and p-mTOR in A-549 cells treated with SC, SCA, SCH, or SCAH at a dose of 200 µg/mL for 48 h. The results presented in Figure 8 suggest that all of the tested fucoidans suppressed levels of p-Akt and p-mTOR as compared to the untreated control. In addition, it was noted that the expression of total Akt (Akt1) did not vary among the different treatments. Our results are similar to previous findings indicating that the commercialized fucoidan extract from *Fucus vesiculosus* suppressed levels of p-Akt and p-mTOR of A-549 cells dose- and time-dependently [73], and commercialized *U. pinnatifida* fucoidan induced apoptosis in A-549 cells via downregulation of phospho-p38 and phospho-PI3K/Akt expression [61]. In summary, the data presented here suggest that Akt/mTOR signaling may play a role in the death of A-549 cells induced by SC, SCA, SCH, and SCAH. Further investigations are needed to elucidate the precise mechanisms and to explore targeting of signaling pathways in lung cancer, especially using in vivo models.

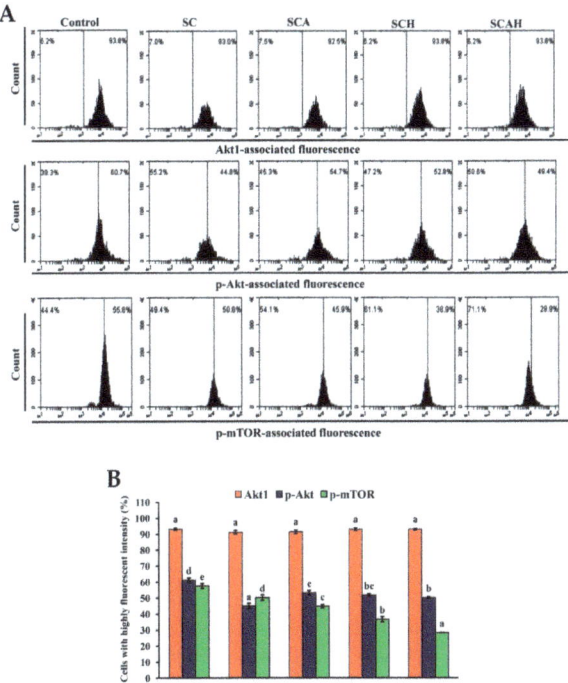

Figure 8. Effects of SC, SCA, SCH, and SCAH treatments on the levels of Akt serine/threonine kinase 1 (Akt1), p-Akt, and p-mammalian target of rapamycin (mTOR) in A-549 cells. Flow-cytometric analysis of A-549 cells treated without and with 200 µg/mL SC, SCA, SCH, and SCAH for 48 h: (**A**) histograms; (**B**) bar chart. Bars in the same Akt1, p-Akt, or p-mTOR group bearing different letters (in a, b, c, d, and e) significantly differ at the level of 0.05. Experiments were repeated three times.

3. Materials and Methods

3.1. Materials

Samples of *S. crassifolium*, a type of brown seaweed, were collected from Kenting (Pingtung, Taiwan), and, after washing and drying, they were sealed in aluminum foil bags and kept at 4 °C until use. Dextrans (5, 50, 150, and 670 kDa), L-fucose, D-glucuronic acid, dimethyl sulfoxide (DMSO), potassium bromide (KBr), 2,2,2-trifluoroacetic acid (TFA), and 3-(4,5-dimethylthiazol-2-yl)-2,5-diphenyltetrazolium bromide (MTT) were obtained from Sigma-Aldrich (St. Louis, MO, USA). Ham's F12K medium, Dulbecco's Modified Eagle Medium (DMEM) medium, trypsin/ethylenediaminetetraacetic acid (EDTA), fetal bovine serum (FBS), penicillin, and streptomycin were obtained from Gibco Laboratories (Grand Island, NY, USA). TMRE and fluorescein isothiocyanate (FITC)-labeled anti-Bcl-2 antibodies were obtained from Molecular Probes, Invitrogen Corp. (Carlsbad, CA, USA).

3.2. Extrusion Process

The extrusion process was done according to the method reported by Huang et al. [15] with minor modification. In brief, a single-screw laboratory extruder (Tsung Hsing Co. Ltd., Kaohsiung, Taiwan) equipped with screw diameter 74 mm, L/D ratio 3.07:1, and rounded die head with a diameter of 5 mm was used. The algal sample was used as the raw material and was preconditioned to a moisture content of 35%. The feed rate was constant at 10.4 kg/h. Other extrusion parameters were set with barrel temperature at 115 °C and screw speed at 360 rpm. The algal extrudate was dried at 55 °C for 30 min, cooled to room temperature (RT), ground into particles that could pass through a 20-mesh screen, and stored at 4 °C for further extraction experiments.

3.3. Water Extraction Procedure

The extraction of native fucoidan from *S. crassifolium* was done according to the method reported by Huang et al. [23]. In brief, the algal sample was mixed with 95% ethanol (w/v = 1:10), shaken for 1 h at room temperature to remove pigments and lipid, and then centrifuged at 970× g for 10 min. The residue was then collected, mixed with double distilled water (w/v = 1:10), and placed in a water bath kept at 85 °C for 1 h with shaking to extract the polysaccharides. The mixture was centrifuged at 3870× g for 10 min, and the supernatant was collected. Ethanol (95%) was added into the supernatant to give a final ethanol concentration of 20% in order to precipitate alginic acid. The mixture was centrifuged at 9170× g for 30 min, the supernatant was collected, and 95% ethanol was added until a final ethanol concentration of 50% was reached in order to obtain fucoidan precipitate. The ethanol-precipitated fucoidan was then recovered by centrifugation at 9170× g for 30 min, dried at 40 °C, milled, and stored at 4 °C for further use. Extraction yield was calculated using the following equation:

$$\text{Extraction yield (\%)} = (\text{weight of the extracted solid, dry basis/weight of the sample, dry basis}) \times 100 \quad (1)$$

3.4. Preparation of Degraded Fucoidans

A sample of native fucoidan weighing 0.2 g was dissolved into 20 mL of distilled water and mixed with 10 mmol/L AA, 10 mmol/L H_2O_2, or a mixed solution of 10 mmol/L H_2O_2 and 10 mmol/L AA. The native fucoidan was degraded at RT for 16 h. Then, the degraded fucoidan was precipitated using 75% ethanol, collected, and dried for further use [24].

3.5. Intrinsic Viscosity Analysis

The viscosity measurements were performed using an Ubbelohde viscometer at 25 ± 1 °C. The pure solvent was ddH$_2$O, and the intrinsic viscosity (η_r) was determined using the following equation:

$$\eta_r = (\ln t/t_0)/c \qquad (2)$$

where t = efflux time for solution (s), t_0 = efflux time for the pure solvent (s), and c = concentration of solution (g/mL).

3.6. Molecular Weight Analysis

The average molecular weights of the fucoidans were determined using a size-exclusion HPLC column Superdex 200 (300 mm × 10 mm inner diameter (ID), GE Healthcare, Piscataway, NJ, USA) using a Shimadzu HPLC system (Shimadzu, Kyoto, Japan) equipped with a refractive index detector. The chromatography conditions were as follows: eluent 0.2 M NaCl; flow rate 0.4 mL/min, sample concentration 10 mg/mL; injection volume 0.15 mL; temperature 25 °C. The column was calibrated with dextrans of different molecular weight (5, 50, 150, and 670 kDa).

3.7. Analytical Methods

The fucose was estimated using the protocol described by Gibbons [74], and L-fucose was utilized as the standard. Total sugar content was assayed using a phenol–sulfuric acid method using L-fucose as the standard. The sulfate content was determined according to the protocol described by Yang et al. [22]. Polyphenols were analyzed by the Folin–Ciocalteu method, and gallic acid was used as the standard [75].

3.8. Monosaccharide Composition Analysis

The monosaccharide composition of fucoidan was determined according to a previously reported method [23] using six monosaccharides (L-fucose, D-galactose, D-glucuronic acid, D-galacturonic acid, D-xylose, and D-mannose) as standards.

3.9. FTIR Spectroscopy

The FTIR spectra were analyzed according to a protocol described elsewhere [41] using an FT-730 instrument (Horiba, Kyoto, Japan). A KBr pellet was prepared by mixing 1 mg of fucoidan with 50 mg of potassium bromide. The spectrum was read between 400 and 4000 cm^{-1}.

3.10. NMR Spectroscopy

The polysaccharide sample was dissolved with 99.9% D$_2$O in an NMR tube, and the NMR spectra were read on a Varian VNMRS-700 NMR spectrometer (Varian, Lexington, MA, USA).

3.11. Cell Culture

BEAS-2B (human bronchial epithelial cells, ATCC CRL-9609, Manassas, VA, USA) and A-549 (human lung carcinoma, BCRC 60074, Hsinchu, Taiwan) were obtained from the ATCC (American Type Culture Collection) (Manassas, VA, USA) and the BCRC (Bioresource Collection and Research Center) (Hsinchu, Taiwan), respectively. A-549 cells were cultured in complete Ham's F12K medium and BEAS-2B was maintained in complete DMEM medium. The complete medium was prepared by supplementing plain medium with 10% FBS, 100 µg/mL streptomycin, and 100 units/mL penicillin. All cells were cultured in a 37 °C humidified 5% CO$_2$ atmosphere. The cells were passaged every 2–3 days.

3.12. Evaluation of Cytotoxic Activity

The cytotoxic activity of the fucoidan extracts was measured using the MTT assay. Briefly, cells were cultured in growth medium with 37 °C humidified 5% CO_2 atmosphere for 24 h. All fucoidan extracts were prepared as a 20 mg/mL stock solution by thoroughly dissolving fucoidan powder in phosphate-buffered saline (PBS). The medium was then removed, and the cells were treated with various concentrations of fucoidan extracts. Final concentrations of 0, 50, 100, 200, 300, 400, and 500 µg/mL were obtained by diluting the stock solution with serum-free medium to prevent the fucoidan extract from potentially losing its potency in the presence of serum. After 48 h of treatment, cells were washed with PBS once, and MTT stock solution was added to each culture so that the final concentration of MTT in the medium was 0.1 mg/mL. After 2–4 h of incubation, the formazan was solubilized by adding isopropanol and measured by absorption at 560 nm. The cell viability was expressed as a percentage of MTT reduction.

3.13. Flow Cytometry-Based Analyses

In all flow cytometry-based analyses, cells (4×10^4 cells/mL) were incubated without (as a non-treated control, cells were in serum-free medium) and with 200 µg/mL SC, SCA, SCH, or SCAH (these fucoidan extracts were prepared as a 20 mg/mL stock solution by thoroughly dissolving fucoidan powder in PBS; a final concentration of 200 µg/mL was obtained by diluting the stock solution with serum-free medium) for 48 h, and then cells were de-attached by trypsin and rinsed two times in cold PBS to obtain cell samples. Then, each flow cytometry-based analysis was performed according to the protocols below.

For the MMP analysis, the assay was conducted according to the method of Yang et al. [22]. Briefly, single-cell suspensions were washed twice with PBS and incubated, in the dark, for 20 min at 37 °C with TMRE (100 nM). After labeling, cells were washed and re-suspended for flow-cytometric measurement in staining solution.

For Bcl-2 expression analysis, single-cell suspensions were fixed using fixation buffer at 37 °C for 20 min. Then, the cells were permeabilized using permeabilization buffer and incubated, in the dark, for 1 h at RT with FITC-labeled anti-Bcl-2 antibody (1:25, *v/v*). After labeling, cells were washed and re-suspended for flow-cytometric measurement in staining solution.

The analysis of cytochrome c release was conducted by following the method of Huang et al. [41]. Briefly, single-cell suspensions were fixed using fixation buffer at 37 °C for 20 min. Then, the cells were permeabilized using permeabilization buffer and incubated, in the dark, for 1 h at RT with FITC-labeled anti-cytochrome c antibody (1:10, *v/v*). After labeling, cells were washed and re-suspended for flow-cytometric measurement in staining solution.

For activated caspase -9 and -3 analyses, the method of Huang et al. was used [41]. Briefly, single-cell suspensions were incubated, in the dark, for 1 h at 37 °C with FITC/LEHD/FMK solution (for caspase-9 detection) or FITC/DEVD/FMK solution (for caspase-3 detection). After labeling, cells were washed and re-suspended for flow-cytometric measurement in staining solution.

The annexin V-FITC/PI staining analysis was conducted using an annexin V-FITC apoptosis detection kit according to the method of Yang et al. [22]. Briefly, single-cell suspensions were incubated, in the dark, for 15 min at RT with annexin V-FITC (1:20, *v/v*) and PI (1:20, *v/v*). After labeling, cells were washed and re-suspended for flow-cytometric measurement in staining solution.

For phosphorylated Akt and mTOR analyses, the assays of phosphorylated Akt and mTOR were conducted using the method of Huang et al. [76]. In brief, single0cell suspensions were fixed using fixation buffer at 37 °C for 1 h. Then, the cells were incubated, in the dark, for 1 h at RT with allophycocyanin (APC)-conjugated anti-Akt1 antibody (1:50, *v/v*), FITC-conjugated anti-phospho-Akt (Ser473) antibody (1:20, *v/v*), or phycoerythrin (PE)-conjugated anti-phospho-mTOR (Ser2448) antibody (1:20, *v/v*). After labeling, cells were washed and re-suspended for flow-cytometric measurement in staining solution. All of the flow-cytometric analyses described above were conducted using a BD Accuri C6 flow cytometer (San Jose, CA, USA).

3.14. Statistical Analysis

All data are expressed as means ± SD (n = 3). Comparisons between different groups were performed by ANOVA followed by the Duncan multiple range test or the Student's t-test. A p-value <0.05 was considered statistically significant.

4. Conclusions

In this paper, a native fucoidan (SC) was extracted from *S. crassifolium* pretreated by single-screw extrusion. The extrusion pretreatment process augmented the extraction yield of fucoidan as compared to the non-extruded sample. Three degraded fucoidans (SCA, SCH, and SCAH) were obtained by degrading SC with different combinations of degradation reagents. Among SC, SCA, SCH, and SCAH, the chemical compositions varied but their structural features were similar, as illustrated by the results of FTIR and NMR analyses. In vitro anti-lung cancer studies revealed that SC, SCA, SCH, and SCAH decreased MMP, decreased Bcl-2 expression, increased the release of cytochrome c, increased activation of caspase-9 and -3, and increased late apoptosis of A-549 cells. In general, SCA has a high amount of low-molecular-weight fraction and the highest fucose content, is highly cytotoxic to A-549 cells, and shows a high ability to suppress Bcl-2 expression, to induce cytochrome c release, to promote activation of caspase-9, and to induce late apoptosis of A-549 cells. Therefore, SCA demonstrated excellent potential for development as an adjuvant treatment of lung cancer. Additional in vitro experiments showed that the Akt/mTOR signaling pathway is involved in SC-, SCA-, SCH-, and SCAH-induced apoptosis of A-549 cells. Further experiments are warranted to elucidate the precise signaling mechanisms involved, especially using in vivo studies.

Supplementary Materials: ^{1}H-NMR spectra and ^{13}C-NMR spectra for SC, SCA, SCH, and SCAH are available online at http://www.mdpi.com/1660-3397/18/6/334/s1.

Author Contributions: Conceptualization, T.-C.W. and C.-H.K.; methodology, Y.-H.T.; software, S.-L.H.; validation, R.-H.H., Y.-H.H., and C.-Y.H.; formal analysis, R.-H.H. and Y.-H.H.; investigation, Y.-H.T., C.-H.K., and Y.-H.H.; resources, C.-H.K. and S.-L.H.; data curation, R.-H.H. and T.-C.W.; writing—original draft preparation, T.-C.W., Y.-H.H., and C.-H.K.; writing—review and editing, C.-H.K. and C.-Y.H.; supervision, Y.-H.H.; project administration, C.-Y.H.; funding acquisition, T.-C.W., Y.-H.H., and C.-Y.H. All authors read and agreed to the published version of the manuscript.

Funding: This research received no external funding.

Acknowledgments: This study was supported by a grant from the Kaohsiung Medical University Hospital (KMUH107-M729) to Tien-Chiu Wu, as well as by the Ministry of Science and Technology, Taiwan, grant number MOST 107-2320-B-992-001, which was awarded to Chun-Yung Huang. The authors thank the Ministry of Education, Taiwan, for supporting this study (grant number MOE-RSC-108RSN0005), awarded to Yong-Han Hong.

Conflicts of Interest: The authors declare no conflicts of interest.

References

1. Siegel, R.L.; Miller, K.D.; Jemal, A. Cancer statistics, 2017. *CA Cancer J. Clin.* **2017**, *67*, 7–30. [CrossRef] [PubMed]
2. Davidson, M.R.; Gazdar, A.F.; Clarke, B.E. The pivotal role of pathology in the management of lung cancer. *J. Thorac. Dis.* **2013**, *5*, S463–S478. [PubMed]
3. Shen, D.J.; Jiang, Y.H.; Li, J.Q.; Xu, L.W.; Tao, K.Y. The RNA-binding protein RBM47 inhibits non-small cell lung carcinoma metastasis through modulation of AXIN1 mRNA stability and Wnt/β-catentin signaling. *Surg. Oncol.* **2020**, *34*, 31–39. [CrossRef]
4. Ministry of Health and Welfare. Taiwan, Statistics of Causes of Death. Available online: http://dep.mohw.gov.tw/DOS/lp-4472-113.html (accessed on 1 May 2020).
5. Rabik, C.A.; Dolan, M.E. Molecular mechanisms of resistance and toxicity associated with platinating agents. *Cancer Treat. Rev.* **2007**, *33*, 9–23. [CrossRef]
6. Kim, E.J.; Park, S.Y.; Lee, J.Y.; Park, J.H.Y. Fucoidan present in brown algae induces apoptosis of human colon cancer cells. *BMC gastroenterol.* **2010**, *10*, 96. [CrossRef]

7. Wang, Y.; Xing, M.; Cao, Q.; Ji, A.; Liang, H.; Song, S. Biological activities of fucoidan and the factors mediating its therapeutic effects: A review of recent studies. *Mar. Drugs* **2019**, *17*, 183. [CrossRef]
8. Luthuli, S.; Wu, S.; Cheng, Y.; Zheng, X.; Wu, M.; Tong, H. Therapeutic effects of Fucoidan: A review on recent studies. *Mar. Drugs* **2019**, *17*, 487. [CrossRef]
9. Wang, J.; Zhang, Q.; Li, S.; Chen, Z.; Tan, J.; Yao, J.; Duan, D. Low molecular weight fucoidan alleviates diabetic nephropathy by binding fibronectin and inhibiting ECM-receptor interaction in human renal mesangial cells. *Int. J. Biol. Macromol.* **2020**, *150*, 304–314. [CrossRef]
10. Huang, C.Y.; Kuo, C.H.; Lee, C.H. Antibacterial and antioxidant capacities and attenuation of lipid accumulation in 3T3-L1 adipocytes by low-molecular-weight fucoidans prepared from compressional-puffing-pretreated *Sargassum crassifolium*. *Mar. Drugs* **2018**, *16*, 24. [CrossRef]
11. Xu, Y.; Xu, J.; Ge, K.; Tian, Q.; Zhao, P.; Guo, Y. Anti-inflammatory effect of low molecular weight fucoidan from *Saccharina japonica* on atherosclerosis in apoE-knockout mice. *Int. J. Biol. Macromol.* **2018**, *118*, 365–374. [CrossRef]
12. Bachelet, L.; Bertholon, I.; Lavigne, D.; Vassy, R.; Jandrot-Perrus, M.; Chaubet, F.; Letourneur, D. Affinity of low molecular weight fucoidan for P-selectin triggers its binding to activated human platelets. *Biochim. Biophys. Acta* **2009**, *1790*, 141–146. [CrossRef]
13. Chen, J.; Wang, W.; Zhang, Q.; Li, F.; Lei, T.; Luo, D.; Zhou, H.; Yang, B. Low molecular weight fucoidan against renal ischemia - reperfusion injury via inhibition of the MAPK signaling pathway. *PLoS ONE* **2013**, *8*, e56224. [CrossRef] [PubMed]
14. Camire, M.E.; Camire, A.; Krumhar, K. Chemical and nutritional changes in foods during extrusion. *Crit. Rev. Food Sci. Nutr.* **1990**, *29*, 35–57. [CrossRef] [PubMed]
15. Huang, C.Y.; Kuo, J.M.; Wu, S.J.; Tsai, H.T. Isolation and characterization of fish scale collagen from tilapia (*Oreochromis* sp.) by a novel extrusion-hydro-extraction process. *Food Chem.* **2016**, *190*, 997–1006. [CrossRef] [PubMed]
16. Duque, A.; Manzanares, P.; Ballesteros, M. Extrusion as a pretreatment for lignocellulosic biomass: Fundamentals and applications. *Renew. Energ.* **2017**, *114*, 1427–1441. [CrossRef]
17. Chen, W.H.; Xu, Y.Y.; Hwang, W.S.; Wang, J.B. Pretreatment of rice straw using an extrusion/extraction process at bench-scale for producing cellulosic ethanol. *Bioresour. Technol.* **2011**, *102*, 10451–10458. [CrossRef] [PubMed]
18. Huang, C.Y.; Tsai, Y.H.; Hong, Y.H.; Hsieh, S.L.; Huang, R.H. Characterization and antioxidant and angiotensin I-converting enzyme (ACE)-inhibitory activities of gelatin hydrolysates prepared from extrusion-pretreated milkfish (*Chanos chanos*) scale. *Mar. Drugs* **2018**, *16*, 346. [CrossRef]
19. Jing, Y.; Chi, Y.J. Effects of twin-screw extrusion on soluble dietary fibre and physicochemical properties of soybean residue. *Food Chem.* **2013**, *138*, 884–889. [CrossRef]
20. Huang, Y.L.; Ma, Y.S. The effect of extrusion processing on the physiochemical properties of extruded orange pomace. *Food Chem.* **2016**, *192*, 363–369. [CrossRef]
21. Zhang, Y.; Li, T.; Shen, Y.; Wang, L.; Zhang, H.; Qian, H.; Qi, X. Extrusion followed by ultrasound as a chemical-free pretreatment method to enhance enzymatic hydrolysis of rice hull for fermentable sugars production. *Ind. Crop. Prod.* **2020**, *149*, 112356. [CrossRef]
22. Yang, W.N.; Chen, P.W.; Huang, C.Y. Compositional characteristics and in vitro evaluations of antioxidant and neuroprotective properties of crude extracts of fucoidan prepared from compressional puffing-pretreated *Sargassum crassifolium*. *Mar. Drugs* **2017**, *15*, 183. [CrossRef] [PubMed]
23. Huang, C.Y.; Wu, S.J.; Yang, W.N.; Kuan, A.W.; Chen, C.Y. Antioxidant activities of crude extracts of fucoidan extracted from *Sargassum glaucescens* by a compressional-puffing-hydrothermal extraction process. *Food Chem.* **2016**, *197*, 1121–1129. [CrossRef] [PubMed]
24. Zhang, Z.; Wang, X.; Mo, X.; Qi, H. Degradation and the antioxidant activity of polysaccharide from *Enteromorpha linza*. *Carbohydr. Polym.* **2013**, *92*, 2084–2087. [CrossRef] [PubMed]
25. Pozharitskaya, O.N.; Shikov, A.N.; Faustova, N.M.; Obluchinskaya, E.D.; Kosman, V.M.; Vuorela, H.; Makarov, V.G. Pharmacokinetic and tissue distribution of fucoidan from *Fucus vesiculosus* after oral administration to rats. *Mar. Drugs* **2018**, *16*, 132. [CrossRef] [PubMed]
26. Pozharitskaya, O.N.; Shikov, A.N.; Obluchinskaya, E.D.; Vuorela, H. The pharmacokinetics of fucoidan after topical application to rats. *Mar. Drugs* **2019**, *17*, 687. [CrossRef]

27. Petit, A.C.; Noiret, N.; Sinquin, C.; Ratiskol, J.; Guezennec, J.; Colliec-Jouault, S. Free-radical depolymerization with metallic catalysts of an exopolysaccharide produced by a bacterium isolated from a deep-sea hydrothermal vent polychaete annelid. *Carbohydr. Polym.* **2006**, *64*, 597–602. [CrossRef]
28. Ale, M.T.; Mikkelsen, J.D.; Meyer, A.S. Important determinants for fucoidan bioactivity: A critical review of structure-function relations and extraction methods for fucose-containing sulfated polysaccharides from brown seaweeds. *Mar. Drugs* **2011**, *9*, 2106–2130. [CrossRef]
29. Zhu, Z.; Zhang, Q.; Chen, L.; Ren, S.; Xu, P.; Tang, Y.; Luo, D. Higher specificity of the activity of low molecular weight fucoidan for thrombin-induced platelet aggregation. *Thromb. Res.* **2010**, *125*, 419–426. [CrossRef]
30. Pozharitskaya, O.N.; Obluchinskaya, E.D.; Shikov, A.N. Mechanisms of bioactivities of fucoidan from the brown seaweed *Fucus vesiculosus* L. of the Barents Sea. *Mar. Drugs* **2020**, *18*, 275. [CrossRef]
31. Hou, Y.; Wang, J.; Jin, W.; Zhang, H.; Zhang, Q. Degradation of *Laminaria japonica* fucoidan by hydrogen peroxide and antioxidant activities of the degradation products of different molecular weights. *Carbohydr. Polym.* **2012**, *87*, 153–159. [CrossRef]
32. Tissot, B.; Salpin, J.-Y.; Martinez, M.; Gaigeot, M.-P.; Daniel, R. Differentiation of the fucoidan sulfated L-fucose isomers constituents by CE-ESIMS and molecular modeling. *Carbohydr. Res.* **2006**, *341*, 598–609. [CrossRef] [PubMed]
33. Wang, C.Y.; Wu, T.C.; Hsieh, S.L.; Tsai, Y.H.; Yeh, C.W.; Huang, C.Y. Antioxidant activity and growth inhibition of human colon cancer cells by crude and purified fucoidan preparations extracted from *Sargassum cristaefolium*. *J. Food Drug Anal.* **2015**, *23*, 766–777. [CrossRef] [PubMed]
34. Tomsik, P.; Soukup, T.; Cermakova, E.; Micuda, S.; Niang, M.; Sucha, L.; Rezacova, M. L-rhamnose and L-fucose suppress cancer growth in mice. *Central Eur. J. Biol.* **2011**, *6*, 1–9. [CrossRef]
35. Jin, W.; Zhang, Q.; Wang, J.; Zhang, W. A comparative study of the anticoagulant activities of eleven fucoidans. *Carbohydr. Polym.* **2013**, *91*, 1–6. [CrossRef] [PubMed]
36. Li, B.; Lu, F.; Wei, X.J.; Zhao, R.X. Fucoidan: Structure and bioactivity. *Molecules* **2008**, *13*, 1671–1695. [CrossRef] [PubMed]
37. Hu, M.; Cui, N.; Bo, Z.; Xiang, F. Structural determinant and its underlying molecular mechanism of STPC2 related to anti-angiogenic activity. *Mar. Drugs* **2017**, *15*, 48. [CrossRef] [PubMed]
38. Movasaghi, Z.; Rehman, S.; ur Rehman, D.I. Fourier transform infrared (FTIR) spectroscopy of biological tissues. *Appl. Spectrosc. Rev.* **2008**, *43*, 134–179. [CrossRef]
39. Shao, P.; Pei, Y.P.; Fang, Z.X.; Sun, P.L. Effects of partial desulfation on antioxidant and inhibition of DLD cancer cell of *Ulva fasciata* polysaccharide. *Int. J. Biol. Macromol.* **2014**, *65*, 307–313. [CrossRef]
40. Palanisamy, S.; Vinosha, M.; Marudhupandi, T.; Rajasekar, P.; Prabhu, N.M. Isolation of fucoidan from *Sargassum polycystum* brown algae: Structural characterization, *in vitro* antioxidant and anticancer activity. *Int. J. Biol. Macromol.* **2017**, *102*, 405–412. [CrossRef]
41. Huang, C.Y.; Kuo, C.H.; Chen, P.W. Compressional-puffing pretreatment enhances neuroprotective effects of fucoidans from the brown seaweed *Sargassum hemiphyllum* on 6-hydroxydopamine-induced apoptosis in SH-SY5Y cells. *Molecules* **2018**, *23*, 78. [CrossRef]
42. Synytsya, A.; Bleha, R.; Synytsya, A.; Pohl, R.; Hayashi, K.; Yoshinaga, K.; Nakano, T.; Hayashi, T. Mekabu fucoidan: Structural complexity and defensive effects against avian influenza A viruses. *Carbohydr. Polym.* **2014**, *111*, 633–644. [CrossRef] [PubMed]
43. Bilan, M.I.; Grachev, A.A.; Shashkov, A.S.; Nifantiev, N.E.; Usov, A.I. Structure of a fucoidan from the brown seaweed *Fucus serratus* L. *Carbohydr. Res.* **2006**, *341*, 238–245. [CrossRef] [PubMed]
44. Tako, M.; Nakada, T.; Hongou, F. Chemical characterization of fucoidan from commercially cultured *Nemacystus decipiens* (Itomozuku). *Biosci. Biotechnol. Biochem.* **1999**, *63*, 1813–1815. [CrossRef] [PubMed]
45. Immanuel, G.; Sivagnanavelmurugan, M.; Marudhupandi, T.; Radhakrishnan, S.; Palavesam, A. The effect of fucoidan from brown seaweed *Sargassum wightii* on WSSV resistance and immune activity in shrimp *Penaeus monodon* (Fab). *Fish Shellfish Immunol.* **2012**, *32*, 551–564. [CrossRef] [PubMed]
46. Jégou, C.; Kervarec, N.; Cérantola, S.; Bihannic, I.; Stiger-Pouvreau, V. NMR use to quantify phlorotannins: The case of *Cystoseira tamariscifolia*, a phloroglucinol-producing brown macroalga in Brittany (France). *Talanta* **2015**, *135*, 1–6. [CrossRef] [PubMed]

47. Ermakova, S.; Sokolova, R.; Kim, S.M.; Um, B.H.; Isakov, V.; Zvyagintseva, T. Fucoidans from brown seaweeds *Sargassum hornery*, *Eclonia cava*, *Costaria costata*: Structural characteristics and anticancer activity. *Appl. Biochem. Biotechnol.* **2011**, *164*, 841–850. [CrossRef]
48. Bilan, M.I.; Grachev, A.A.; Ustuzhanina, N.E.; Shashkov, A.S.; Nifantiev, N.E.; Usov, A.I. A highly regular fraction of a fucoidan from the brown seaweed *Fucus distichus* L. *Carbohydr. Res.* **2004**, *339*, 511–517. [CrossRef]
49. Kumar, T.V.; Lakshmanasenthil, S.; Geetharamani, D.; Marudhupandi, T.; Suja, G.; Suganya, P. Fucoidan - A α-d-glucosidase inhibitor from *Sargassum wightii* with relevance to type 2 diabetes mellitus therapy. *Int. J. Biol. Macromol.* **2015**, *72*, 1044–1047. [CrossRef]
50. Vishchuk, O.S.; Ermakova, S.P.; Zvyagintseva, T.N. Sulfated polysaccharides from brown seaweeds Saccharina japonica and Undaria pinnatifida: Isolation, structural characteristics, and antitumor activity. *Carbohydr. Res.* **2011**, *346*, 2769–2776. [CrossRef]
51. Imbs, T.I.; Ermakova, S.P.; Malyarenko, O.S.; Isakov, V.V.; Zvyagintseva, T.N. Structural elucidation of polysaccharide fractions from the brown alga *Coccophora langsdorfii* and *in vitro* investigation of their anticancer activity. *Carbohydr. Polym.* **2016**, *135*, 162–168. [CrossRef]
52. Chen, H.M.; Lee, M.J.; Kuo, C.Y.; Tsai, P.L.; Liu, J.Y.; Kao, S.H. *Ocimum gratissimum* aqueous extract induces apoptotic signalling in lung adenocarcinoma cell A549. *Evid. Based Complement. Alternat. Med.* **2011**, *2011*, 739093. [CrossRef] [PubMed]
53. Tschoeke, S.K.; Hellmuth, M.; Hostmann, A.; Robinson, Y.; Ertel, W.; Oberholzer, A.; Heyde, C.E. Apoptosis of human intervertebral discs after trauma compares to degenerated discs involving both receptor-mediated and mitochondrial-dependent pathways. *J. Orthop. Res.* **2008**, *26*, 999–1006. [CrossRef] [PubMed]
54. Riedl, S.J.; Salvesen, G.S. The apoptosome: Signalling platform of cell death. *Nat. Rev. Mol. Cell Biol.* **2007**, *8*, 405–413. [CrossRef] [PubMed]
55. Ly, J.D.; Grubb, D.R.; Lawen, A. The mitochondrial membrane potential ($\Delta\psi m$) in apoptosis; an update. *Apoptosis* **2003**, *8*, 115–128. [CrossRef] [PubMed]
56. Penninger, J.M.; Kroemer, G. Mitochondria, AIF and caspases - rivaling for cell death execution. *Nat. Cell Biol.* **2003**, *5*, 97–99. [CrossRef] [PubMed]
57. Gottlieb, E.; Armour, S.M.; Harris, M.H.; Thompson, C.B. Mitochondrial membrane potential regulates matrix configuration and cytochrome c release during apoptosis. *Cell Death Differ.* **2003**, *10*, 709–717. [CrossRef]
58. Jiang, X.; Wang, X. Cytochrome-c-mediated apoptosis. *Annu. Rev. Biochem.* **2004**, *73*, 87–106. [CrossRef]
59. Paul, J. Anticancer potential of fucoidan extracted from *Padina distromatica* Hauck (brown seaweed) from Hare Island, Thoothukudi, TamilNadu, India. *Asian J. Pharm. Sci. Technol.* **2014**, *4*, 217–221.
60. Marudhupandi, T.; Kumar, T.T.A.; Lakshmanasenthil, S.; Suja, G.; Vinothkumar, T. In vitro anticancer activity of fucoidan from *Turbinaria conoides* against A549 cell lines. *Int. J. Biol. Macromol.* **2015**, *72*, 919–923. [CrossRef]
61. Boo, H.J.; Hyun, J.H.; Kim, S.C.; Kang, J.I.; Kim, M.K.; Kim, S.Y.; Cho, H.; Yoo, E.S.; Kang, H.K. Fucoidan from *Undaria pinnatifida* induces apoptosis in A549 human lung carcinoma cells. *Phytother. Res.* **2011**, *25*, 1082–1086. [CrossRef]
62. Burris, H.A. Overcoming acquired resistance to anticancer therapy: Focus on the PI3K/AKT/mTOR pathway. *Cancer Chemother. Pharmacol.* **2013**, *71*, 829–842. [CrossRef]
63. Liu, P.; Cheng, H.; Roberts, T.M.; Zhao, J.J. Targeting the phosphoinositide 3-kinase pathway in cancer. *Nat. Rev. Drug Discov.* **2009**, *8*, 627–644. [CrossRef] [PubMed]
64. Polivka Jr, J.; Janku, F. Molecular targets for cancer therapy in the PI3K/AKT/mTOR pathway. *Pharmacol. Ther.* **2014**, *142*, 164–175. [CrossRef] [PubMed]
65. Dienstmann, R.; Rodon, J.; Serra, V.; Tabernero, J. Picking the point of inhibition: A comparative review of PI3K/AKT/mTOR pathway inhibitors. *Mol. Cancer Ther.* **2014**, *13*, 1021–1031. [CrossRef]
66. Shiao, W.C.; Kuo, C.H.; Tsai, Y.H.; Hsieh, S.L.; Kuan, A.W.; Hong, Y.H.; Huang, C.Y. *In vitro* evaluation of anti-colon cancer potential of crude extracts of fucoidan obtained from *Sargassum glaucescens* pretreated by compressional-puffing. *Appl. Sci.* **2020**, *10*, 3058. [CrossRef]
67. Slomovitz, B.M.; Coleman, R.L. The PI3K/AKT/mTOR pathway as a therapeutic target in endometrial cancer. *Clin. Cancer Res.* **2012**, *18*, 5856–5864. [CrossRef]
68. Gil, E.M.C. Targeting the PI3K/AKT/mTOR pathway in estrogen receptor-positive breast cancer. *Cancer Treat. Rev.* **2014**, *40*, 862–871.

69. Morgan, T.M.; Koreckij, T.D.; Corey, E. Targeted therapy for advanced prostate cancer: Inhibition of the PI3K/Akt/mTOR pathway. *Curr. Cancer Drug Targets* **2009**, *9*, 237–249. [CrossRef]
70. Marinov, M.; Ziogas, A.; Pardo, O.E.; Tan, L.T.; Dhillon, T.; Mauri, F.A.; Lane, H.A.; Lemoine, N.R.; Zangemeister-Wittke, U.; Seckl, M.J. AKT/mTOR pathway activation and BCL-2 family proteins modulate the sensitivity of human small cell lung cancer cells to RAD001. *Clin. Cancer Res.* **2009**, *15*, 1277–1287. [CrossRef]
71. Fumarola, C.; Bonelli, M.A.; Petronini, P.G.; Alfieri, R.R. Targeting PI3K/AKT/mTOR pathway in non small cell lung cancer. *Biochem. Pharmacol.* **2014**, *90*, 197–207. [CrossRef]
72. Mabuchi, S.; Kuroda, H.; Takahashi, R.; Sasano, T. The PI3K/AKT/mTOR pathway as a therapeutic target in ovarian cancer. *Gynecol. Oncol.* **2015**, *137*, 173–179. [CrossRef] [PubMed]
73. Lee, H.; Kim, J.-S.; Kim, E. Fucoidan from seaweed *Fucus vesiculosus* inhibits migration and invasion of human lung cancer cell via PI3K-Akt-mTOR pathways. *PLoS ONE* **2012**, *7*, e50624. [CrossRef]
74. Gibbons, M.N. The determination of methylpentoses. *Analyst* **1955**, *80*, 268–276. [CrossRef]
75. Meda, A.; Lamien, C.E.; Romito, M.; Millogo, J.; Nacoulma, O.G. Determination of the total phenolic, flavonoid and proline contents in Burkina Fasan honey, as well as their radical scavenging activity. *Food Chem.* **2005**, *91*, 571–577. [CrossRef]
76. Huang, C.Y.; Wu, T.C.; Hong, Y.H.; Hsieh, S.L.; Guo, H.R.; Huang, R.H. Enhancement of cell adhesion, cell growth, wound healing, and oxidative protection by gelatins extracted from extrusion-pretreated tilapia (*Oreochromis* sp.) fish scale. *Molecules* **2018**, *23*, 2406. [CrossRef]

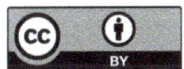

© 2020 by the authors. Licensee MDPI, Basel, Switzerland. This article is an open access article distributed under the terms and conditions of the Creative Commons Attribution (CC BY) license (http://creativecommons.org/licenses/by/4.0/).

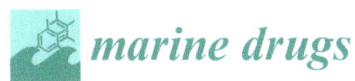

Article

Fucoidan from *Ascophyllum nodosum* Suppresses Postprandial Hyperglycemia by Inhibiting Na$^+$/Glucose Cotransporter 1 Activity

Xindi Shan [1,2,†], Xueliang Wang [1,2,†], Hao Jiang [1,2], Chao Cai [1,2], Jiejie Hao [1,2,*] and Guangli Yu [1,2,*]

1. Key Laboratory of Marine Drugs of Ministry of Education, Shandong Provincial Key Laboratory of Glycoscience and Glycotechnology, School of Medicine and Pharmacy, Ocean University of China, Qingdao 266003, China; shanxindi@hotmail.com (X.S.); wangsun13141314@126.com (X.W.); haojiang@ouc.edu.cn (H.J.); caic@ouc.edu.cn (C.C.)
2. Laboratory for Marine Drugs and Bioproducts, Pilot National Laboratory for Marine Science and Technology (Qingdao), Qingdao 266237, China
* Correspondence: 2009haojie@ouc.edu.cn (J.H.); glyu@ouc.edu.cn (G.Y.); Tel./Fax: +86-532-8203-1609 (G.Y.)
† These authors contributed equally to this work.

Received: 13 August 2020; Accepted: 19 September 2020; Published: 22 September 2020

Abstract: We previously demonstrated that fucoidan with a type II structure inhibited postprandial hyperglycemia by suppressing glucose uptake, but the mechanism remains elusive. Here, we aimed to assess whether the effect of glucose absorption inhibition was related to the basic structure of fucoidans and preliminarily clarified the underlying mechanism. Fucoidans with type II structure and type I structure were prepared from *Ascophyllum nodosum* (AnF) or *Laminaria japonica* (LjF) and *Kjellmaniella crassifolia* (KcF), respectively. The effects of various fucoidans on suppressing postprandial hyperglycemia were investigated using in vitro (Caco-2 monolayer model), semi-in vivo (everted gut sac model), and in vivo (oral glucose tolerance test, OGTT) assays. The results showed that only AnF with a type II structure, but not LjF or KcF with type I structure, could inhibit the glucose transport in the Caco-2 monolayer and everted gut sac models. A similar result was seen in the OGTT of Kunming mice and leptin receptor-deficient (db/db) mice, where only AnF could effectively inhibit glucose transport into the bloodstream. Furthermore, AnF (400 mg/kg/d) treatment decreased the fasting blood glucose, HbA1c, and fasting insulin levels, while increasing the serum glucagon-like peptide-1 (GLP-1) level in obese leptin receptor-deficient (db/db) mice. Furthermore, surface plasmon resonance (SPR) analysis revealed the specific binding of AnF to Na$^+$/glucose cotransporter 1 (SGLT1), which indicated the effect of AnF on postprandial hyperglycemia could be due to its suppression on SGLT1 activity. Taken together, this study suggests that AnF with a type II structure can be a promising candidate for hyperglycemia treatment.

Keywords: fucoidan from *Ascophyllum nodosum*; postprandial hyperglycemia; in vitro and in vivo evaluation; SGLT1

1. Introduction

Diabetes mellitus (DM) is a group of metabolic disorders that are characterized by hyperglycemia [1]. Hyperglycemia is caused by the combined action of insulin deficiency and/or insulin resistance in diabetic patients [2]. Long-term hyperglycemia is associated with microvascular complications and leads to cardiovascular disease, diabetic nephropathy, and other severe complications, which are the major causes of death in diabetic patients [3]. In the early stages of DM, the effective control and strict management of postprandial blood glucose levels are crucial for alleviating DM. The current effective ways to reduce postprandial blood glucose level are as follows: (I) inhibit the activities of digestive enzymes, such as glucosidases and α-amylase, which can produce glucose from starch and other carbohydrates [4]; (II) promote the secretion of insulin, such as by inhibiting dipeptidyl peptidase 4 (DPP-4) and elevating glucagon-like peptide 1 (GLP-1) activities [5,6]; (III) reduce glucose reabsorption in the kidney by inhibiting Na$^+$/glucose cotransporter 2 (SGLT2) activity [7]; (IV) suppress the glucose absorption into the bloodstream via the small intestinal by inhibiting the function of Na$^+$/glucose cotransporter 1 (SGLT1) [8].

Although there are several oral hypoglycemic agents that can reduce the blood glucose level in DM, these agents are mainly chemically synthetic, costly, and can cause severe adverse side-effects (e.g., serious hypoglycemia and kidney damage) [9,10]. Thus, the discovery of effective, safer, and affordable drugs for DM patients has attracted significant research attention. Research suggests that certain natural herbal products can exert hypoglycemic effects and are safer and easier to obtain than other synthetic chemicals [11]. Convincing evidence suggests that bioactive compounds (e.g., proteins, polyphenols, tannins, and phenolic acids) can directly affect intestinal glucose uptake by competitive inhibition of the glucose transporter SGLT1 [12–14]. In the small intestine, SGLT1 is expressed in the apical cell membrane constituting the brush border [15], which is of primary importance for glucose absorption from the lumen to the epithelial cells of the intestine [16,17]. Ina et al. demonstrate that rice albumin could alleviate postprandial hyperglycemia by inhibiting SGLT1 function via in vivo and in vitro assays [18]. Müller et al. confirmed that the extracts of guava leaves and fruits, which contain polysaccharides, polyphenols, and other bioactive substances, can effectively reduce intestinal glucose transport by inhibiting the function of SGLT1 in vivo [19].

An increasing number of studies have demonstrated that non-toxic biological macromolecules, especially polysaccharides, possess prominent efficacies for treating DM and other metabolic diseases [20–24]. In addition, Tang et al. reported that water-soluble polysaccharides from *Lycium barbarum* have a conspicuously inhibitory effect on glucose uptake in vitro [25], which may have been due to the inhibitory effect on the intestinal glucose transporter SGLT1. Fucoidan is a family of sulfated fucan predominantly existing in the cell walls of brown algae and several marine invertebrates (e.g., sea cucumbers and sea urchins) [26]. These water-soluble heteropolysaccharides are composed of various percentages of L-fucose and sulfate ester groups. Fucoidans from natural sources are usually composed of two types of chain structures, type I, with α (1→3)-linked fucose, and type II, made up of alternating α (1→3)- and α (1→4)-linked fucose molecules [27]. In recent years, fucoidans isolated from different sources have been extensively studied due to their diverse biological activities, including anticoagulant, anti-inflammatory, antivirus, antitumor, lipid-lowering, antidiabetic nephropathy, antimetabolic syndrome, and prebiotic effects [26,28]. Due to their promising therapeutic effects and availability from various kinds of cheap brown algae, an increasing number of studies have been devoted to the development and utilization of fucoidans in the fields of drugs and functional foods. Although the application prospects of fucoidans are promising, it is worth noting that the bioactivities of fucoidans are probably highly dependent on their structural properties (such as type of glycosidic linkages, molecular weight (MW), and branches) [26,29] and little attention has been devoted to determining the effects of fucoidans with various structure on attenuating postprandial hyperglycemia and its underlying mechanism.

We reported that fucoidan from *Fucus vesiculosus* (FvF) with a type II structure can significantly inhibit α-glucosidase and the glucose transport activities in the small intestine, and regulate glucose consumption and lipid metabolism via reactive oxygen species (ROS)-mediated c-Jun N-terminal kinase (JNK) and protein kinase B (Akt) signaling pathways, thus improving postprandial hyperglycemia in diabetic mice [30,31]. To explore the relationship between the inhibitory effect of glucose absorption and fucoidan, it is necessary to rule out the other factors related to antihyperglycemia. Therefore, we prepared three fucoidans as follows: fucoidan from *Ascophyllum nodosum* (AnF) with a type II structure [32] and mild inhibition of α-glucosidase [31], and fucoidans from *Laminaria japonica* (LjF) and *Kjellmaniella crassifolia* (KcF) with type I structures [33,34]. Additionally, we investigated the pharmacological effects of the above fucoidans on alleviating postprandial hyperglycemia using in vitro (Caco-2 monolayer model), semi-in vivo (everted gut sac model), and in vivo (oral glucose tolerance test (OGTT) in Kunming and leptin receptor-deficient (db/db) mice) assays. Based on previous studies [25,30], we also focused on evaluating the binding affinity of various fucoidans to SGLT1 via surface plasmon resonance (SPR). Taken together, as we have previously reported, FvF with a type II structure could alleviate the postprandial hyperglycemia. Thus, this study aimed to evaluate the effects of fucoidans with different types of fucosidic linkages on alleviating postprandial hyperglycemia and preliminarily elucidated the underlying mechanism.

2. Results

2.1. Physicochemical Properties of Fucoidans from Various Sources

The basic physicochemical properties of AnF, LjF, and KcF were determined and are summarized in Table 1. The sulfate content ranged from 22% to 28%, and the sulfate content of AnF was lower compared with that of LjF or KcF. The MWs of AnF and LjF were similar, which were both much lower than that of KcF ($p < 0.05$). According to our monosaccharide composition analysis, these three fucoidans were mainly composed of fucose, and the contents of fucose were similar in AnF and LjF, while KcF had a much higher fucose content ($p < 0.05$). The above results were consistent with that reported in previous literatures [32–34]. In general, the main differences between these three fucoidans were the type of glycosidic linkages, MWs, and fucose content. The bioactivities of fucoidans with various physicochemical properties can be different. Therefore, we further investigated the effects of these three fucoidans on alleviating postprandial hyperglycemia in vitro and in vivo.

Table 1. Compositions of fucoidans from various sources.

Sample	Source	Linkage Mode	SO_4^{2-} (%)	MW (kDa)	Monosaccharide Composition (%)							
					Man	GlcN	Rha	GlcA	Glc	Gal	Xyl	Fuc
AnF	*Ascophyllum nodosum*	1→3/1→4	22.7	210	7.5	0.6	0.3	3.3	8.0	3.8	17.9	58.5
LjF	*Laminaria japonica*	1→3	26.0	200	9.3	2.0	3.9	4.1	5.1	19.6	4.1	52.0
KcF	*Kjellmaniella crassifolia*	1→3	27.6	940	11.0	1.4	0.8	6.3	1.7	3.9	2.9	72.1
FvF [31]	*Fucus vesiculosus*	1→3/1→4	26.3	1039	ND	ND	ND	ND	1.0	1.9	2.3	94.8

AnF: fucoidan from *Ascophyllum nodosum*; LjF: fucoidan from *Laminaria japonica*; KcF: fucoidan from *Kjellmaniella crassifolia*; FvF: fucoidan from *Fucus vesiculosus*; MW, molecular weight; Man, mannose; GlcN, glucosamine; Rha, rhamnose; GlcA, glucuronic acid; Glc, glucose; Gal, galactose; Xyl, xylose; Fuc, fucose.

2.2. Effect of Fucoidans on Inhibiting Glucose Transport in a Caco-2 Monolayer Cell Model

Here, we used a Caco-2 monolayer cell model to evaluate the influences of various fucoidans on intestinal glucose transport. The Caco-2 monolayer cell model is a well-established in vitro model for studying the transport of substrates (e.g., glucose, nutrients, and drugs) through the intestine [35]. The prerequisite for the simulation of in vivo intestinal processes is the differentiation of the Caco-2 monolayer cell, which expresses a tissue-typical cell membrane and transport proteins. In addition, it has been verified that there is a high expression of endogenous SGLT1 in polarized Caco-2 cells [36]. As shown in Figure 1A, the transepithelial electrical resistance (TEER) value rose rapidly from 49 Ω^*cm^2 on the fourth day to about 476 Ω^*cm^2 after a 16-day incubation. Then, this cell monolayer model tended to be completed, and the resistance value changed little on the 21st day compared to that on the 16th day, which indicated that the cells started to differentiate. Moreover, the activities of alkaline phosphatase (ALP) on both sides of the transwell chamber were measured to judge the degree of cell differentiation and the success of the cell model [37]. As shown in Figure 1B, the ratio of ALP activities significantly increased to about 8 during the 21 days incubation, which indicated that the degree of differentiation in Caco-2 cells was high, and the cells displayed obvious polarization. The above results indicated that a Caco-2 monolayer cell model was successfully constructed, which was then used to study the effects of fucoidans on the transmembrane transport of glucose. The inhibitory activity of specific fucoidan on the transport of 2-Deoxy-2-[(7-nitro-2,1,3-benzoxadiazol-4-yl) amino]-D-glucose (2-NBDG) using the Caco-2 monolayer model is shown in Figure 1C. These results showed that only 400 µg/mL of an AnF solution could significantly inhibit the transport of 2-NBDG in this Caco-2 monolayer cell model compared with the Control group ($p < 0.05$), while the same concentration of LjF and KcF could not. Compared to the effects of AnF and LjF on 2-NBDG transport, our results indicate that the type of glycosidic linkages may play a crucial role in inhibiting glucose transport. In addition, both LjF and KcF had no marked effects on glucose transport in the Caco-2 monolayer cell model, which indicated that MW and fucose content may not play a pivotal role in that. We have previously reported that FvF could significantly reduce glucose transport in a Caco-2 monolayer cell mode [30]. In general, only AnF and FvF, with type II structures, could inhibit the glucose transport in a Caco-2 monolayer cell model, which indicated the importance of the type of glycosidic linkages in inhibiting glucose transport.

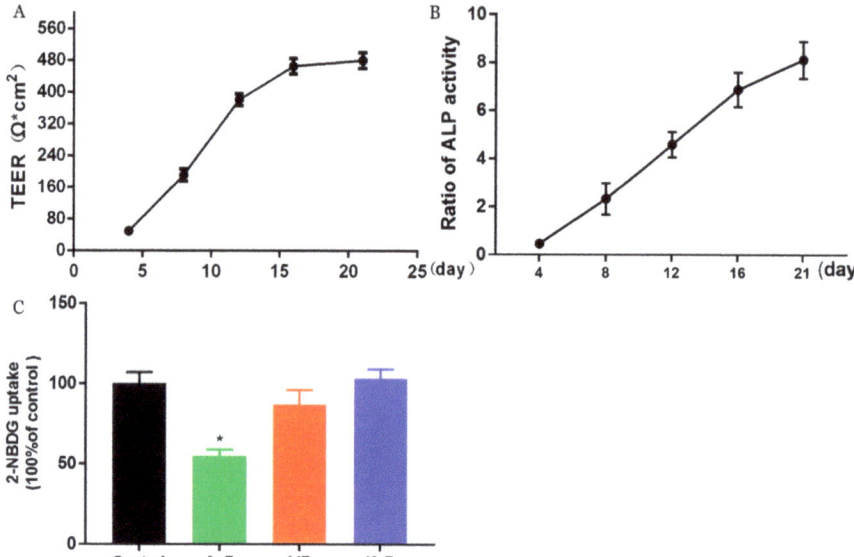

Figure 1. Inhibitory effects of fucoidans on 2-Deoxy-2-[(7-nitro-2,1,3-benzoxadiazol-4-yl) amino]-D-glucose (2-NBDG) transport in a Caco-2 monolayer cell model. The transepithelial electrical resistance (TEER) of Caco-2 monolayer cell model (**A**); alkaline phosphatase (ALP) activity ratio of Caco-2 monolayer cell model (**B**), calculated by the ratio of ALP activities on the apical side to the basolateral side; inhibitory effects of fucoidans on 2-NBDG transport (**C**). Control, Caco-2 monolayer cell model treated with HBSS buffer; *Ascophyllum nodosum* (AnF), Caco-2 monolayer cell model treated with 400 µg/mL of AnF; or *Laminaria japonica* (LjF): Caco-2 monolayer cell model treated with 400 µg/mL of LjF; *Kjellmaniella crassifolia* (KcF): Caco-2 monolayer cell model treated with 400 µg/mL of KcF. Data are expressed as the mean ± SEM. * $p < 0.05$, compared with the Control group.

2.3. Effect of Fucoidans on Intestinal Glucose Uptake Using an Everted Gut Sac Model

Glucose can be transported from the intestinal lumen into small intestinal enterocytes by SGLT1, which is located at the apical brush border [38]. SGLT1 was originally expressed on the serous side of the intestine and was moved to the outside in an everted gut sac model. Thus, the everted gut sac model can be used as an efficient semi-in vivo tool for studying substrates and drug absorption mechanisms, as well as the role of compounds on regulating SGLT1 activity in the intestine [39,40]. Therefore, the inhibition of glucose absorption was evaluated using the everted gut sac model to explore the inhibitory effect on SGLT1 activity. As shown in Figure 2, 100 µg/mL of AnF could effectively decrease the glucose absorption compared with the Control group ($p < 0.05$), and this inhibitory effect was elevated with an increased AnF concentration, while LjF and KcF showed no significant inhibitory effect in the range from 100 µg/mL to 600 µg/mL. All in all, the above results demonstrated that only AnF with a type II structure had a marked inhibition on glucose intake in a dose-dependent manner via inhibiting SGLT1 activity, which was consistent with the results in Section 2.2. Once again, the type of glycosidic linkages was shown to play an important role in suppressing glucose absorption from the intestinal lumen.

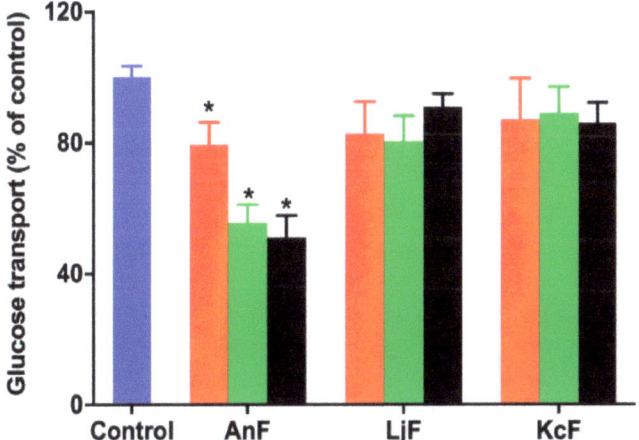

Figure 2. Inhibition rate of different concentrations of fucoidans on glucose uptake in an everted gut sac model. Control, the everted gut sac model treated with Krebs–Ringer bicarbonate buffer; AnF, the everted gut sac model treated with various concentrations of AnF; LjF, the everted gut sac model treated with various concentrations of LjF; KcF, the everted gut sac model treated with various concentrations of KcF. Red represents the results of treatment with 100 µg/mL of specific fucoidan; green represents the results of treatment with 400 µg/mL of specific fucoidan; black represents the result of treatment with 600 µg/mL of fucoidan. Data are expressed as the mean ± SEM. * $p < 0.05$, specific concentration of AnF treated group compared with the Control group.

2.4. Effects of Fucoidans on OGTT in Kunming Mice

Intestinal glucose absorption is mediated by SGLT1 [41]. First, the carbohydrates in food are degraded to monosaccharides (such as glucose, galactose, etc.) through the action of various glycosidases. Next, glucose is then transported into the cells on the mucosal side by SGLT1. In addition, it has been confirmed that fucoidans have a certain inhibitory effect on α-glucosidase [42] and cannot be digested by gastric and pancreatic enzymes [43]. Therefore, the OGTT was used to explore the inhibitory effects of fucoidans on glucose absorption via inhibiting SGLT1 activity, which can avoid the influence of glucosidase. As shown in Figure 3, the administration of 200 mg/kg of AnF effectively suppressed the elevation in the postprandial blood glucose level and the areas under curve after glucose loading in Kunming mice compared with the Control group ($p < 0.05$), while LjF and KcF treatments could not. The above results verified the efficient decrease in postprandial blood glucose conferred by AnF treatment, as compared to LjF and KcF in Kunming mice, which was consistent with our results from in vitro and semi-in vivo assays (shown in Sections 2.2 and 2.3). Thus, we further investigated and evaluated the hypoglycemic effect of AnF in db/db mice.

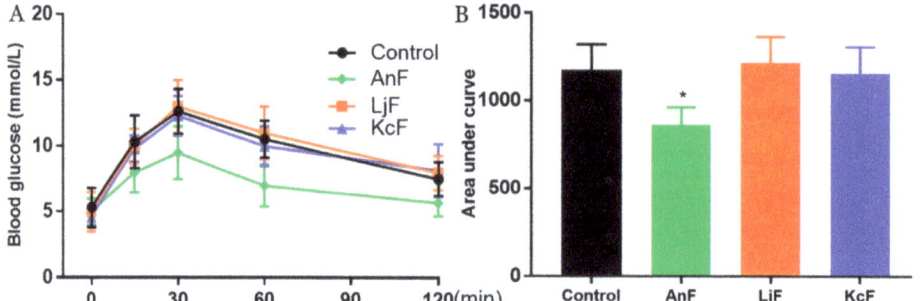

Figure 3. Effects of fucoidans on the oral glucose tolerance test (OGTT) in Kunming mice. Curve of OGTT (**A**) and area under curve (**B**). Control, Kunming mice gavaged with PBS; AnF, Kunming mice gavaged with 200 mg/kg of AnF; LjF: Kunming mice gavaged with 200 mg/kg of LjF; KcF: Kunming mice gavaged with 200 mg/kg of KcF. Data are expressed as the mean ± SEM. * $p < 0.05$, compared with the Control group. Six mice of each group were analyzed.

2.5. Effects of AnF on the OGTT in db/db Mice

OGTT is the gold standard for DM diagnosis [44] and is used to evaluate the function of β cells and the individual ability to regulate postprandial blood glucose levels. Thus, a glucose solution was gavaged after 15 h of fasting at the end of a 4-week feeding trial in db/db mice. The AnF group showed remarkable suppression of OGTT and the area under curve in db/db mice ($p < 0.05$), which was comparable to the effects of metformin (Metf) (Figure 4). This result indicated that AnF can improve blood glucose homeostasis in mice with diabetes.

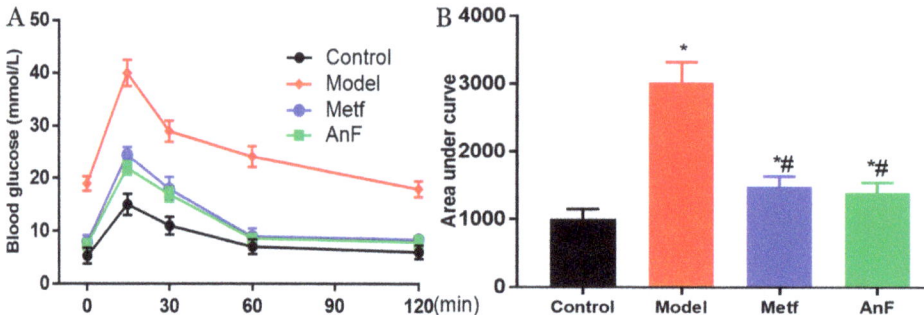

Figure 4. Effects of AnF on OGTT in leptin receptor-deficient (db/db) mice. Curve of OGTT (**A**) and area under curve (**B**). Control, C57BL/6J mice; Model, db/db mice; metformin (Metf), db/db mice with 200 mg/kg/d of metformin; AnF: db/db mice with 200 mg/kg/d of AnF. Data are expressed as the mean ± SEM. * $p < 0.05$, compared with the Control group; # $p < 0.05$, compared with the Model group. Six mice of each group were analyzed.

2.6. Effects of AnF on Body Weight in db/db Mice

During the 4-weeks feeding trial, db/db mice gained much more weight compared to normal C57BL/6J mice ($p < 0.05$) (Figure 5), while both AnF and metformin induced a trend of weight loss in db/db mice. In addition, another study in our lab showed that AnF significantly reduced the body weight gain of mice, which were fed with a high-fat diet [28]. The above results indicated that AnF could effectively lower the body weight in mice with DM.

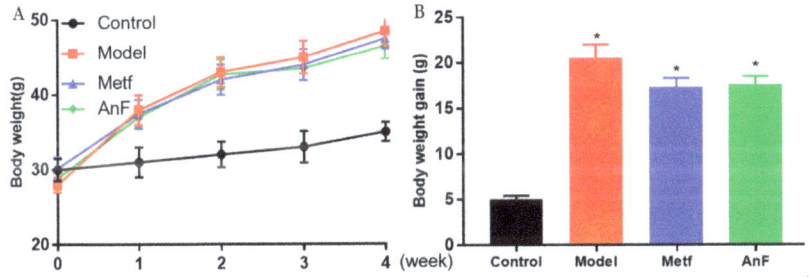

Figure 5. Effect of AnF on body weight change in db/db mice. Body weight change (**A**) and body weight gain (**B**). Control, C57BL/6J mice; Model, db/db mice; Metf, db/db mice with 200 mg/kg/d of metformin; AnF, db/db with 200 mg/kg/d AnF. Data are expressed as the mean ± SEM. * $p < 0.05$, compared with the Control group. Six mice of each group were analyzed.

2.7. Effects of AnF on Glucose-Insulin Homeostasis in db/db Mice

DM is characterized by hyperglycemia and systemic insulin resistance [45]. Thus, we investigated the effect of AnF on glucose-insulin homeostasis in db/db mice. As shown in Figure 6A, AnF significantly alleviated fasting hyperglycemia compared with the Model group ($p < 0.05$). The administration of AnF as well as metformin, resulted in an effective decrease in hemoglobin A1c (HbA1c) level ($p < 0.05$) compared with the Model group (Figure 6B), which indicated that AnF had a long-term effect on alleviating hyperglycemia. As shown in Figure 6C,D, the results showed the significant effect of AnF on suppressing hyperinsulinemia and lowering the homeostasis model assessment-insulin resistance (HOMA-IR) index in db/db mice ($p < 0.05$). All of these analyses confirmed the glucose–insulin homeostasis effects of AnF in db/db mice.

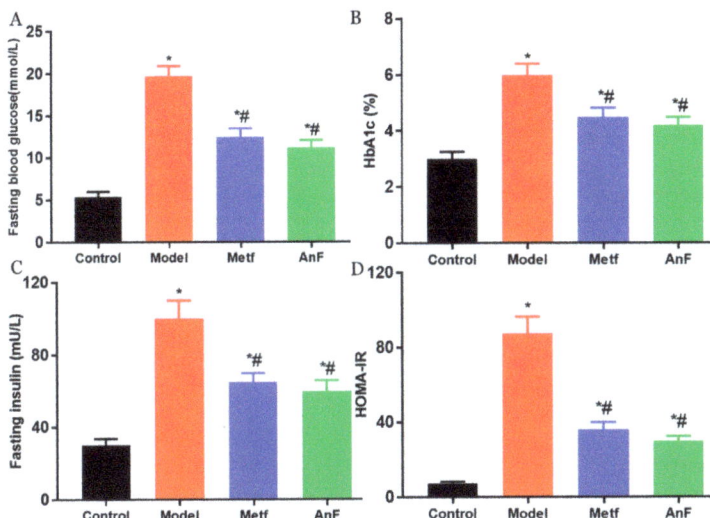

Figure 6. Effects of AnF on glucose-insulin homeostasis in db/db mice. Fasting blood glucose (**A**); hemoglobin A1c (HbA1c) (**B**); Fasting insulin (**C**); homeostasis model assessment-insulin resistance (HOMAI-IR) (**D**). Control, C57BL/6J mice; Model, db/db mice; Metf, db/db mice with 200 mg/kg/d of metformin; AnF, db/db with 200 mg/kg/d AnF. Data are expressed as the mean ± SEM. * $p < 0.05$, compared with the Control group; # $p < 0.05$, compared with the Model group. Six mice of each group were analyzed.

2.8. Effects of AnF on GLP-1 Level in db/db Mice

Increasingly, studies have demonstrated that SGLT1 in the intestine serves as a sensor for the acute glucose-induced GLP-1 secretion [46,47]. The short-term inhibition of SGLT1 in the intestine can delay the absorption of glucose, and this unabsorbed glucose can stimulate L cells to secrete GLP-1 [48,49]. GLP-1 can act on pancreatic β cells to increase insulin release in a glucose-dependent manner and decrease pancreatic glucagon secretion, which both contribute to the antihyperglycemic effect [50]. Studies have indicated that the inhibition of SGLT1 in the intestine can not only increase the content of serum active GLP-1 (aGLP-1) level but also significantly increase the serum total GLP-1 (tGLP-1) level [51,52]. The effects of AnF on inhibiting postprandial blood glucose level by in vitro (Caco-2 monolayer model), semi-in vivo (everted gut sac model), and in vivo assays indicate that AnF can inhibit SGLT1 activity. Thus, we investigated the effect of AnF on the level of GLP-1 in db/db mice further. As shown in Figure 7, AnF effectively increased the serum content of tGLP-1 and aGLP-1 compared with the Model group, but this was still lower compared to the normal levels ($p < 0.05$), which indicated the moderate inhibition of SGLT1 by AnF can cause GLP-1 release without side effects on the digestive system.

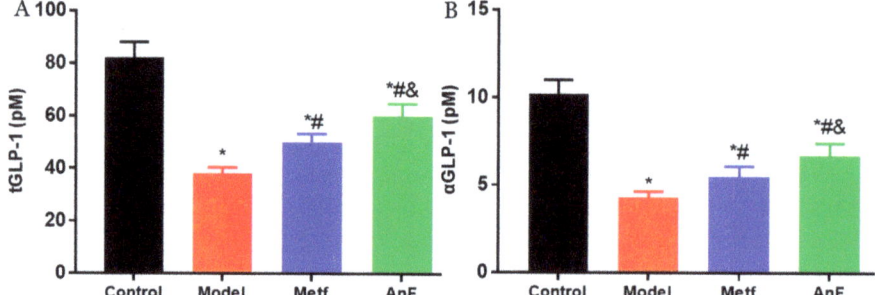

Figure 7. Effects of AnF on serum total glucagon-like peptide-1 (tGLP-1) and active GLP-1 (aGLP-1) levels in db/db mice. tGLP-1 (**A**) and aGLP-1 (**B**) levels. Control, C57BL/6J mice; Model, db/db mice; Metf, db/db mice with 200 mg/kg/d of metformin; AnF, db/db with 200 mg/kg/d AnF. Data are expressed as the mean ± SEM. * $p < 0.05$, compared with the Control group; # $p < 0.05$, compared with the Model group; and & $p < 0.05$, compared with the Metf group. Six mice of each group were analyzed.

2.9. Interaction Study between Fucoidans and SGLT1

Our in vitro and in vivo assays demonstrated that AnF could effectively decrease the glucose transport and postprandial blood glucose levels, while LjF and KcF could not, which may have been due to the various inhibitions of SGLT1 activity by fucoidans. Thus, we validated the binding affinities between these three fucoidans (AnF, LjF, and KcF) and SGLT1 protein further using SPR. The response units were recorded in real-time as sensor grams using the BIAcore system (Figure 8), and the kinetic parameters (such as the binding constant (K_a, $M^{-1}s^{-1}$), dissociation constant (Kd, 1/s), and average dissociation constant (K_D, M)) were also summarized. These results showed that AnF and FvF with type II structures bound directly to SGLT1, and the K_D was 3.4×10^{-6} M and 9.696×10^{-6} M, respectively. In contrast, no significant affinity was detected between KcF/LjF and SGLT1. Therefore, we concluded that the inhibitory effect of AnF on SGLT1 was due to the strong binding between them, which could effectively block the glucose transport capacity of SGLT1. As expected, AnF and FvF, with type II structures, bound directly to SGLT1, while KcF and LjF, with type I structures, could not, which was consistent with the effects of these respective molecules on glucose transport and postprandial blood glucose levels in vitro and in vivo assays and our previous study [30]. As SGLT1 is a crucial factor for regulating glucose transport and postprandial blood glucose levels, these data indicated that SGLT1 was probably a potential target for fucoidans with type II structure to exert the hypoglycemic effects.

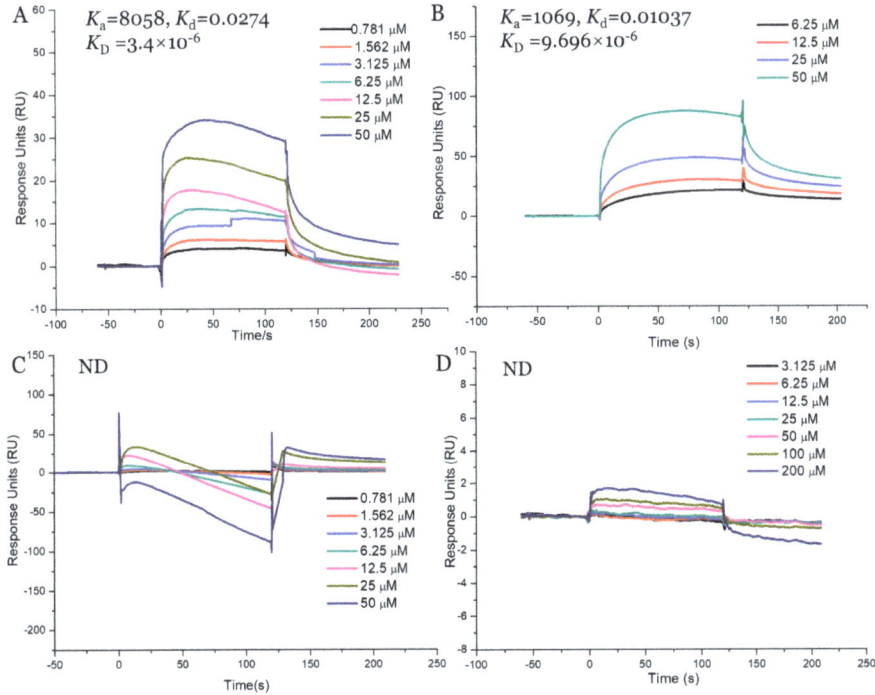

Figure 8. Surface plasmon resonance (SPR) kinetic binding analysis of the interactions of Na$^+$/glucose cotransporter 1 (SGLT1) with AnF (**A**), FvF (**B**), KcF (**C**), and LjF (**D**). ND, not detected.

3. Discussion

Postprandial hyperglycemia is a key factor in the formation and development of DM, and abnormally elevated intestinal SGLT1 activity is the main cause in DM patients with postprandial hyperglycemia. As SGLT1 is crucial for intestinal glucose absorption, important strategies in the prevention and treatment of hyperglycemia include exploring compounds with significantly inhibitory effects on SGLT1 activity [53]. In our previous studies, we found that fucoidan with a type II structure exhibited significant inhibition of α-glucosidase activity in vitro, rather than fucoidan with a type I structure [31]. In addition, AnF reduced α-glucosidase activity to about 30%, whereas the application of FvF resulted in a 90% decrease in α-glucosidase activity relative to that of the control. And we also elucidated that FvF increased glucose consumption and relieved insulin resistance via ROS-mediated JNK and Akt signaling pathways by using HepG2 cell line. In vivo, FvF could regulate lipid metabolism to attenuate metabolic syndrome [30]. For clarifying the mechanism of inhibiting glucose absorption of type II structure fucoidan, another type II fucoidan, AnF with lower α-glucosidase inhibition was used to rule out other factors. Furthermore, it is encouraging to develop potential antihyperglycemic polysaccharide compounds from natural resources. Thus, we assessed the effects of AnF (type II structure), LjF (type I structure), and KcF (type I structure) on postprandial blood glucose levels, and found that only AnF could effectively alleviate postprandial hyperglycemia. The underlying mechanism might be that only AnF and FvF, with type II structures, exhibited effective binding affinity to SGLT1 via SPR, which further indicated that fucoidans with type II structures could reduce postprandial hyperglycemia by suppression of SGLT1 activity.

SGLT1 is pivotal for the absorption of glucose in the intestinal tract [54]. The inhibitory activities of fucoidans on SGLT1 activity were evaluated by in vitro (Caco-2 monolayer model), semi-in vivo (everted gut sac model), and in vivo (OGTT in Kunming mice) assays, which demonstrated that only AnF could significantly decrease the transport of glucose by inhibiting the activity of SGLT1, while LjF and KcF could not. It has been verified that the bioactivity of fucoidans depends highly on their structural properties [21]. Both LjF and KcF had no marked effects on glucose transport, which indicated that MW and fucose content may not play a pivotal role in this ability. In addition, the various effects of AnF and LjF on glucose transport indicated that the type of fucosidic linkages may play a more crucial role. Combined with the result that FvF with a type II structure could conspicuously reduce the transport of glucose, these results indicate the importance of the type of glycosidic linkages in inhibiting glucose transport.

It was also reported that type II fucoidans could be a promising α-glucosidase inhibitor to reduce blood glucose levels [31]. Thus, OGTT was used to evaluate the effects of fucoidans on SGLT1 activity in vivo, avoiding the influence of α-glucosidase, and the absorption of glucose in the intestinal tract can only be realized through the transport of the SGLT1 protein. OGTT results in Kunming mice and db/db mice further confirmed the effect of AnF on decreasing postprandial blood glucose, improving glucose tolerance and insulin sensitivity. In addition, AnF with a type II structure effectively increased the GLP-1 levels, which further confirmed the inhibition of AnF on SGLT1 [51,52]. Moreover, fucoidans cannot be digested by gastric enzymes in the gastrointestinal tract and exhibit extremely low bioavailability after oral administration [43], which indicated that fucoidans, with type II structures, can play an effective and lasting role in inhibiting SGLT1 activity in vivo. Additionally, it has been reported that the in vivo effect of fucoidan on blood coagulation was not obvious, probably due to its low intestinal absorption [55]. However, it is necessary to assess the cytotoxicity and blood-thinning properties (e.g., activated partial thromboplastin time (APTT)) of various fucoidans for developing as potential nutraceuticals or dietary supplements for treating the hyperglycemia. All in all, we will pay more attention to the toxicity of various fucoidans in future studies.

4. Materials and Methods

4.1. Preparation of Fucoidans

Three different brown seaweeds, *Ascophyllum nodosum* (collected from the Irish Sea), *Laminaria Japonica* (collected from the South China Sea), and *Kjellmaniella crassifolia* (collected from the South China Sea), were purchased from Kunshan Yihong Seaweed Co. Ltd. (Kunshan, Jiangsu, China). The extraction and purification processes of AnF, LjF, and KcF were carried out according to the method, as previously described [30,56]. Briefly, brown algae were dried, powdered, and then pass through a 12-mesh net, followed by delipidating (60 °C, 4 h, 95% ethanol, 1:20) and two cycles of extraction with double-distilled water (ddH$_2$O) (80 °C, 3 h, 1:20). After centrifugation at 5000 rpm for 10 min, the supernatants were combined and concentrated, and then anhydrous ethanol was added to achieve a final concentration of 80%, and the supernatants were left overnight at 4 °C. After centrifugation at 5000 rpm for 10 min, the crude fucoidans were obtained. Then, the precipitate was redissolved in ddH$_2$O, and 3 M of CaCl$_2$ solution was added to remove alginate completely until no precipitation occurred. The solution was centrifuged at 8000 rpm for 10 min to remove precipitates, and the supernatant containing fucoidan was dialyzed in a dialysis bag with a 7000 Da MW cutoff, then lyophilized to obtain the refined fucoidans. Chemicals reagents were obtained from the Sigma Chemical Co. (Sigma–Aldrich, St. Louis, MO, USA) unless otherwise stated.

4.2. Physicochemical Properties Analysis of Fucoidans

The sulfate content was determined by the BaCl$_2$-gelatin method as follows [57]. Fucoidan (3 mg/mL) was degraded in 1 M of HCl at 110 °C for 6 h, then the absorbance of the degraded solution was determined at 400 nm after mixing with an equal volume of BaCl$_2$-gelatin. The sulfate content was calculated based on a standard curve, which was established with a Na$_2$SO$_4$ standard. The monosaccharide composition was analyzed with the acid hydrolysis method described previously [58]. In brief, the monosaccharide composition was determined using a 1-phenyl-3-methyl-5-pyrazolone precolumn derivatization HPLC on an

Agilent Eclipse XDB-C18 Column (Agilent, Santa Clara, CA, USA). Sample (10 μL) was eluted with 0.1 mol/L phosphate buffer (pH 6.7) and acetonitrile (83:17 volume fraction) at a flow rate of 1 mL/min at 30 °C. Then, a UV detector was used to detect the signal at 245 nm. MW was determined using high-performance gel permeation chromatography coupled with a multi-angle laser light scattering instrument. The MWs of fucoidans were determined using an Agilent 1260 HPLC system (Agilent Technologies, CA, USA) on the Shodex Ohpak SB-HQ 804 column in series with an SB-HQ 803 column (TosoHaas Corp., Tosoh, Japan) detected with a Wyatt Dawn Heleos II multi-angle laser scattering system (Wyatt Technology, Santa Barbara, CA, USA) and refractive index detector. One hundred microliters of sample was eluted with 0.1 M of Na_2SO_4 solution at a flow rate of 0.6 mL/min at 35 °C. MWs were calculated using Astra 5.3.4.20 software (Wyatt Technology, Santa Barbara, CA, USA). The type of glycosidic linkages of fucoidans was determined by the published papers, i.e., FvF (31), AnF (32), KcF (33), and LjF (34).

4.3. Effects of Fucoidans on Glucose Absorption Using Caco-2 Monolayer Model

The inhibitory effects of fucoidans on glucose uptake in vitro were measured using a human colon cancer cell line monolayer model (Caco-2 cells, from the Cell Bank of the Chinese Academy of Sciences, Shanghai, China) incubated with 2-NBDG (MedChem Express, Monmouth, NJ, USA) in various conditions. Caco-2 cells were cultured in Dulbecco's Modified Eagle Medium (DMEM) with 10% FBS, 1% penicillin/streptomycin, 25 mM HEPES, and 0.35 g/L sodium bicarbonate (Gibco, Carlsbad, CA, USA) at 37 °C with 5% CO_2. A Caco-2 monolayer model was established as follows [59]. Briefly, Caco-2 cells were adjusted to 2×10^5 cells/mL, and 100 μL of this cell suspension was inoculated in the upper layer of a transwell compartment (0.4 μm, 1.12 cm^2, PET) (Corning Inc., Corning, NY, USA) and incubated at 37 °C for 2 min. Then, 500 μL of DMEM was added to the upper layer, while 1.5 mL DMEM was added to the lower layer for Caco-2 cells to differentiate into enterocyte-like cells at 37 °C. Then, the TEER was measured, which could evaluate the integrity of the Caco-2 monolayer cells. In addition, another index to evaluate the successful construction of the Caco-2 monolayer model was to determine the ALP activity ratio of the apical side to the basolateral side. In the Caco-2 monolayer cell model, the apical side located to the upper side of the transwell had higher ALP activity, while the basolateral side located to the lower side had lower ALP activity. The enzyme activities of both sides of the transwell were measured using the ALP ELISA kit (Shanghai Enzyme-linked Biotechnology Co. Ltd., Shanghai, China) according to the manufacturer's recommended protocol on the 4th, 8th, 12th, 16th, and 21st-day post-induction, respectively. Then, the ALP activity ratio was calculated. The 2-NBDG uptake in the Caco-2 monolayer model was conducted as previously described [60]. Briefly, the culture medium was removed from each well and replaced with 100 μL of HBSS buffer in the presence of 2-NBDG (100 μM) or 2-NBDG (100 μM) together with 400 μg/mL of specific fucoidan. Then the cells were incubated at 37 °C for 30 min. Finally, the fluorescence intensity (Ex/Em = 485/535 nm) in the lower layer was measured using a Spark 10M (Tecan Trading AG, Männedorf, Switzerland).

4.4. Effects of Fucoidans on OGTT in Kunming Mice and Glucose Transport Using Everted Gut Sac Model

An everted gut sac model was established as previously described [40]. Briefly, six-week-old male Kunming mice were purchased from the Vital River Laboratory Animal Technology Co. Ltd. (Beijing, China). The mice were raised in ventilated cages, maintained in a light-dark cycle of 12 h at 23 °C–25 °C, with free access to water and food. After a two-week adaptive period, the mice were randomly divided into four groups of six each. OGTT was performed as follows [61,62]. The mice of each group were fasted for 15 h, then the experimental groups were given the specific fucoidan by gavage at a dose of 200 mg/kg, while the Control group was given the same volume of saline. Then, mice were given a 20% glucose solution at a dose of 2 g/kg by oral gavage in 15 min. Next, blood glucose levels were detected using a standard glucometer (Johnson & Johnson, New Brunswick, NJ, USA) at 0, 30, 60, 90, and 120 min by cutting the tail tip. In addition, the increment of plasma glucose following glucose loading was expressed in terms of the area under curve, using the trapezoidal rule. The jejunum was separated from the Kunming mice one week after the OGTT experiment. Mice were euthanized by pentobarbital sodium injection (80 mg/kg) accompanied by isoflurane inhalation to maintain anesthesia. The jejunum was cut into 5-cm segments and quickly transferred into cold Krebs–Ringer buffer in the state of oxygen maintenance. Due to the overturning of the intestinal sac, SGLT1 protein originally on the serosal side moved to the outside, so the intestinal epithelial cells could absorb glucose from the outside to the inside in. Thus, Krebs–Ringer buffer was injected into the intestinal capsule of the everted gut sac model, then placed in Krebs–Ringer buffer (containing 30 mM D-glucose) with various concentrations of specific fucoidan in the experimental groups, while the group treated with Krebs–Ringer buffer (containing 30 mM D-glucose) was used as the Control. After incubation for 30 min at 37 °C, the glucose concentrations of the inside and outside of the intestinal capsule were determined using the glucose oxidase-peroxidase method with a glucose oxidase kit (Applygen Technologies Inc., Beijing, China) [63]. Additionally, the glucose intake ratio was calculated by the glucose concentration of the inside, divided by the glucose concentration of the outside. All animal procedures were approved by the Committee of Experimental Animals of School of Medicine and Pharmacy, Ocean University of China (OUCSMP-18081201), and conformed to the Guide for the Care and Use of Laboratory Animals published by the United States National Institutes of Health (NIH Publication No 85-23, revised 1996).

4.5. Effects of AnF on Alleviating Hyperglycemia in db/db Mice

Briefly, eight-week-old male db/db mice were provided by the Model Animal Research Center of Nanjing University (Nanjing, China). In addition, eight-week-old male C57BL/6J mice were purchased from the Vital River Laboratory Animal Technology Co. Ltd. (Beijing, China) as a Control group. The mice were raised as described in the methods in Section 4.4. After a two-week acclimation period, the db/db mice were randomly divided into three groups as follows, with six mice in each group: the Metf and AnF groups received either metformin (200 mg/kg/d dissolved in saline) or AnF (200 mg/kg/d dissolved in saline) by gavage for four weeks, while the Model group was given an equal amount of saline. Body weights were measured every week. OGTT was conducted at the end of the trial as follows: mice were fasted for 15 h, and the fasting blood glucose levels were detected. Then, the mice were given a 20% glucose solution by gavage at a dose of 2 g/kg body weight. The changes in blood glucose levels were detected, as described in Section 4.4. All animal procedures were approved by the Committee of Experimental Animals of School of Medicine and Pharmacy, Ocean University of China (OUCSMP-18081201), and conformed to the Guide for the Care and Use of Laboratory Animals published by the United States National Institutes of Health (NIH Publication No 85-23, revised 1996).

4.6. Effects of AnF on Biochemical Indexes in db/db Mice

Db/db mice with various treatments were finally euthanized by pentobarbital sodium injection (80 mg/kg) accompanied by isoflurane inhalation to maintain anesthesia after being fasted for 15 h. Blood samples were collected via retro-orbital bleeding, then centrifuged at $2000\times g$ for 15 min to obtain serum for serological assays. The levels of fasting insulin and HbA1c in serum were determined using a mouse insulin ELISA kit and a mouse HbA1c ELISA kit from Omnimabs (Alhambra, CA, USA) according to the manufacturer's instructions, respectively. HOMA-IR was calculated as fasting insulin (mU/L) × fasting glucose (mM)/22.5. For tGLP-1 and aGLP-1 contents detection, a DPP-4 inhibitor was quickly added into the blood samples and mixed evenly. Then, the blood was centrifuged for 10 min at $2000\times g$ to obtain the supernatant for assays. The contents of tGLP-1 and aGLP-1 were determined using mouse ELISA kits (Linco, St. Charles, MO, USA) according to the manufacturer's instructions, respectively.

4.7. Binding Kinetics Analysis of Interaction between SGLT1 and Fucoidans

The binding kinetics between various fucoidans and SGLT1 protein was determined by an SPR biomacromolecule interaction analyzer BIAcore T200 (General Electric Company, Boston, MA, USA), as previously described [64,65]. After washing the surface of the CM5 chip (General Electric Company, Boston, MA, USA) with PBS-P running buffer (General Electric Company, Boston, MA, USA), the surface of the chip was activated with 0.4 M EDC/0.1 M NHS for 420 s at a flow rate of 10 μL/min. Immediately after activation, an SGLT1 solution (20 μg/mL) (ab152683, Abcam, Cambridge, UK) in sodium acetate buffer (pH 4.5) was added onto the chip surface for 30 s at a flow rate of 10 μL/min. After that, the chip surface was sealed by incubating with 1 M of ethanolamine (pH = 8.5) for 30 min. PBS-P buffer was running for at least 2 h to stabilize the baseline. To assess the real-time binding of fucoidans to SGLT1, varying concentrations of specific fucoidan were injected over the sensor chip surface at a flow-rate of 30 μL/min for 120 s, followed by another 900 s dissociation period. The sensor surface was regenerated by 0.1 mM NaOH for 10 s. The response was monitored as a function of time (sensor gram) at 25 °C and subtracted from the response of the reference surface. The binding constant (Ka), dissociation constant (K_d), and average dissociation constant ($K_D = K_d/Ka$) of the interaction between various fucoidans and SGLT1 protein could be calculated from curve fitting. Kinetic parameters were evaluated using the BIAcore T200 evaluation software 3.1 (General Electric Company, Boston, MA, USA).

4.8. Statistical Analysis

Data are presented as the mean ± standard error of the mean (SEM). The difference between groups was analyzed using SPSS software (v.20.0; IBM, Armonk, NY, USA) via one-way ANOVA with Student's *t*-test. And, Tukey's honest significant difference test was used for the analysis of multiple comparisons. Difference was considered to be statistically significant between various groups when $p < 0.05$. The results were interpreted using GraphPad Prism software (v.7.0; GraphPad Software Inc., San Diego, CA, USA).

5. Conclusions

For the first time, in vitro (Caco-2 monolayer and SPR assay), semi-in vivo (everted gut sac), and in vivo (Kunming mice and db/db mice) models were used to evaluate the effects of various fucoidans on suppressing hypoglycemia, especially postprandial hyperglycemia. Our data indicated the potential effects of AnF on the regulation of blood glucose levels by direct inhibition of glucose transport via SGLT1, therefore, remarkably reducing glucose transport and relieving postprandial hyperglycemia. In conclusion, fucoidans with type II structures (such as FvF and AnF) have the potential to be a promising candidate compound in the treatment of postprandial hyperglycemia via its direct binding to SGLT1 and inhibition of its glucose transport activity, while KcF and LjF with type I structures cannot. Our study demonstrates that the type of glycosidic linkages of fucoidans may play a more crucial role in their hypoglycemic effects via inhibiting SGLT1 activity. However, further research is still necessary to clarify the exact structure–activity relationship of fucoidans as SGLT1 inhibitors and the precise molecular binding mode between fucoidans and SGLT1 protein.

Author Contributions: X.S. performed the major experiments. X.W. performed the SPR experiment and wrote the manuscript. X.W., H.J., and C.C. revised the manuscript. X.W. and H.J. analyzed experimental data. G.Y. and J.H. conceived the project and designed the experiments. All authors have read and agreed to the published version of the manuscript.

Funding: This work was supported by the National Natural Science Foundation of China (31670811, 81991522, 81402982), National Major Science and Technology Project of China (2018ZX09735-004), NSFC-Shandong Joint Fund for Marine Science Research Centers (U1606403), Shandong Provincial Major Science and Technology Innovation Project (2018SDKJ0404), and Natural Science Foundation of Shandong Province (ZR2017BC007).

Acknowledgments: The authors are grateful to all members of the laboratory for their continuous technical advice and helpful discussion.

Conflicts of Interest: The authors declare no competing financial interest.

Abbreviations

DM: diabetes mellitus; SGLT1: Na$^+$/glucose cotransporter 1; OGTT: oral glucose tolerance test; AnF: fucoidan from *Ascophyllum nodosum*; KcF: fucoidan from *Kjellmaniella crassifolia*; LjF: fucoidan from *Laminaria japonica*; 2-NBDG: 2-Deoxy-2-[(7-nitro-2,1,3-benzoxadiazol-4-yl) amino]-D-glucose; SPR: surface plasmon resonance; ALP: alkaline phosphatase; GLP-1: glucagon-like peptide 1; DPP-4: dipeptidyl peptidase 4; aGLP-1: active GLP-1; tGLP-1: total GLP-1; HOMA-IR: homeostasis model assessment-insulin resistance; HbA1c: hemoglobin A1c; ddH2O: double-distilled water; DMEM: Dulbecco's Modified Eagle Medium; TEER: transepithelial electrical resistance; MEM: minimum Eagle's medium; BSA: bovine serum albumin; FvF: fucoidan from *Fucus vesiculosus*, MW: molecular weight; UAs: uronic acids; DMEM: Dulbecco's Modified Eagle Medium; Metf: metformin; db/db: leptin receptor-deficient; APTT: activated partial thromboplastin time; ROS: reactive oxygen species; JNK: c-Jun N-terminal kinase; Akt: protein kinase B.

References

1. Maritim, A.C.; Sanders, R.A.; Watkins, J.B. Diabetes, oxidative stress, and antioxidants: A review. *J. Biochem. Mol. Toxicol.* **2003**, *17*, 24–38. [CrossRef]
2. DeFronzo, R.A. From the triumvirate to the ominous octet: A new paradigm for the treatment of type 2 diabetes mellitus. *Diabetes* **2009**, *58*, 773–795. [CrossRef]
3. Loghmani, E. Diabetes mellitus: Type 1 and type 2. In *Guidelines for Adolescent Nutrition Services*; Scientific Research Publishing: Irvine, CA, USA, 2005; pp. 167–182.
4. Heo, S.J.; Hwang, J.Y.; Choi, J.I.; Han, J.S.; Kim, H.J.; Jeon, Y.J. Diphlorethohydroxycarmalol isolated from *Ishige okamurae*, a brown algae, a potent α-glucosidase and α-amylase inhibitor, alleviates postprandial hyperglycemia in diabetic mice. *Eur. J. Pharmacol.* **2009**, *615*, 252–256. [CrossRef] [PubMed]
5. Rizzo, M.; Rizvi, A.A.; Spinas, G.A.; Rini, G.B.; Berneis, K. Glucose lowering and anti-atherogenic effects of incretin-based therapies: GLP-1 analogues and DPP-4-inhibitors. *Expert Opin. Investig. Drugs* **2009**, *18*, 1495–1503. [CrossRef] [PubMed]
6. MacDonald, P.E.; El-kholy, W.; Riedel, M.J.; Salapatek, A.M.F.; Light, P.E.; Wheeler, M.B. The multiple actions of GLP-1 on the process of glucose-stimulated insulin secretion. *Diabetes* **2002**, *51*, 434–442. [CrossRef] [PubMed]
7. Katsuno, K.; Fujimori, Y.; Takemura, Y.; Hiratochi, M.; Itoh, F.; Komatsu, Y.; Fujikura, H.; Isaji, M. Sergliflozin, a novel selective inhibitor of low-affinity sodium glucose cotransporter (SGLT2), validates the critical role of SGLT2 in renal glucose reabsorption and modulates plasma glucose level. *J. Pharmacol. Exp. Ther.* **2007**, *320*, 323–330. [CrossRef]
8. Dobbins, R.L.; Greenway, F.L.; Chen, L.; Liu, Y.; Breed, S.L.; Andrews, S.M.; Wald, J.A.; Walker, A.; Smith, C.D. Selective sodium-dependent glucose transporter 1 inhibitors block glucose absorption and impair glucose-dependent insulinotropic peptide release. *Am. J. Physiol.-Gastr. Liver Physiol.* **2015**, *308*, 946–954. [CrossRef]
9. Tahrani, A.A.; Bailey, C.J.; Del Prato, S.; Barnett, A.H. Management of type 2 diabetes: New and future developments in treatment. *Lancet* **2011**, *378*, 182–197. [CrossRef]
10. Guthrie, R.M. Evolving therapeutic options for type 2 diabetes mellitus: An overview. *Postgrad. Med.* **2012**, *124*, 82–89. [CrossRef]
11. Deng, R. A review of the hypoglycemic effects of five commonly used herbal food supplements. *Recent Pat. Food Nutr. Agric.* **2012**, *4*, 50–60. [CrossRef]
12. Fawaz, A.; Hoi-Man, C.; Preedy, V.R.; Sharp, P.A. Regulation of glucose transporter expression in human intestinal Caco-2 cells following exposure to an anthocyanin-rich berry extract. *PLoS ONE* **2013**, *8*, e78932.
13. Manzano, S.; Williamson, G. Polyphenols and phenolic acids from strawberry and apple decrease glucose uptake and transport by human intestinal Caco-2 cells. *Mol. Nutr. Food Res.* **2010**, *54*, 1773–1780. [CrossRef] [PubMed]
14. Schulze, C.; Bangert, A.; Kottra, G.; Geillinger, K.E.; Schwanck, B.; Vollert, H.; Blaschek, W.; Daniel, H. Inhibition of the intestinal sodium-coupled glucose transporter 1 (SGLT1) by extracts and polyphenols from apple reduces postprandial blood glucose levels in mice and humans. *Mol. Nutr. Food Res.* **2014**, *58*, 1795–1808. [CrossRef] [PubMed]
15. Vrhovac, I.; Eror, D.B.; Klessen, D.; Burger, C.; Breljak, D.; Kraus, O.; Radović, N.; Jadrijević, S.; Aleksic, I.; Walles, T. Localizations of Na$^+$-D-glucose cotransporters SGLT1 and SGLT2 in human kidney and of SGLT1 in human small intestine, liver, lung, and heart. *Pflügers Arch.-Eur. J. Physiol.* **2015**, *467*, 1881–1898. [CrossRef] [PubMed]

16. Martín, M.G.; Turk, E.; Lostao, M.P.; Kerner, C.; Wright, E.M. Defects in Na$^+$/glucose cotransporter (SGLT1) trafficking and function cause glucose-galactose malabsorption. *Nat. Genet.* **1996**, *12*, 216–220. [CrossRef]
17. Turk, E.; Zabel, B.; Mundlos, S.; Dyer, J.; Wright, E. Glucose/galactose malabsorption caused by a defect in the Na$^+$/glucose cotransporter. *Nature* **1991**, *350*, 354–356. [CrossRef]
18. Ina, S.; Hamada, A.; Nakamura, H.; Yamaguchi, Y.; Kumagai, H.; Kumagai, H. Rice (*Oryza sativa japonica*) albumin hydrolysates suppress postprandial blood glucose elevation by adsorbing glucose and inhibiting Na$^+$-d-glucose cotransporter SGLT1 expression. *J. Funct. Foods* **2020**, *64*, 103603. [CrossRef]
19. Müller, U.; Stübl, F.; Schwarzinger, B.; Sandner, G.; Iken, M.; Himmelsbach, M.; Schwarzinger, C.; Ollinger, N.; Stadlbauer, V.; Höglinger, O. In vitro and in vivo inhibition of intestinal glucose transport by guava (*Psidium guajava*) extracts. *Mol. Nutr. Food Res.* **2018**, *62*, 1701012. [CrossRef]
20. Wang, P.C.; Zhao, S.; Yang, B.Y.; Wang, Q.H.; Kuanga, H.X. Anti-diabetic polysaccharides from natural sources: A review. *Carbohydr. Polym.* **2016**, *148*, 86–97. [CrossRef]
21. Wang, X.L.; Wang, X.; Jiang, H.; Cai, C.; Li, G.Y.; Hao, J.J.; Yu, G.L. Marine polysaccharides attenuate metabolic syndrome by fermentation products and altering gut microbiota: An overview. *Carbohydr. Polym.* **2018**, *195*, 601–612. [CrossRef]
22. Wang, X.L.; Yang, Z.M.; Xu, X.; Jiang, H.; Cai, C.; Yu, G.L. Odd-numbered agaro-oligosaccharides alleviate type 2 diabetes mellitus and related colonic microbiota dysbiosis in mice. *Carbohydr. Polym.* **2020**, *240*, 116261. [CrossRef] [PubMed]
23. Wang, X.L.; Jiang, H.; Zhang, N.; Cai, C.; Li, G.Y.; Hao, J.J.; Yu, G.L. Anti-diabetic activities of agaropectin-derived oligosaccharides from *Gloiopeltis furcata* via regulation of mitochondrial function. *Carbohydr. Polym.* **2020**, *229*, 115482. [CrossRef] [PubMed]
24. Necyk, C.; Zubach-Cassano, L. Natural health products and diabetes: A practical review. *Can. J. Diabetes* **2017**, *41*, 642–647. [CrossRef] [PubMed]
25. Tang, H.L.; Chen, C.; Wang, S.K.; Sun, G.J. Biochemical analysis and hypoglycemic activity of a polysaccharide isolated from the fruit of *Lycium barbarum* L. *Int. J. Biol. Macromol.* **2015**, *77*, 235–242. [CrossRef] [PubMed]
26. Li, B.; Lu, F.; Wei, X.J.; Zhao, R.X. Fucoidan: Structure and bioactivity. *Molecules* **2008**, *13*, 1671–1695. [CrossRef] [PubMed]
27. Albana, C.; Ushakova, N.A.; Preobrazhenskaya, M.E.; Armida, D.I.; Antonio, P.; Licia, T.; Nicola, T.; Morozevich, G.E.; Berman, A.E.; Bilan, M.I. A comparative study of the anti-inflammatory, anticoagulant, antiangiogenic, and antiadhesive activities of nine different fucoidans from brown seaweeds. *Glycobiology* **2007**, *17*, 541–552.
28. Shang, Q.S.; Song, G.R.; Zhang, M.F.; Shi, J.J.; Xu, C.Y.; Hao, J.J.; Li, G.Y.; Yu, G.L. Dietary fucoidan improves metabolic syndrome in association with increased *Akkermansia* population in the gut microbiota of high-fat diet-fed mice. *J. Funct. Foods* **2017**, *28*, 138–146. [CrossRef]
29. Shang, Q.S.; Shan, X.D.; Cai, C.; Hao, J.J.; Li, G.Y.; Yu, G.L. Dietary fucoidan modulates the gut microbiota in mice by increasing the abundance of *Lactobacillus* and *Ruminococcaceae*. *Food Funct.* **2016**, *7*, 3224–3232. [CrossRef]
30. Wang, X.L.; Shan, X.D.; Dun, Y.L.; Cai, C.; Hao, J.J.; Li, G.Y.; Cui, K.Y.; Yu, G.L. Anti-metabolic syndrome effects of fucoidan from *Fucus vesiculosus* via reactive oxygen species-mediated regulation of JNK, Akt, and AMPK signaling. *Molecules* **2019**, *24*, 3319. [CrossRef]
31. Shan, X.D.; Liu, X.; Hao, J.J.; Cai, C.; Fan, F.; Dun, Y.L.; Zhao, X.L.; Liu, X.X.; Li, C.X.; Yu, G.L. In vitro and in vivo hypoglycemic effects of brown algal fucoidans. *Int. J. Biol. Macromol.* **2016**, *82*, 249–255. [CrossRef]
32. Foley, S.A.; Szegezdi, E.; Mulloy, B.; Samali, A.; Tuohy, M.G. An unfractionated fucoidan from *Ascophyllum nodosum*: Extraction, characterization, and apoptotic effects in vitro. *J. Nat. Prod.* **2011**, *74*, 1851–1861. [CrossRef] [PubMed]
33. Wu, J.D.; Lv, Y.J.; Liu, X.X.; Zhao, X.L.; Jiao, G.L.; Tai, W.J.; Wang, P.P.; Zhao, X.; Cai, C.; Yu, G.L. Structural study of sulfated fuco-oligosaccharide branched glucuronomannan from *Kjellmaniella crassifolia* by ESI-CID-MS/MS. *J. Carbohydr. Chem.* **2015**, *34*, 303–317. [CrossRef]
34. Wang, J.; Zhang, Q.B.; Zhang, Z.S.; Song, H.F.; Li, P.C. Potential antioxidant and anticoagulant capacity of low molecular weight fucoidan fractions extracted from *Laminaria japonica*. *Int. J. Biol. Macromol.* **2010**, *46*, 6–12. [CrossRef] [PubMed]
35. Hilgers, A.R.; Conradi, R.A.; Burton, P.S. Caco-2 cell monolayers as a model for drug transport across the intestinal mucosa. *Pharm. Res.* **1990**, *7*, 902–910. [CrossRef] [PubMed]

36. Kipp, H.; Khoursandi, S.; Scharlau, D.; Kinne, R.K. More than apical: Distribution of SGLT1 in Caco-2 cells. *Am. J. Physiol.-Cell Physiol.* **2003**, *285*, 737–749. [CrossRef]
37. Matsumoto, H.; Erickson, R.H.; Gum, J.R.; Yoshioka, M.; Gum, E.; Kim, Y.S. Biosynthesis of alkaline phosphatase during differentiation of the human colon cancer cell line Caco-2. *Gastroenterology* **1990**, *98*, 1199–1207. [CrossRef]
38. Wright, E.M. Intestinal sugar transport. In *Physiology of the Gastrointestinal Tract*; Academic Press: Manhattan, NY, USA, 1994; pp. 1751–1772.
39. Alam, M.A.; Al-Jenoobi, F.I.; Al-mohizea, A.M. Everted gut sac model as a tool in pharmaceutical research: Limitations and applications. *J. Pharm. Pharmacol.* **2012**, *64*, 326–336. [CrossRef]
40. Hamilton, K.L.; Butt, A.G. Glucose transport into everted sacs of the small intestine of mice. *Adv. Physiol. Educ.* **2013**, *37*, 415–426. [CrossRef]
41. Röder, P.V.; Geillinger, K.E.; Zietek, T.S.; Thorens, B.; Koepsell, H.; Daniel, H. The role of SGLT1 and GLUT2 in intestinal glucose transport and sensing. *PLoS ONE* **2014**, *9*, e89977. [CrossRef]
42. Kim, K.T.; Rioux, L.E.; Turgeon, S.L. Alpha-amylase and alpha-glucosidase inhibition is differentially modulated by fucoidan obtained from *Fucus vesiculosus* and *Ascophyllum nodosum*. *Phytochemistry* **2014**, *98*, 27–33. [CrossRef]
43. Nagamine, T.; Nakazato, K.; Tomioka, S.; Iha, M.; Nakajima, K. Intestinal absorption of fucoidan extracted from the brown seaweed, *Cladosiphon okamuranus*. *Mar. Drugs* **2015**, *13*, 48–64. [CrossRef] [PubMed]
44. Alberti, K.G.M.M.; Zimmet, P.Z. Definition, diagnosis and classification of diabetes mellitus and its complications. Part 1: Diagnosis and classification of diabetes mellitus. Provisional report of a WHO consultation. *Diabet. Med.* **1998**, *15*, 539–553. [CrossRef]
45. McCulloch, D.K.; Robertson, R.P. *Pathogenesis of Type 2 Diabetes Mellitus*; UpTo-Date [consultado 12 Fev 2013]; Available online: http://www.uptodate.com/contents/pathogenesis-of-type-2-diabetes-mellitus (accessed on 10 October 2019).
46. Gribble, F.M. The gut endocrine system as a coordinator of postprandial nutrient homoeostasis. *Proc. Nutr. Soc.* **2012**, *71*, 456–462. [CrossRef] [PubMed]
47. Moriya, R.; Shirakura, T.; Ito, J.; Mashiko, S.; Seo, T. Activation of sodium-glucose cotransporter 1 ameliorates hyperglycemia by mediating incretin secretion in mice. *Am. J. Physiol.-Endocrinol. Metab.* **2009**, *297*, 1358–1365. [CrossRef]
48. Baggio, L.L.; Drucker, D.J. Biology of Incretins: GLP-1 and GIP. *Gastroenterology* **2007**, *132*, 2131–2157. [CrossRef]
49. Hjøllund, K.R.; Deacon, C.F.; Holst, J.J. Dipeptidyl peptidase-4 inhibition increases portal concentrations of intact glucagon-like peptide-1 (GLP-1) to a greater extent than peripheral concentrations in anaesthetised pigs. *Diabetologia* **2011**, *54*, 2206–2208. [CrossRef]
50. Drucker, D.J. Incretin action in the pancreas: Potential promise, possible perils, and pathological pitfalls. *Diabetes* **2013**, *62*, 3316–3323. [CrossRef]
51. Powell, D.R.; Smith, M.; Greer, J.; Harris, A.; Zhao, S.; Dacosta, C.; Mseeh, F.; Shadoan, M.K.; Sands, A.; Zambrowicz, B. LX4211 increases serum glucagon-like peptide 1 and peptide YY levels by reducing sodium/glucose cotransporter 1 (SGLT1)-mediated absorption of intestinal glucose. *J. Pharmacol. Exp. Ther.* **2013**, *345*, 250–259. [CrossRef]
52. Shibazaki, T.; Tomae, M.; Ishikawa-Takemura, Y.; Fushimi, N.; Itoh, F.; Yamada, M.; Isaji, M. KGA-2727, a novel selective inhibitor of a high-affinity sodium glucose cotransporter (SGLT1), exhibits antidiabetic efficacy in rodent models. *J. Pharmacol. Exp. Ther.* **2012**, *342*, 288–296. [CrossRef]
53. Timo, R.; Volker, V. Development of SGLT1 and SGLT2 inhibitors. *Diabetes* **2018**, *61*, 2079–2086.
54. Gorboulev, V.; Schürmann, A.; Vallon, V.; Kipp, H.; Jaschke, A.; Klessen, D.; Friedrich, A.; Scherneck, S.; Rieg, T.; Cunard, R. Na^+-D-glucose cotransporter SGLT1 is pivotal for intestinal glucose absorption and glucose-dependent incretin secretion. *Diabetes* **2012**, *61*, 187–196. [CrossRef] [PubMed]
55. Irhimeh, M.R.; Fitton, J.H.; Lowenthal, R.M. Pilot clinical study to evaluate the anticoagulant activity of fucoidan. *Blood Coagul. Fibrinolysis* **2009**, *20*, 607–610. [CrossRef] [PubMed]
56. Ponce, N.M.A.; Pujol, C.A.; Damonte, E.B.; Flores, M.A.L.; Stortz, C.A. Fucoidans from the brown seaweed *Adenocystis utricularis*: Extraction methods, antiviral activity and structural studies. *Carbohyd. Res.* **2003**, *338*, 153–165. [CrossRef]

57. Dodgson, K.; Price, R. A note on the determination of the ester sulphate content of sulphated polysaccharides. *Biochem. J.* **1962**, *84*, 106–110. [CrossRef]
58. Stevenson, T.T.; Furneaux, R.H. Chemical methods for the analysis of sulphated galactans from red algae. *Carbohydr. Res.* **1991**, *210*, 277–298. [CrossRef]
59. Peng, L.; Li, Z.R.; Green, R.S.; Holzman, I.R.; Lin, J. Butyrate enhances the intestinal barrier by facilitating tight junction assembly via activation of AMP-activated protein kinase in Caco-2 cell monolayers. *J. Nutr.* **2009**, *139*, 1619–1625. [CrossRef]
60. Blodgett, A.B.; Kothinti, R.K.; Kamyshko, I.; Petering, D.H.; Kumar, S.; Tabatabai, N.M. A fluorescence method for measurement of glucose transport in kidney cells. *Diabetes Technol. Ther.* **2011**, *13*, 743–751. [CrossRef]
61. He, Y.L.; Wang, Y.; Bullock, J.M.; Deacon, C.F.; Holst, J.J.; Dunning, B.E.; Ligueros-Saylan, M.; Foley, J.E. Pharmacodynamics of vildagliptin in patients with type 2 diabetes during OGTT. *J. Clin. Pharmacol.* **2007**, *47*, 633–641. [CrossRef]
62. Nagy, C.; Einwallner, E. Study of in vivo glucose metabolism in high-fat diet-fed mice using oral glucose tolerance test (OGTT) and insulin tolerance test (ITT). *JoVE-J. Vis. Exp.* **2018**, *131*, e56672. [CrossRef]
63. Barham, D.; Trinder, P. An improved colour reagent for the determination of blood glucose by the oxidase system. *Analyst* **1972**, *97*, 142–145. [CrossRef]
64. Li, J.; Cai, C.; Wang, L.H.; Yang, C.D.; Jiang, H.; Li, M.M.; Xu, D.; Li, G.Y.; Li, C.X.; Yu, G.L. Chemoenzymatic synthesis of heparan sulfate mimetic glycopolymers and their interactions with the receptor for advanced glycation end-product. *ACS Macro Lett.* **2019**, *8*, 1570–1574. [CrossRef]
65. Terada, Y.; Seto, H.; Hoshino, Y.; Murakami, T.; Shinohara, S.; Tamada, K.; Miura, Y. SPR study for analysis of a water-soluble glycopolymer interface and molecular recognition properties. *Polym. J.* **2017**, *49*, 255–262. [CrossRef]

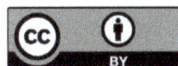

© 2020 by the authors. Licensee MDPI, Basel, Switzerland. This article is an open access article distributed under the terms and conditions of the Creative Commons Attribution (CC BY) license (http://creativecommons.org/licenses/by/4.0/).

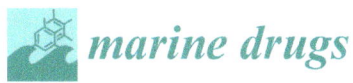

Article

Incorporation of FGF-2 into Pharmaceutical Grade Fucoidan/Chitosan Polyelectrolyte Multilayers

Natalie L. Benbow [1], Samuel Karpiniec [2], Marta Krasowska [1,*] and David A. Beattie [1,*]

[1] Future Industries Institute, University of South Australia, Mawson Lakes, SA 5095, Australia
[2] Marinova, Cambridge, TAS 7170, Australia
* Correspondence: Marta.Krasowska@unisa.edu.au (M.K.); David.Beattie@unisa.edu.au (D.A.B.)

Received: 14 September 2020; Accepted: 22 October 2020; Published: 26 October 2020

Abstract: Biopolymer polyelectrolyte multilayers are a commonly studied soft matter system for wound healing applications due to the biocompatibility and beneficial properties of naturally occurring polyelectrolytes. In this work, a popular biopolymer, chitosan, was combined with the lesser known polysaccharide, fucoidan, to create a multilayer film capable of sequestering growth factor for later release. Fucoidan has been shown to act as a heparin-mimic due to similarities in the structure of the two molecules, however, the binding of fibroblast growth factor-2 to fucoidan has not been demonstrated in a multilayer system. This study assesses the ability of fucoidan to bind fibroblast growth factor-2 within a fucoidan/chitosan polyelectrolyte multilayer structure using attenuated total internal reflectance infrared spectroscopy and quartz crystal microbalance with dissipation monitoring. The fibroblast growth factor-2 was sequestered into the polyelectrolyte multilayer as a cationic layer in the uppermost layers of the film structure. In addition, the diffusion of fibroblast growth factor-2 into the multilayer has been assessed.

Keywords: fucoidan; chitosan; fibroblast growth factor-2; polyelectrolyte multilayer; infrared spectroscopy; quartz crystal microbalance

1. Introduction

The use of growth factors in tissue engineering has been widely studied due to their ability to encourage healing and tissue growth [1]. A key example of an application where growth factors could provide significant benefit is for enhancing healing of chronic wounds. Chronic wounds are a significant issue in healthcare, severely affecting quality of life of affected people and contributing 2% to the total health care expenditure in countries such as Australia, the U.K. and the U.S.A. [2,3]. Applying growth factors to a wound site could promote healing by mimicking a healthy body's natural response to injury, i.e., by delivering the growth factors to a wound bed, the migration and proliferation of cells will be promoted. Of particular interest is fibroblast growth factor-2 (FGF-2) which is one of several biomolecules that are responsible for signalling cell migration and proliferation in the body [4]. FGF-2 is part of the 22-member FGF-family and has been shown to promote angiogenesis, cell proliferation, migration, and differentiation [5]. FGF-2 is commonly studied as a model growth factor in materials science studies for wound healing applications [6–10] and has been shown to reduce healing time [11,12]. However, there are limitations in regards to the delivery of growth factors, i.e., the growth factor must be protected from degradation and delivered at the optimal stage of healing at the right dose and for the correct duration [13].

Polyelectrolyte multilayers (PEMs) are surface coatings that offer potential advantages for delivering growth factors in many biomedical applications, such as vascular repair [14] and also in wound healing. When deployed for wound treatment, the architecture of the PEM film can be designed to give a burst release [15–17] or slow diffusion of the peptides from the film [18].

Delivery of target molecules can be partially controlled through changing the conditions of multilayer assembly including ionic strength [19], pH [16,20,21], temperature [22] and polyelectrolyte species [8]. In addition, PEMs can be applied to many surfaces including flat planes [23], nanoparticles [24] and nanocapsules [25,26], and three-dimensional (3D) porous scaffolds [27]. Furthermore, growth factors often show no conformational change or reorganisation upon binding to polyelectrolytes in PEMs when absorbed from solution at room temperature [5,28,29].

The goal of our study into growth factor-loaded PEM films was two-fold. First, to create a multilayer that will act as a natural matrix for the growth factor. Second, to create a multilayer host film that could have potential for synergistic therapeutic effect. Both of these goals were addressed through the choice of the polymers used to create the multilayers. Our work has made use of two naturally occurring biopolymers as the two major multilayer components; fucoidan and chitosan. The latter of these two polymers finds widespread application and study in the area of would healing, due to its properties: non-toxic, biocompatible, biodegradable, and anti-fungal. Past studies have also shown that chitosan promotes fibroblast proliferation [30,31]

Fibroblast growth factor-2 (FGF-2) needs to be embedded within the PEM to ensure it is protected from degradation but can remain biologically active [32]. The heparin binding site of FGF-2 is a highly positive environment due to the basic amino acid groups present [28] and can interact with negatively charged sulfate groups in heparin and heparin-mimics, including fucoidan [33–38] to create a ternary complex with the growth factor cell receptors. This complex is required for FGF-2 to be bioactive [33] and has been shown to improve skin healing [39]. Combining fucoidan and growth factors has been attempted by other groups, and has been shown to improve angiogenesis [40,41] and cell proliferation [42]. A single previous example exists of fucoidan combined with a growth factor (vascular endothelial growth factor) in a multilayer film [43]. This study found improved anti-thrombic properties and re-endothelialisation of a decellurised heart valve in response to interaction with this multilayer system.

Furthermore, fucoidan can be pro-angiogenic [38], anti-inflammatory, anti-viral, and promotes anti-bacterial activity of other molecules [44,45]. In addition, it can be pro- or anti-coagulant depending on molecular weight [46], promotes cell proliferation and migration [35,39,47] and can be immuno-modulating depending on the molecular weight and structure [48–50]. Fucoidan also inhibits MMP-2 (matrix metalloproteinase-2), an enzyme that degrades type IV collagen, a major component of basement membranes upon which the epithelium is constructed [51]. Meanwhile, chitosan has been shown to offer protection of FGF-2 against denaturation from heat, proteolysis and acid [52]. Chitosan has been shown to accelerate healing in diabetic mice (chronic wound models), acting as a delivery method for FGF-2 to further promote healing [52,53].

We have used attenuated total internal reflectance Fourier transform infrared spectroscopy and quartz crystal microbalance with dissipation monitoring to investigate the fucoidan/chitosan polyelectrolyte multilayers as a potential reservoir for FGF-2. Additionally, the permeation of FGF-2 into the multilayer was compared to the permeation of lysozyme. Lysozyme is a small protein of similar size and charge to FGF-2 and has been shown to permeate into these multilayers in our previous work [54]. Our overall aim has been to determine how FGF-2 can be incorporated into multilayer films, either pre-prepared for deployment in biomaterials applications, or as a sink within a biofluid environment to harvest and protect released FGF-2, to allow it to survive for longer in the environment in which it needs to act.

2. Results

2.1. QCM-D

Gorouhi et al. found that epidermal growth factor was still effective at promoting cell proliferation when covered by two bilayers in a PEM [32], thus, FGF-2 was placed at bilayer 6 of 8 in our study. Quartz crystal microbalance with dissipation (QCM-D) monitoring experiments were performed to monitor the build-up of the multilayers, either with, or without, the inclusion of the growth factor. In the case of a growth factor-embedded film, the PEM was constructed with sequential exposure of the substrate to the two polysaccharides until bilayer 5.5 (fucoidan terminating). The PEM was then exposed to PBS (phosphate buffer solution) for 5 min followed by 15 min FGF-2 25 µg·mL^{-1} solution, then a 5 min rinse with PBS to remove any unbound FGF-2. This PBS/FGF-2/PBS cycle substituted as the 6th CS (chitosan) layer. The PEM construction was continued as normal from the fucoidan terminating seventh bilayer, until 8 bilayers were deposited. For the non-embedded/blank system (i.e., without growth factor incorporation), the multilayer was exposed to PBS at the 5.5. bilayer formation point, and then chitosan was added in place of the growth factor, prior to continuing the formation until 8 bilayers were formed. Two independent experiments were performed with a total of two sensors for each condition. A representative measurement is shown in Figure 1, whilst the average Sauerbrey thickness, average hydrated mass and average dissipation can be found in Figure 2.

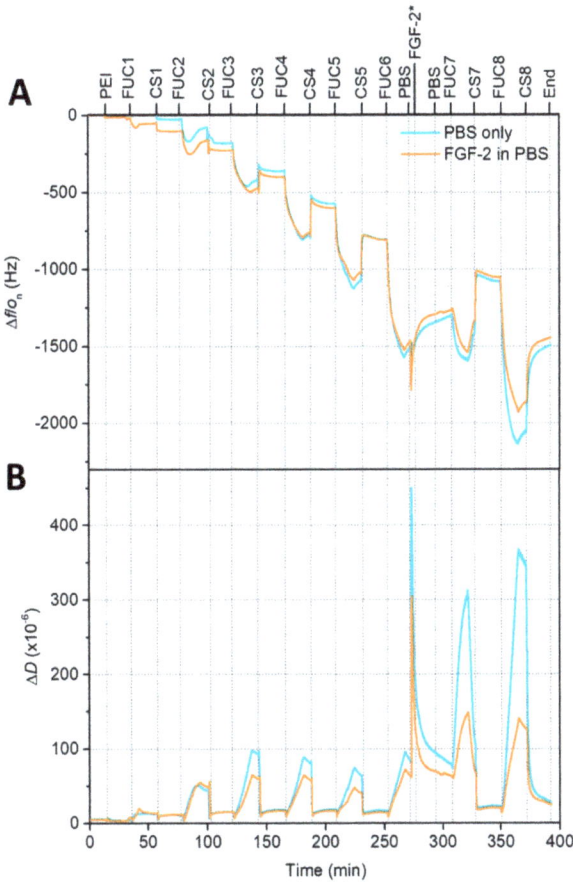

Figure 1. A representative QCM-D (Quartz crystal microbalance with dissipation) plot of frequency (**A**) and dissipation (**B**) for build-up of 8 bilayers for FUC/CS (fucoidan/chitosan) multilayers on gold sensors (5th overtone) where the PEM (polyelectrolyte multilayer) exposed to FGF-2 (fibroblast growth factor-2) are indicated by an orange line, whilst the control PEM exposed to only PBS (phosphate buffer solution) is marked with a blue line. The vertical dashed lines indicate the start of the adsorption step of each polymer. * Indicates were FGF-2 adsorption began for the data set presented in orange.

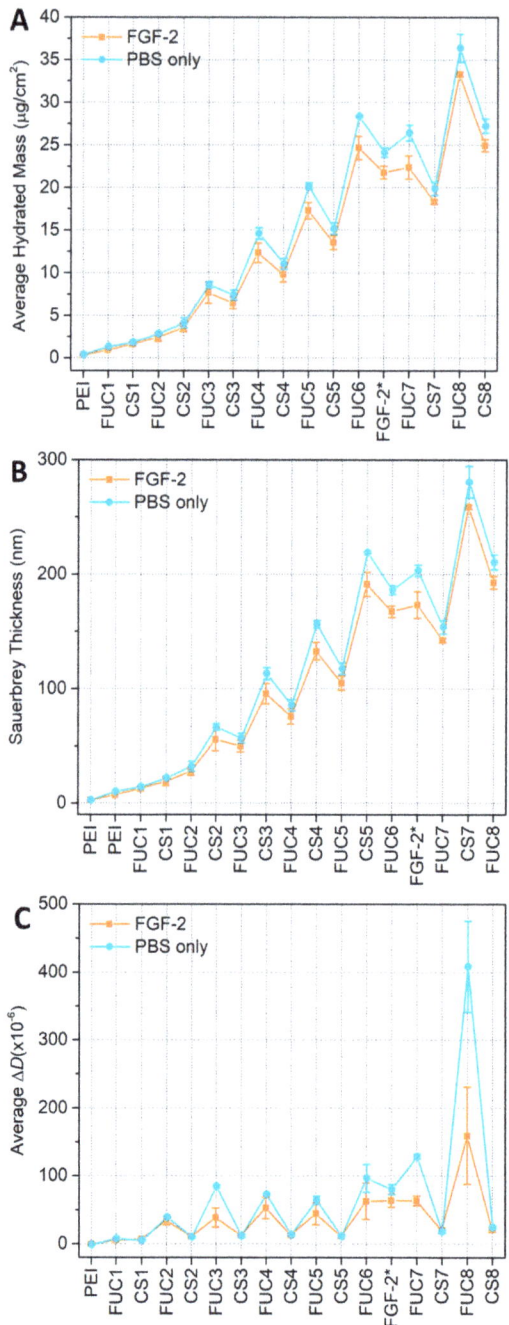

Figure 2. QCM-D calculations for (**A**) the average hydrated Sauerbrey mass, (**B**) the average Sauerbrey thickness; and (**C**) the average dissipation of the 8 bilayer FUC/CS PEM with embedded FGF-2 (orange with square markers–and highlighted with an asterisk on the x-axis) and PBS without FGF-2 (blue with circle markers).

The QCM-D data presented in Figure 1 indicate that the fucoidan layers show an increase in both frequency magnitude and dissipation, which becomes larger with increasing layer number, reflecting the supra-linear growth of the multilayer. The chitosan layers show a sharp decrease in both frequency magnitude and dissipation. In both panels of Figure 1 a sharp spike can be seen when the multilayer is initially exposed to PBS. The frequency magnitude and dissipation then decrease to values less than the 6 bilayer fucoidan-terminating PEM within 5 min for both multilayers exposed to FGF-2 in PBS and PBS only. There is a small but continual decrease in the frequency when the film is exposed to PBS (both with FGF-2 and without) indicating a mass loss during this time. However, QCM-D cannot distinguish between polymer mass and water mass loss. Our previous work has shown that 10 bilayer fucoidan/chitosan multilayers experience both a degree of mass loss and swelling when exposed to PBS [54]. However, any swelling occurring here (Figure 1) cannot be seen in the frequency measurements after the initial spike, in fact, a decrease in thickness is observed (see Figure 2).

The pattern seen in the early layers, of lower frequency and dissipation for chitosan layers, and a sharp increase in both frequency magnitude and dissipation for fucoidan layers, continues after PBS exposure with some differences, the first fucoidan layer after PBS exposure shows the same frequency as the previous fucoidan layer. The dissipation increases sharply with the fucoidan adsorption after PBS. The seventh and eighth chitosan layers show a decrease from the previous reported fucoidan layers in the frequency magnitude and dissipation values. The hydrated mass calculated using the Sauerbrey relation and the Sauerbrey thickness (panel A and B of Figure 2), show that the incorporation of FGF-2 does not have a significant impact on these two attributes of the multilayer compared to a PEM only exposed to PBS. The hydrated mass can be seen to follow a linear profile up to bilayer 3 where a saw-tooth profile emerges, with the chitosan layers having a lower hydrated mass than the previous fucoidan layers. Upon exposure to PBS the hydrated mass can be seen to decrease, following this exposure the continued build-up of the multilayer again shows a saw-tooth profile similar to before the PBS/FGF-2/PBS cycle. The PEM that was only exposed to PBS appears to show a marginally higher adsorbed mass, however, this was present prior to PBS exposure so is likely caused by a variation in the samples themselves.

Similarly, the thickness data in panel B of Figure 2, show a similar profile to the mass calculations prior to PBS exposure, where the linear profile ends at bilayer 3 and the saw-tooth begins. Again, when chitosan is adsorbed to the fucoidan-terminating multilayer the film becomes thinner, when the next layer of fucoidan is adsorbed the entire multilayer become thicker. When exposed to PBS, the thickness of the multilayer increases, upon the adsorption of the first subsequent bilayer pair, consisting of fucoidan then chitosan, the thickness decreases. These changes in thickness and mass show a swelling and deswelling profile. No polymer is added during the PBS only rinse and very little mass is added during the PBS/FGF-2/PBS cycle, yet the mass and thickness both increase.

The average dissipation data is presented in panel C of Figure 2, the PEMs with and without growth factor have very similar dissipations after being exposed to FGF-2 in PBS or only PBS. Though, this small difference may be due to variation in the samples that exists prior to the PBS exposure. For the seventh layer of fucoidan, there was a significant difference in the dissipation with the PBS only system having a much greater dissipation than the multilayer with embedded FGF-2, the eighth fucoidan layer shows a similar difference. However, the dissipation of the seventh and eighth chitosan layers are the same for both the multilayer with embedded FGF-2 and the multilayer that was only exposed to PBS.

2.2. ATR FTIR

The ATR FTIR (attenuated total reflectance Fourier transform infrared) spectroscopy build-up and growth factor embedding experiments were performed with two independent repeats on a ZnSe IRE (internal reflection element). The spectra in Figure 3 show the PEM build-up proceeded as expected up to 5.5 bilayers (some of the later layer spectra have been offset vertically for clarity). The spectra show the characteristic peaks of fucoidan and chitosan (assigned previously [55–57]).

The characteristic peaks assigned to chitosan are the amide I/C=O at 1633 cm^{-1} and amide II at 1535 cm^{-1}. While the characteristic peaks attributed to the sulfate stretching vibration are at 1249 cm^{-1} and 1220 cm^{-1}. Other peaks of interest include the overlapping peaks at 1167 cm^{-1} assigned to C–O–C stretching vibration fucoidan and 1152 cm^{-1} assigned to C–O–C/C–N stretching vibrations of chitosan. The glycosidic linkages and skeletal C–O stretching vibrations is encompassed by the peaks at 1090 cm^{-1}, 1051 cm^{-1} and 1025 cm^{-1} for both polysaccharides. A complete list of peak positions and assignments can be found in Table 1.

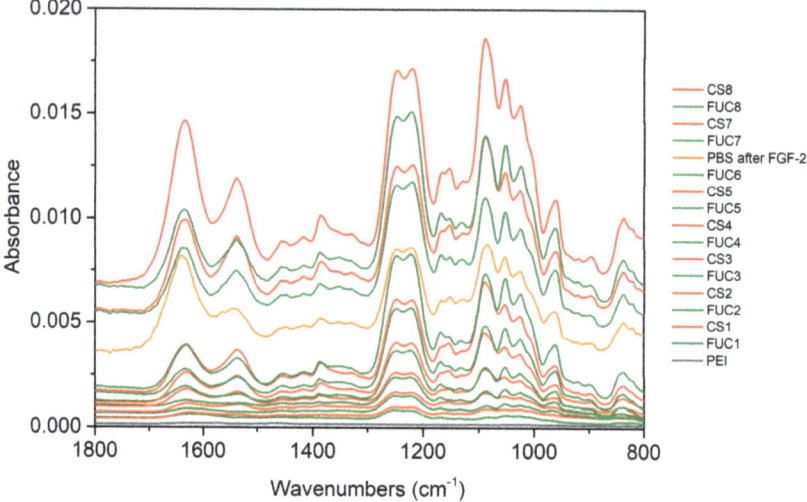

Figure 3. ATR FTIR (attenuated total reflectance Fourier transform infrared) spectra of build-up of a 8 bilayer FUC/CS PEM on a ZnSe IRE, where FGF-2 was embedded at bilayer 6. The grey line represents the spectrum of PEI, green lines represent FUC layers, red lines represent CS, and the orange line shows the spectrum of FGF-2 after a 5 min PBS rinse.

During the individual layer adsorption steps, when fucoidan was adsorbed an increase in the sulfonate stretching band at 1238 cm^{-1} is clearly seen along with increases in the lower wavenumbers of the glycosidic linkage region (1100–950 cm^{-1}). As chitosan adsorbs the greatest differences are increases in the entire glycosidic linkage region and in the amide I and II bands. These amide bands decrease slightly upon subsequent fucoidan adsorption. This decrease is the result of stripping of chitosan from the multilayer upon adsorption of fucoidan. Stripping of polyelectrolytes has been observed in fucoidan/chitosan multilayers in past work from this group (and is commonly observed more broadly with polyions of dissimilar molecular weights), when fucoidan of much lower molecular weight has been used (see [56] and references contained therein).

The spectrum of the PBS rinse after FGF-2 adsorption displays some significant changes. At 5.5 bilayers the PEM has been calculated to be 192 ± 10 nm thick using the Sauerbrey equation from the QCM-D measurements presented in Figure 2, panel B. When the film was exposed to PBS/FGF-2/PBS the Sauerbrey thickness decreased to 168 ± 5 nm, despite an initial spike caused by PBS. The significant decrease in absorbance after the PBS/FGF-2/PBS cycle indicates mass loss of polysaccharides from the film. The peak heights of the sulfonate bands and the glycosidic region match that of the 5th bilayer, chitosan terminating film suggesting much of the previously adsorbed fucoidan layer has been removed. In addition, increases in the amide I/II bands indicating that FGF-2 adsorbed to the multilayer.

Table 1. Assignment of bands observed for ATR FTIR (attenuated total reflectance Fourier transform infrared) spectra of (i) a 9.5 bilayer fucoidan/chitosan polyelectrolyte multilayer on a Ge IRE (internal reflection element) and (ii) an 8 bilayer fucoidan/chitosan polyelectrolyte multilayer with FGF-2 embedded at bilayer 6 built on a ZnSe IRE [27,30–40]. Annotations: ν is stretching vibration, ν_{as} is asymmetric stretching vibration, ν_s is symmetric stretching vibration, γ is out-of-plane bending vibration, δ is in-plane bending vibration.

Peak Assignment	9.5 BL Chitosan/Fucoidan (Ge IRE)	8 BL Chitosan/Fucoidan with FGF-2 Embedded at BL 6 (ZnSe IRE)
ν_s(C-O-S)	838	838
ν_s(C-H)	898	898
ν(C-O), ν_s(C-O-S)	961	961
ν(C-O-C), ν(C-O), ν(C-C)	1025	1024
ν(C-O-C), ν(C-O), ν(S=O)	1052	1052
	1089	1091
ν(C-N), γ(C-O-C)	1155	1155
γ(C-O-C)	1167	1167
ν_{as}(S=O)	1222	1220
	1248	1248
γ(CH$_3$)	1386	1386
δ(CH$_2$)	1416	1416
δ(CH$_2$)	1454	1454
Amide II, δ(N-H), ν_{as}(COO$^-$)	1538	1536
Amide I, δ(O-H)	1632	1635

Following the PBS/FGF-2/PBS cycle the multilayer build-up was continued. The first fucoidan layer after this cycle has the same peak heights as the preceding fucoidan layer that was diminished by the adsorption of the FGF-2 layer (and associated PBS rinse cycles). The characteristic peaks in the next chitosan layer spectra increase very little, whilst the next bilayer appears to return to a more typical build-up as seen with the early layers prior to PBS/FGF-2 exposure. There is one additional difference in the final chitosan layer; the sulfate band attributed to fucoidan increases, likely due to underlying chitosan peaks in the spectrum and the large amount of chitosan that appears to be adsorbing to this layer. It is unlikely to be a result of the penetration depth of the evanescent wave as the d_p of the ZnSe IRE is approximately 850 nm ($\tilde{n}$ = 1650 cm^{-1}) and the Sauerbrey thickness of the multilayer at the time of formation of the eighth chitosan layer is 193 ± 5 nm for the film with embedded FGF-2 (see the supporting information of our previous work [54] for calculations of d_p).

The spectra presented in Figure 4, show more clearly the spectral change associated with the adsorption step of the growth factor. The amide I/II bands characteristic of proteins, in this case FGF-2, are sharp and clear, and are found at peak maxima of 1642 cm^{-1} and 1541 cm^{-1}, respectively. The amide I/II bands increase over the 15 min adsorption. It is clear that FGF-2 has adsorbed to the surface of the multilayer. The subsequent PBS rinse showed no further change in the polysaccharide peaks or the amide bands suggesting the FGF-2 remained bound onto the multilayer surface and no further mass loss of the polysaccharides occurred. The FGF-2 exposure spectra will also include some contribution from the bulk solution above the PEM as well as any FGF-2 adsorbed to the PEM.

Finally, it was important to confirm that the FGF-2 remains bound within the PEM after build-up is continued, i.e., it is not removed by polyelectrolyte stripping. The spectra of the layers added after FGF-2 were processed by subtracting the spectra of the PBS rinse after FUC6 in a 1 to 1 ratio from each. These spectra are then processed to remove the O-H bending mode of water lost during this adsorption step, by summing the spectrum with a spectrum of PBS. Representative spectra are presented in Figure 5. Negative changes in the amide bands of the spectra in this figure may show if FGF-2 was desorbing or being removed from the multilayer.

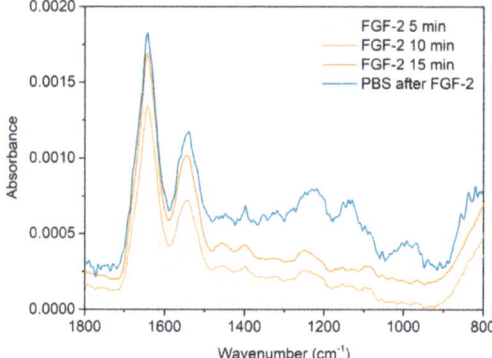

Figure 4. ATR FTIR individual layer spectra of the FGF-2 adsorption every 5 min in orange and the subsequent PBS rinse in blue. FGF-2 spectra are produced by 1 to 1 subtraction of the prior PBS rinse spectrum from each spectrum collected over the adsorption time, followed by subtraction of a PBS spectra to remove the O–H bending mode contribution of water.

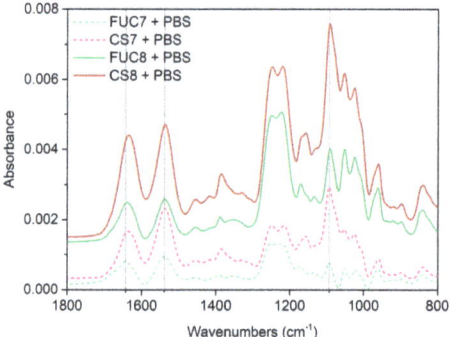

Figure 5. Representative ATR FTIR spectra of the layers added after FGF-2 adsorption. These spectra were produced by subtracting the spectra of the PBS rinse after FUC6 in a 1 to 1 ratio from each, followed by adding a PBS spectra to flatten the region between 1650–1700 cm^{-1} to remove the O–H bending mode of water lost during this adsorption step. Green lines show the fucoidan layers whilst red shows the chitosan layers. The vertical lines indicate the peak maxima of the amide I/II of FGF-2.

The first FUC (seventh bilayer) adsorption after the embedded growth factor contains a clear sulfate band characteristic of fucoidan as would be expected, however, there is significant distortion in the region from 1100–900 cm^{-1} due to the overlapping nature of PBS peaks in this region. In addition, the amide I band peak maxima can be found at 1643 cm^{-1}, whilst the amide II maxima is at 1539 cm^{-1}, these peaks are indicative of FGF-2 remaining bound to the multilayer after fucoidan adsorption. Upon subsequent chitosan adsorption the amide I and II peaks became more rounded and the peak maxima of the amide I shifted to 1638 cm^{-1} but the amide II remained in the same position. Additionally, two peaks increase significantly at 1384 cm^{-1} and 1093 cm^{-1}, assigned to the CH$_3$ deformation and the C-O-C stretching mode of the glycosidic linkage overlapping with the symmetric stretching of phosphate in PBS (see electronic Supplementary Materials Figure S1). These peaks only increase with each chitosan addition. In the next fucoidan layer spectra the amide I band shifts back to 1640 cm^{-1}, and both amide bands greatly reduce in size. This indicates that chitosan is removed from the film as was seen previously, while the shift towards the FGF-2-like amide I band suggests that the growth factor is still trapped within the film. The final adsorption of chitosan sees the amide I shift more dramatically to 1634 cm^{-1} due to significantly larger adsorbed amount.

These spectra also clearly show that the sharp peak at 1093 cm^{-1} is associated with chitosan adsorption. This sharp peak appears at the same wavenumber as the first of the glycosidic linkage peaks of the polyelectrolytes, i.e., the C-O-C and C-O stretching bands. However, this peak also overlaps with the symmetric stretching of phosphate in PBS [58], which is composed of two peaks at 1062 cm^{-1} and 1125 cm^{-1} (see electronic Supplementary Materials Figure S1).

In addition to determining that the FGF-2 does not release upon simple exposure to PBS, it is valuable to determine the likely structure and distribution of the FGF-2 within the multilayer. The presence of FGF-2 as a distinct layer within the multilayer will likely result in a different interaction within a wound environment compared to FGF-2 that is evenly distributed throughout the PEM film. In recently submitted work from our group, we determined that lysozyme was able to adsorb onto and permeate into a multilayer of FUC/CS (fucoidan/chitosan) [54]. Lysozyme and FGF-2 are both small proteins, with similar molecular weights and hydrodynamic radii; for lysozyme the molecular weight is 14.7 kDa and has a hydrodynamic radius of 19.5 Å, whilst FGF-2 has values of 17.2 kDa and 28 Å, respectively [9,28]. In addition, both have an overall positive charge at physiological pH, with isoelectric points at 11.3 for lysozyme and 9.6 for FGF-2. It was therefore our initial hypothesis that FGF-2 would behave similarly when a solution of the growth factor was placed in contact with a multilayer.

To test this hypothesis, ATR FTIR spectroscopy on a Ge IRE was employed to monitor the build-up of a 9.5 bilayer FUC/CS PEM, similar to our previous experiments with lysozyme. The build-up was found to match the data from our earlier work, and is presented in Figure 6. The multilayer was then exposed to PBS solution for 5 min, and then a 25 µg·mL^{-1} FGF-2 solution (in PBS, which was used to maintain the secondary structure of the proteins) was injected into the flowcell and remained stagnant over the film for 15 min and a spectra collected of the bulk solution over the multilayer. The spectra of the protein exposure are presented in Figure 7 panel A, where a ratio of 1 to 1 was used to subtract the spectrum of PBS over FUC10 from the spectrum of 15 min protein exposure. The film was exposed to FGF-2 was exposed to PBS for 2 h and this spectrum is presented in Figure 7 panel B.

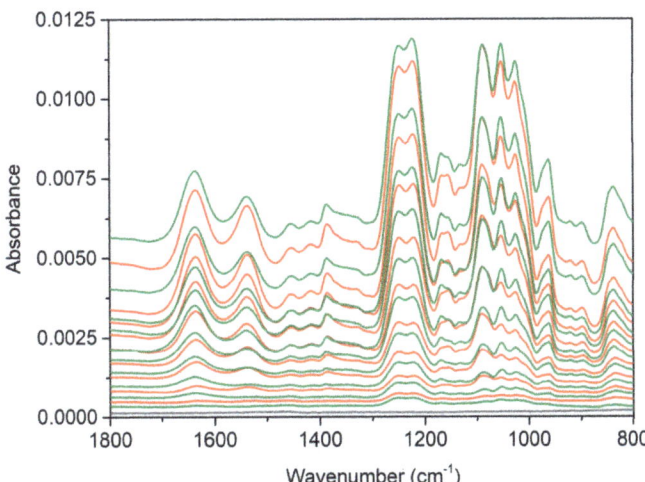

Figure 6. ATR FTIR spectra of the build-up of a 9.5 bilayer PEM on a Ge IRE. The spectra are produced by subtracting a spectrum of the background electrolyte from each spectrum collected after each polymer adsorption/rinse step. The spectrum of PEI is shown in grey, the spectra of the fucoidan layers are shown in green and the chitosan layers are shown in red.

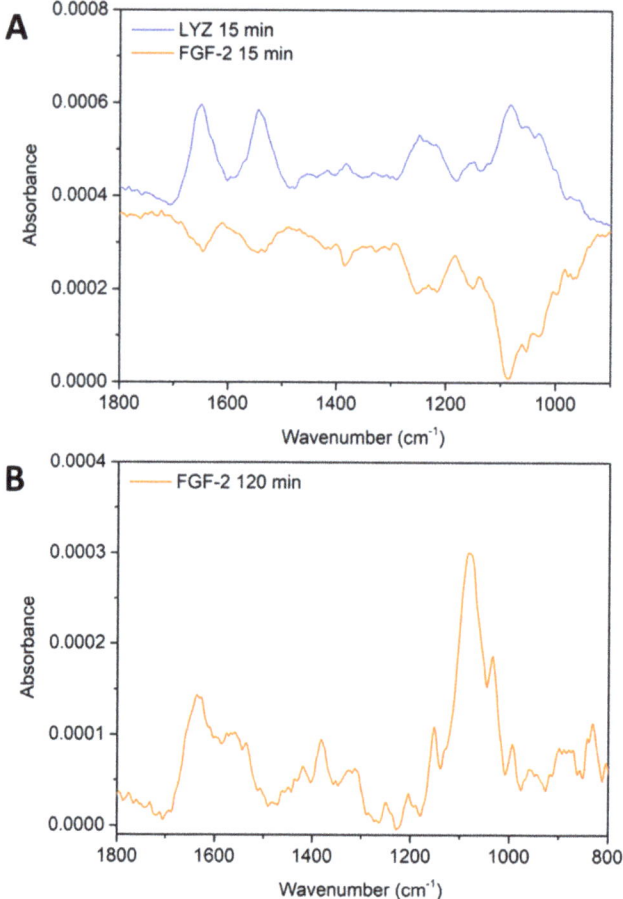

Figure 7. (**A**) ATR FTIR difference spectra of a 9.5 bilayer PEM exposed to PBS for 5 min followed by either lysozyme (dark blue) or FGF-2 (orange) for 15 min. (**B**) ATR FTIR difference spectrum of a 9.5 bilayer PEM exposed to PBS for 5 min followed by FGF-2 (orange) for 120 min. (Difference spectra acquired by subtracting the spectrum of the PBS exposed multilayer from the multilayer exposed to the two biomolecules).

Upon fucoidan adsorption the sulfate peaks increase up to bilayer 4. From bilayer 5 onwards, the sulfate peak increases upon both fucoidan and chitosan adsorption. The amide I/II bands characteristic of chitosan increase upon adsorption of chitosan, but decrease upon subsequent adsorption of fucoidan throughout build-up, however, this becomes more noticeable in the latter layers. This is attributed to mass loss of chitosan via stripping by fucoidan as it adsorbs and swelling of the film. Swelling can be seen in ATR FTIR spectra where the penetration depth of the IRE is not much greater than the thickness of the film. This can also account for the increase in the sulfate peak after chitosan adsorption mentioned above.

The spectra in Figure 7 show that lysozyme can be detected within the multilayer, with amide I and amide II bands clearly visible at 1651 cm^{-1} and 1547 cm^{-1}. In addition, the glycosidic linkage region of the polysaccharides can also be seen with a maxima at 1084 cm^{-1}, as well as the sulfonate stretching band characteristic of FUC at 1215–1252 cm^{-1}. In contrast, the FGF-2 spectrum shows negative bands at 1647 cm^{-1} and 1547 cm^{-1} assigned to the amide I/II of CS, as well as the negative sulfonate stretching band and the glycosidic linkage region with minima at 1215–1252 cm^{-1}, and 1084 cm^{-1}, respectively.

The refractive index of the Ge prism upon which these experiments were performed was n_{Ge} = 4.0, within the $\tilde{n}$ = 700–3450 cm^{-1} range [59]. A high refractive index means that the penetration depth (d_p) of the evanescent wave from the surface of the IRE in an aqueous environment is small, where d_p = 414 nm at $\tilde{n}$ = 1540 cm^{-1} and d_p = 505 nm at $\tilde{n}$ = 1250 cm^{-1} (see our previous work for all calculated d_p values and graphs of refractive indices for ZnSe and Ge IREs in the mid-IR range). In our earlier work, AFM measurements were used to determine the thickness of the 9.5 bilayer PEM in KCl electrolyte (377 ± 10 nm) and when exposed to PBS (432 ± 14 nm) [54]. These thickness measurements show that the multilayer is thicker than the penetration depth of the evanescent wave from a Ge IRE in the region of the amide I/II bands. Therefore, the spectra in Figure 7 shows that the film allows lysozyme to penetrate, as indicated by the amide I/II bands, and the PEM deswells as expected (and visualized by the increase in the polysaccharide peaks). However, the FGF-2 does not interact with the PEM in the same manner, the spectra indicates that the PEM is continuing to swell (likely due to the PBS) and is not counteracted by protein sorption (no positive amide I/II bands can be seen).

The FGF-2 bulk solution was allowed to remain on the film for 2 h (Figure 7 panel B), after this time the characteristic peaks of chitosan could be seen at 1636 cm^{-1} and 1558 cm^{-1}, plus the glycosidic linkage region centred around 1080 cm^{-1}. However, there appeared to be no amide I/II bands that matched the shape/ratios of the protein or any sulfate stretching bands indicative of fucoidan. This indicates that FGF-2 did not permeate into the film over this time frame and the film de-swelled into the evanescent wave. Specifically, a region/layer with high chitosan content, or that chitosan is diffusing through the PEM into the lower layers closer to the IRE surface. This diffusion may be facilitated by the long exposure to PBS meaning that the film remains in the swollen state during this time. Therefore, the chitosan may be freer to diffuse due to the higher degree of extrinsic versus intrinsic charge compensation and the 'looser' structure of the swollen PEM.

Since the our previous work determined that the PEM was able to exclude proteins based on size [54], the spectra presented in Figure 7 indicate that FGF-2 must interact via a different mechanism than lysozyme (LYZ) with the multilayer components since the difference in molecular weight and hydrodynamic radii between LYZ and FGF-2 is small. It must be also noted that heparin-like glycosaminoglycans (GAGs) (i.e., fucoidan) support dimerisation of FGF-2 which contributes to the potency of the growth factor in vivo [60]. However, our experiments could not distinguish between dimerised FGF-2 in contact with the fucoidan surface of the PEM, or whether monomers of FGF-2 were binding to the fucoidan on the films without dimerisation occurring.

3. Discussion

The data in this study clearly shows that FGF-2 does not permeate into the multilayer but can be embedded irreversibly at a desired location within the film. Both observations are likely due to the specific interactions between FGF-2 and heparin/or heparin-like mimics, i.e., fucoidan [33,61]. The FGF-2 protein has heparin-specific binding regions on the protein surface that contain lysine residues [62]. Under physiological conditions lysine residues are positively charged and can act as hydrogen bond donors [63]. The FGF family of growth factors all have different heparan sulfate glycosaminoglycan (HSGAG) binding domains [61]. The binding of FGF to HSGAGs is vital for binding to the tyrosine kinase receptors (FGFR) on cell surfaces as a ternary complex and regulating signalling [61]. FGF binding to an HSGAG oligosaccharide has been shown to involve both ionic and van der Waals forces, and was optimal due to the conformational changes of the HSGAG backbone that occur from protein binding, where the HSGAG kinks across 3 specific monosaccharide units, glucosamine-iduronate-glucosamine [61]. More recent work has shown that that binding of FGF to HSGAGs requires 3-O-sulfated glucosamine saccharide units, not specifically iduronate which has an additional carboxylate group in the 6-O-position [64]. *Fucus vesiculosus* fucoidan is predominantly comprised of long chains of 2-O-sulfated glucosamine units with some 3-O-sulfated glucosamines [50].

Thus, it is likely able to form the kinked structure around FGF proteins in a similar manner to the HSGAGs studied by Raman et al. [61]. The specificity of heparin binding domains in proteins such as FGF-2 result in quite different behaviour when compared to other proteins of similar size and charge that lack the specific heparin binding domains, i.e., lysozyme [65]. Another factor to consider is the oligermisation states of FGF-2, Kwan et al. reported that HSGAGs induced dimerisation of FGF-2 via surface-exposed cystine residues [60]. The HSGAGs stabilise the FGF-2 dimers and the dimers have a more potent effect than the monomeric form. If the FGF-2 is dimerising when in contact with fucoidan at the surface of the multilayer, this may contribute to the lack of diffusion into the lower layers of the film.

The work by Masuoka et al. showed that chitosan was able to protect FGF-2 from heat and enzymatic degradation at pH 7.3 (in PBS) but had no protective effect against acid degradation (pH < 5) [52]. This suggests that chitosan at or above its isoelectric point may be able to bind to FGF-2 as well. The amine groups of chitosan have an isoelectric point of 6.5 [66,67]. So, in PBS solution (pH 7.3) almost 50% of the amine groups will lose their positive charge. In our multilayers, if FGF-2 were binding to chitosan then when the pH is reduced to pH 5 upon return to the background electrolyte some loss of FGF-2 may be expected. However, this does not appear to be the case.

Other authors have seen similar results with other multilayer systems [68] where LYZ is able to permeate but FGF-2 does not, but, this is not always the case, and it is dependent on a multilayer structure [8,69–71]. Hsu et al. have published two works of interest, where either LYZ or FGF-2 were incorporated into the PEM structure as a component in a tetralayer [69]. In the first study, CS/poly(β-L-malic acid) (PMLA)/CS or LYZ/PMLA tetralayers were investigated with varying degrees of click crosslinking introduced via modified PMLA components to minimise interlayer diffusion and thus, control release of therapeutics [69]. Here, LYZ was used as a model protein, and was trapped in the lower part of the PEM by a cross-linked layer of PMLA. This barrier layer was able to suppress the burst release of protein and made the release duration longer, going from 2 to 3 days. Hsu's second work, utilised the same PEM system with LYZ and FGF-2 [69]. In this study, they replaced LYZ with FGF-2 in the tetralayer PEM and found that more than six times less FGF-2 was incorporated than in similar LYZ films [69]. In addition, the loading of FGF-2 was linear with respect to film thickness. The release of FGF-2 had a similar profile to that of LYZ from the same films however, was of longer duration. The FGF-2 released from the films was found to have a greater proliferative activity than 'as-received' FGF-2, likely due to the co-release of chitosan, which may offer protective effects against heat denaturization [69].

Another group of authors who have created a body of work on the topic is Macdonald et al. who investigated PEMs comprised of a variety of synthetic and natural polyelectrolytes and their interactions with LYZ [70], FGF-2 [8] and BMP-2 [71]. In their 2008 paper, lysozyme was utilised as the polyanion in a tetralayer structure (polyX/polyanion/LYZ/polyanion)$_n$ where, n = 10–80 and polyX was one of two synthesised cationic poly(β-aminoesters), whilst the polyanion was, either heparin (HEP) or chondroitin [70]. The amount of LYZ incorporated was linear with film thickness. The same films were investigated with FGF-2 as the embedded protein in the tetralayer structure. It was found that poly2/HEP films contained the most FGF-2, partly due to the hydrophobicity of poly2 vs. poly1 which would result in less intrinsic charge compensation (poly2 films are thicker than poly1 due to this). In addition, films containing HEP can sequester more FGF-2 than the equivalent films containing chondroitin. It was proposed that the specific interactions between HEP and FGF-2 may be the dominant factor, however, in their previous work the HEP films were also able to load more LYZ than the chondroitin films [70]. So, the specific interactions between FGF-2 and HEP may not be the only reason why HEP multilayers were able to load more FGF-2 than the chondroitin films.

These studies correlate with our data confirming that heparin-specific binding sites play an important role in the uptake of FGF-2 to fucoidan/chitosan multilayer films and that fucoidan is likely acting as a heparin-mimic even when it is within a multilayer structure.

This is further confirmed by the FUC7 + PBS spectra in Figure 5, which shows that FGF-2 remains bound within the multilayer upon fucoidan adsorption, however, it is less clear in the subsequent spectra due to the overlapping amide bands of chitosan and FGF-2. Yet, it is still possible to assume the FGF-2 remains bound since upon addition of the seventh chitosan layer the amide I band does not shift as low as previously seen in earlier studies from our group [54] (to 1630 cm^{-1}) and when the eighth fucoidan layer is adsorbed (and some chitosan is stripped) there is a shift in the amide I to higher wavenumbers i.e., closer to the peak maximum of FGF-2.

The sharp peak (Figure 5) assigned to the symmetric stretching of phosphate in PBS [58] (see electronic Supplementary Materials Figure S1) could suggest that some phosphate remains bound via ionic interactions to chitosan after the electrolyte is changed back to KCl. Laucirica et al. have shown that amine-phosphate interactions are specific and that this binding becomes apparent under physiologically relevant conditions [72]. In addition, the same work showed that the divalent HPO_4^{2-} has an affinity for amino-groups that is five times greater than the monovalent $H_2PO_4^{1-}$ ion due to the hydrogen bonding between the protons on the amine and the charged oxygen species of phosphate ions [72]. Peng et al. found similar results with molecular dynamics that showed that phosphate ions adsorb on to amino-terminated self-assembled monolayers but chloride ions do not [73].

4. Materials and Methods

4.1. Materials

Protosan UP CL 213, a chitosan salt that dissolves in water (CS, 75–90% deacetylated, 150–400 kDa) was sourced from NovaMatrix (Sandvika, Norway). Pharmaceutical grade *Fucus vesiculosus* fucoidan (FUC, Batch no. DPFVF2015505 from the Maritech ®® range, 98% purity, 1.4% uronic acid, 56.9 kDa, 26.6% sulfate 50.7% fucose) was supplied by Marinova Pty Ltd. (Cambridge, TAS, Australia). The purification of fucoidan to remove pyrogens produces a highly pure material that is acceptable for medical use. Human fibroblast growth factor-basic (FGF-2, 154 a.a.) was supplied by Peprotech-Lonza, Mt Waverley, VIC, Australia. Lysozyme from chicken egg white (LYZ, dialyzed, lyophilized, powder, 100000 U·mg^{-1}) and polyethylenimine (PEI, branched, 25 kDa) and were obtained from Sigma-Aldrich, Australia.

Potassium chloride (KCl, 99%, AR) was purchased from Chem-Supply (Gillman, SA, Australia). The KCl was further purified to remove surface active impurities, by calcination at 550 °C for 8 h, followed by recrystalisation and finally, another calcination. Phosphate buffered saline (Dulbecco A) was obtained from Thermo Fisher Scientific, Adelaide, SA, Australia and used as supplied. HCl and KOH (both volumetric grade) were sourced from Merck KGaA, Darmstadt, Germany. Reagents used for cleaning surfaces include; ethanol 100% undenatured (AR, Chem-Supply, Gillman, SA, Australia), Hellmanex (Hellma Analytics, Müllheim, Germany), pH 7 Tickopur R 30 and OP-U colloidal silica suspension (Struers, Ballerup, Denmark).

4.2. Solution Preparation

Milli-Q water (resistivity: 18.2 MΩ·cm; interfacial tension: 72.4 mN·m^{-1} at 22 °C; total organic carbon content: < 4 mg·L^{-1}) was used to prepare all solutions and for cleaning of surfaces and glassware. The background electrolyte for the polyelectrolyte solutions was pH 5 0.1 M KCl solution (pH adjusted prior to making other solutions). PEI (500 ppm) was prepared in background electrolyte, stirred overnight and used within one week. Solutions of CS and FUC (both 500 ppm) were prepared in background electrolyte and stirred overnight. The polysaccharide solutions were used within 24 h of preparation. The background electrolyte, FUC and CS solutions were pH adjusted with volumetric grade KOH and HCl solutions to pH 5 before experiments. All pH adjustments were performed to give a value of ± 0.05 from the desired pH. PEI was used at its native pH in 0.1 M KCl pH 5 solution. Both LYZ and FGF-2 (both 25 ppm) were prepared the day of the experiment in PBS (pH 7.3) and stirred briefly to dissolve the protein. The concentration of 25 μg·mL^{-1} FGF-2 solution was chosen for two main reasons; (i) physiological concentrations are approximately 50 pg·mL^{-1} in plasma [74], (ii) spectroscopic detection levels were found to be in the range of hundreds of µg·mL^{-1} for solution spectra. Typically, adsorption to a multilayer increases the concentration within the evanescent wave, and thus detection of less than this concentration is possible, it was decided to work in a range that would ensure detection. In addition other authors have found concentrations between 1.65–100 µg·mL^{-1} growth factor solutions sufficient for multilayer studies [8,18,75–77].

4.3. Polyelectrolyte Multilayer Preparation and Growth Factor Adsorption/Incorporation

Multilayers were prepared, in situ, under flow for all experiments. Initially, the system is flushed with KCl background electrolyte, then an anchoring layer of PEI is deposited by flowing the solution over the substrate for 15 min followed by a 5 min rinse with KCl. Following the PEI layer, FUC is adsorbed then CS. Each polymer is adsorbed for 15 min followed by a 5 min KCl rinse. The fucoidan and chitosan layers make one bilayer pair. This bilayer is repeated until the desired bilayer number is reached. Where FGF-2 was embedded in the film, a total of 8 bilayers were used with a FGF-2 layer at bilayer 6 i.e., PEI-(FUC/CS)$_5$-(FUC/FGF-2)-(FUC/CS)$_2$. For the permeation experiments multilayers composed of 9.5 bilayers were used so the film can be described by; PEI-(FUC/CS)$_9$-FUC.

4.4. Attenuated Total Reflectance Fourier Transform Infrared Spectroscopy (ATR FTIR)

Fourier transform infrared experiments were performed on a Varian 670-IR FTIR spectrometer (Agilent Technologies, Mulgrave, VIC, Australia). A Ge internal reflection element (IRE) was used for FGF-2 permeation experiments. A ZnSe IRE was used for the data shown throughout the main manuscript. The IRE was mounted in a Fast IR single reflection ATR accessory (Harrick Scientific, Pleasantville, NY, USA) and fitted with a liquid flow cell attached to a peristaltic pump (Masterflex L/S, John Morris Scientific, Deepdene, VIC, Australia) with Tygon tubing (Masterflex L/S 13, Cole Parmer, Vernon Hills, IL, USA).

The ZnSe/Ge IRE (Harrick Scientific, Pleasantville, NY, USA) was buffed in a figure-of-eight pattern for approximately 5 min with OP-U colloidal silica suspension on a wet, MD-Nap ™ 250 mm polishing pad (both Struers, Ballerup, Denmark), followed by buffing for a further 2 min with Milli-Q water. Each component was sonicated in a surfactant for 30 min; the IRE in 2% pH 7 Tickopur, the flow cell and the tubing were sonicated in 2% Hellmanex - each solution was injected through the tubing 3 times with syringes (Luer slip, 5 cc·mL^{-1}, Terumo, Tokyo, Japan). Each component was rinsed with Milli-Q water and then sonicated in 100% undenatured ethanol for 15 min (tubing was not exposed to ethanol), followed by a further rinse, then sonicated in Milli-Q water for 15 min. Finally, the components were rinsed a last time, dried under a stream of high purity dried nitrogen gas (99.999%, BOC, North Ryde, NSW, Australia) and allowed to dry fully overnight in a covered plastic container before being mounted.

Multilayers were created on the IRE surface under flow by following the protocol outlined above. The FGF-2 adsorption and PBS rinses were performed by flowing PBS over the multilayer for 5 min at 1.000 mL·min^{-1}. Then the tubing was removed and FGF-2 solution was injected directly into the flowcell chamber via a syringe (Luer slip, 1 cc·mL^{-1}, Terumo, Japan). The injection of the solution was staged over the 15 min adsorption, with 0.3 mL injected at 0, 5 and 10 min. For the diffusion study the FGF-2 remained on the multilayer for 2 h. The tubing was reconnected to the flowcell and then flushed with PBS again for 5 min at 1.000 mL·min^{-1}.

Single channel spectra from 256 scans were obtained in the region of 650 cm^{-1} (on the ZnSe IRE) or 780 cm^{-1} (on the Ge IRE) to 4000 cm^{-1}, with 4 cm^{-1} resolution (commonly employed for studies of condensed matter systems, as higher resolution does not provide finer detail of peaks due to the natural linewidth of peaks in such systems) using Agilent Resolutions Pro software v5.2.0.36. Spectra were recorded for each experiment, as follows; (i) a background spectrum in air; (ii) a water vapour (WV) spectrum in air 10 min after the background spectrum; (iii) a spectrum of the background electrolyte after 5 min flow; (iv) then polymer spectra after each successive adsorption/rinse cycle.

Spectra were collected at specific time points, during the PBS/FGF-2/PBS cycle; (i) after the 5 min PBS rinse of the 5.5 bilayer, fucoidan terminating PEM, (ii) every 5 min during FGF-2 adsorption and (iii) after the 5 min PBS rinse after growth factor adsorption. These spectra were processed by subtracting the initial PBS rinse from the FGF-2 and subsequent PBS rinse with a 1 to 1 ratio, then a spectrum of PBS was added to flatten the O-H bending mode of water.

Whilst for the diffusion study on the 9.5 bilayer multilayer, spectra were collected at 15 min FGF-2 adsorption and then after a final 5 min PBS rinse following the 2 h FGF-2 adsorption. These spectra were processed by subtracting the PBS rinse of the multilayer in a 1 to 1 ratio from all subsequent spectra. Each experiment was performed as two independent repeats. Spectral processing was performed with OMNIC software v8.2.0.387 (Thermo Fisher Scientific, Scoresby, VIC, Australia).

The multilayer build-up spectra presented below (Figure 3) and in the electronic supplementary material were produced by subtracting the spectrum of the background electrolyte (KCl) from each spectrum to remove the contribution of water in the O-H bending mode region (~1630 cm^{-1}). In Figures 4 and 5 the spectra were produced by subtracting the spectra of the PBS rinse of the 6th fucoidan layer (PBS rinse after FUC6) in a 1 to 1 ratio from each, followed by adding a PBS spectra to flatten the region between 1650–1700 cm^{-1} to remove the O-H bending mode of water. Finally, manual water vapour correction was performed, followed by automatic baseline correction, for all spectra.

4.5. Quartz Crystal Microbalance with Dissipation Monitoring (QCM-D)

The experiments were performed on a Q-sense E4 instrument (Biolin Scientific, Västra Frölunda, Sweden) under continuous flow conditions. The multilayers are formed on Si-coated 5 MHz AT-cut quartz crystal sensors (SiO$_2$ 50 nm, QSX 303, Q-sense, Biolin Scientific, Sweden). The sensors were cleaned by sonicating in 1 M HCl for 30 min, followed by 2% Hellmanex for 30 min then Milli-Q water for 10 min. The sensors were individually dried under a stream of high purity dried nitrogen and air plasma cleaned for 60 s (Harrick Plasma, Ithaca, NY, USA).

Once cleaned, the sensors were placed into the QCM chambers, where they were allowed to stabilise in background electrolyte prior to measurement for 1 h under flow at 0.050 mL·min^{-1} using a multi-channel peristaltic pump (Ismatec, Cole-Palmer, Wertheim, Germany). Then solutions were pumped through the system following the adsorption protocol described above at rates of 0.100 mL·min^{-1} for polyelectrolyte/protein adsorption and 0.300 mL·min^{-1} for the background electrolyte rinse.

The PBS/FGF-2/PBS cycle was performed using a flow rate of 0.300 mL·min^{-1} for 5 min for the PBS rinse prior to the adsorption of growth factor. The FGF-2 adsorption was performed by flowing the growth factor solution over the multilayer for 1 min at a rate of 0.30 mL·min^{-1}, then for 14 min at a rate of 0.05 mL·min^{-1}. The subsequent PBS flush was performed at 0.05 mL·min^{-1} and 0.30 mL·min^{-1} for 5 min each (the extra slow flush was used to account for the additional exposure time of FGF-2 due to spectra collection in ATR FTIR spectroscopy measurements).

5. Conclusions

The ATR infrared spectra and quartz crystal microbalance measurements presented show that fibroblast growth factor-2 can be embedded into the film structure by adsorbing layers of polyelectrolytes over the FGF-2. In addition, it was found that the overall multilayer structure is altered by PBS exposure during the embedding process, and that the incorporation of growth factor had little disruptive effect on the film build-up. This ability of fucoidan to bind fibroblast growth factor 2 in a multilayer structure could offer new methods for protecting and deploying growth factor in a wound bed. Such deployment as a coating on wound dressing material would allow the growth factor to be active in a wound bed as the polyelectrolyte degrades and exposes/releases the growth factor.

Supplementary Materials: The following are available online at http://www.mdpi.com/1660-3397/18/11/531/s1, Figure S1: ATR FTIR spectrum.

Author Contributions: Conceptualisation: D.A.B., M.K. Data curation: N.L.B., M.K. Formal analysis: N.L.B., D.A.B. Funding acquisition: D.A.B., M.K. Investigation: N.L.B., S.K., M.K. Supervision: S.K., M.K., D.A.B. Writing–original draft: N.B. Writing–review and editing: N.B., S.K., M.K., D.A.B. All authors have read and agreed to the published version of the manuscript.

Funding: The authors would like to acknowledge the support of the Australian Government's Cooperative Research Centres Program. DB acknowledges the financial support from the Australian Research Council (ARC: Future Fellowship FT100100393).

Conflicts of Interest: There are no conflicts of interest to declare.

References

1. Traversa, B.; Sussman, G. The Role of Growth Factors, Cytokines and Proteases in Wound Management. *Prim. Intent. Aust. J. Wound Manag.* **2001**, *9*, 161–167.
2. Graves, N.; Zheng, H. Modelling the direct health care costs of chronic wounds in Australia. *Wound Pract. Res. J. Aust. Wound Manag. Assoc.* **2014**, *22*, 20.
3. Järbrink, K.; Ni, G.; Sönnergren, H.; Schmidtchen, A.; Pang, C.; Bajpai, R.; Car, J. The humanistic and economic burden of chronic wounds: A protocol for a systematic review. *Syst. Rev.* **2017**, *6*, 1–7. [CrossRef] [PubMed]
4. Moura, L.I.; Dias, A.M.; Carvalho, E.; De Sousa, H.C. Recent advances on the development of wound dressings for diabetic foot ulcer treatment—A review. *Acta Biomater.* **2013**, *9*, 7093–7114. [CrossRef] [PubMed]
5. Ornitz, D.M. FGFs, heparan sulfate and FGFRs: Complex interactions essential for development. *BioEssays* **2000**, *22*, 108–112. [CrossRef]
6. Zuo, Q.; Guo, R.; Liu, Q.; Hong, A.; Shi, Y.; Kong, Q.; Huang, Y.; He, L.; Xue, W. Heparin-conjugated alginate multilayered microspheres for controlled release of bFGF. *Biomed. Mater.* **2015**, *10*, 035008. [CrossRef]
7. Sun, X.; Cheng, L.; Zhao, J.; Jin, R.; Sun, B.; Shi, Y.; Zhang, L.; Zhang, Y.; Cui, W. BFGF-grafted electrospun fibrous scaffolds via poly(dopamine) for skin wound healing. *J. Mater. Chem. B* **2014**, *2*, 3636–3645. [CrossRef]
8. Macdonald, M.L.; Rodriguez, N.M.; Shah, N.J.; Hammond, P.T. Characterization of Tunable FGF-2 Releasing Polyelectrolyte Multilayers. *Biomacromolecules* **2010**, *11*, 2053–2059. [CrossRef]
9. King, W.J.; Jongpaiboonkit, L.; Murphy, W.L. Influence of FGF2 and PEG hydrogel matrix properties on hMSC viability and spreading. *J. Biomed. Mater. Res. Part A* **2009**, *9*, 1110–1123. [CrossRef]
10. Almodóvar, J.; Bacon, S.; Gogolski, J.; Kisiday, J.D.; Kipper, M.J. Polysaccharide-Based Polyelectrolyte Multilayer Surface Coatings Can Enhance Mesenchymal Stem Cell Response to Adsorbed Growth Factors. *Biomacromolecules* **2010**, *11*, 2629–2639. [CrossRef]
11. Song, Y.H.; Zhu, Y.T.; Ding, J.; Zhou, F.Y.; Xue, J.X.; Jung, J.H.; Li, Z.J.; Gao, W.Y. Distribution of fibroblast growth factors and their roles in skin fibroblast cell migration. *Mol. Med. Rep.* **2016**, *14*, 3336–3342. [CrossRef] [PubMed]
12. Qu, Y.; Cao, C.; Wu, Q.; Huang, A.; Song, Y.; Li, H.; Zuo, Y.; Chu, C.; Li, J.; Man, Y.; et al. The dual delivery of KGF and bFGF by collagen membrane to promote skin wound healing. *J. Tissue Eng. Regen. Med.* **2018**, *12*, 1508–1518. [CrossRef] [PubMed]
13. Sweitzer, S.; Fann, S.A.; Borg, T.K.; Yost, M.J.; Baynes, J.W. What Is the Future of Diabetic Wound Care? *Diabetes Educ.* **2006**, *32*, 197–210. [CrossRef] [PubMed]
14. Kerdjoudj, H.; Berthelemy, N.; Boulmedais, F.; Stoltz, J.-F.; Menu, P.; Voegel, J.C. Multilayered polyelectrolyte films: A tool for arteries and vessel repair. *Soft Matter* **2010**, *6*, 3722–3734. [CrossRef]
15. Peterson, A.M.; Möhwald, H.; Shchukin, D.G.; Moehwald, H. pH-Controlled Release of Proteins from Polyelectrolyte-Modified Anodized Titanium Surfaces for Implant Applications. *Biomacromolecules* **2012**, *13*, 3120–3126. [CrossRef]
16. Salvi, C.; Lyu, X.; Peterson, A.M. Effect of Assembly pH on Polyelectrolyte Multilayer Surface Properties and BMP-2 Release. *Biomacromolecules* **2016**, *17*, 1949–1958. [CrossRef]
17. Naves, A.F.; Motay, M.; Mérindol, R.; Davi, C.P.; Felix, O.; Catalani, L.H.; Decher, G. Layer-by-Layer assembled growth factor reservoirs for steering the response of 3T3-cells. *Colloids Surfaces B Biointerfaces* **2016**, *139*, 79–86. [CrossRef]
18. Shah, N.J.; Macdonald, M.L.; Beben, Y.M.; Padera, R.F.; Samuel, R.E.; Hammond, P.T. Tunable dual growth factor delivery from polyelectrolyte multilayer films. *Biomaterials* **2011**, *32*, 6183–6193. [CrossRef]

19. Marudova, M.; Exner, G.; Pilicheva, B.; Marinova, A.; Viraneva, A.; Bodurov, I.; Sotirov, S.; Vlaeva, I.; Uzunova, Y.; Yovcheva, T. Effect of assembly pH and ionic strength of chitosan/casein multilayers on benzydamine hydrochloride release. *Int. J. Polym. Mater.* **2018**, *68*, 90–98. [CrossRef]
20. Peterson, A.M.; Pilz-Allen, C.; Kolesnikova, T.; Möhwald, H.; Shchukin, D.G.; Moehwald, H. Growth Factor Release from Polyelectrolyte-Coated Titanium for Implant Applications. *ACS Appl. Mater. Interf.* **2013**, *6*, 1866–1871. [CrossRef]
21. Peterson, A.M.; Pilz-Allen, C.; Möhwald, H.; Shchukin, D.G. Evaluation of the role of polyelectrolyte deposition conditions in growth factor release. *J. Mater. Chem. B* **2014**, *2*, 2680–2687. [CrossRef] [PubMed]
22. Saikaew, R.; Marsal, P.; Grenier, B.; Dubas, S.T. Temperature controlled loading and release of curcumin in polyelectrolyte multilayers thin films. *Mater. Lett.* **2018**, *215*, 38–41. [CrossRef]
23. Webber, J.L.; Benbow, N.L.; Krasowska, M.; Beattie, D.A. Formation and enzymatic degradation of poly-l-arginine/fucoidan multilayer films. *Colloid Surface B* **2017**, *159*, 468–476. [CrossRef] [PubMed]
24. Wang, Z.; Wang, K.; Lu, X.; Li, C.; Han, L.; Xie, C.; Liu, Y.; Qu, S.; Zhen, G. Nanostructured Architectures by Assembling Polysaccharide-Coated BSA Nanoparticles for Biomedical Application. *Adv. Health Mater.* **2015**, *4*, 927–937. [CrossRef] [PubMed]
25. Trushina, D.B.; Bukreeva, T.V.; Borodina, T.N.; Belova, D.D.; Belyakov, S.; Antipina, M.N. Heat-driven size reduction of biodegradable polyelectrolyte multilayer hollow capsules assembled on CaCO3 template. *Colloids Surfaces B Biointerfaces* **2018**, *170*, 312–321. [CrossRef] [PubMed]
26. Adamczak, M.; Hoel, H.; Gaudernack, G.; Barbasz, J.; Szczepanowicz, K.; Warszyński, P. Polyelectrolyte multilayer capsules with quantum dots for biomedical applications. *Colloids Surfaces B Biointerfaces* **2012**, *90*, 211–216. [CrossRef] [PubMed]
27. Losi, P.; Briganti, E.; Errico, C.; Lisella, A.; Sanguinetti, E.; Chiellini, F.; Soldani, G. Fibrin-based scaffold incorporating VEGF- and bFGF-loaded nanoparticles stimulates wound healing in diabetic mice. *Acta Biomater.* **2013**, *9*, 7814–7821. [CrossRef]
28. Amorim, S.; Pires, R.A.; Da Costa, D.S.; Reis, R.L.; Pashkuleva, I. Interactions between Exogenous FGF-2 and Sulfonic Groups: In Situ Characterization and Impact on the Morphology of Human Adipose-Derived Stem Cells. *Langmuir* **2013**, *29*, 7983–7992. [CrossRef]
29. Hammond, P.T. Building biomedical materials layer-by-layer. *Mater. Today* **2012**, *15*, 196–206. [CrossRef]
30. Muzzarelli, R.A.A. Chitins and chitosans for the repair of wounded skin, nerve, cartilage and bone. *Carbohydr. Polym.* **2009**, *76*, 167–182. [CrossRef]
31. Jayakumar, R.; Prabaharan, M.; Kumar, P.S.; Nair, S.; Tamura, H. Biomaterials based on chitin and chitosan in wound dressing applications. *Biotechnol. Adv.* **2011**, *29*, 322–337. [CrossRef] [PubMed]
32. Gorouhi, F.; Shah, N.M.; Raghunathan, V.; Mohabbati, Y.; Abbott, N.L.; Isseroff, R.R.; Murphy, C.J. Epidermal Growth Factor–Functionalized Polymeric Multilayer Films: Interplay between Spatial Location and Bioavailability of EGF. *J. Investig. Dermatol.* **2014**, *134*, 1757–1760. [CrossRef] [PubMed]
33. Chabut, D.; Fischer, A.-M.; Colliec-Jouault, S.; Laurendeau, I.; Matou, S.; Le Bonniec, B.; Helley, D. Low Molecular Weight Fucoidan and Heparin Enhance the Basic Fibroblast Growth Factor-Induced Tube Formation of Endothelial Cells through Heparan Sulfate-Dependent α6 Overexpression. *Mol. Pharmacol.* **2003**, *64*, 696–702. [CrossRef] [PubMed]
34. Matou, S.; Helley, D.; Chabut, D.; Bros, A.; Fischer, A.-M. Effect of fucoidan on fibroblast growth factor-2-induced angiogenesis in vitro. *Thromb. Res.* **2002**, *106*, 213–221. [CrossRef]
35. Lake, A.C.; Vassy, R.; Di Benedetto, M.; Lavigne, D.; Le Visage, C.; Perret, G.Y.; Letourneur, D. Low Molecular Weight Fucoidan Increases VEGF165-induced Endothelial Cell Migration by Enhancing VEGF165Binding to VEGFR-2 and NRP1. *J. Biol. Chem.* **2006**, *281*, 37844–37852. [CrossRef]
36. Ye, X.; Wang, H.; Zhou, J.; Li, H.; Liu, J.; Wang, Z.; Chen, A.; Zhao, Q. The Effect of Heparin-VEGF Multilayer on the Biocompatibility of Decellularized Aortic Valve with Platelet and Endothelial Progenitor Cells. *PLoS ONE* **2013**, *8*, e54622. [CrossRef]
37. Belford, D.A.; Hendry, I.A.; Parish, C.R. Investigation of the ability of several naturally occurring and synthetic polyanions to bind to and potentiate the biological activity of acidic fibroblast growth factor. *J. Cell. Physiol.* **1993**, *157*, 184–189. [CrossRef]
38. Luyt, C.-E.; Meddahi-Pellé, A.; Ho-Tin-Noé, B.; Colliec-Jouault, S.; Guezennec, J.; Louedec, L.; Prats, H.; Jacob, M.-P.; Osborne-Pellegrin, M.; Letourneur, D.; et al. Low-Molecular-Weight Fucoidan Promotes

Therapeutic Revascularization in a Rat Model of Critical Hindlimb Ischemia. *J. Pharmacol. Exp. Ther.* **2003**, *305*, 24–30. [CrossRef]
39. Song, Y.S.; Li, H.; Balcos, M.C.; Yun, H.-Y.; Baek, K.J.; Kwon, N.S.; Choi, H.-R.; Park, K.-C.; Kim, D.-S. Fucoidan Promotes the Reconstruction of Skin Equivalents. *Korean J. Physiol. Pharmacol.* **2014**, *18*, 327–331. [CrossRef]
40. Kim, B.S.; Park, J.; Kang, H.-J.; Kim, H.-J.; Lee, J. Fucoidan/FGF-2 induces angiogenesis through JNK- and p38-mediated activation of AKT/MMP-2 signalling. *Biochem. Biophys. Res. Commun.* **2014**, *450*, 1333–1338. [CrossRef]
41. Nakamura, S.; Nambu, M.; Ishizuka, T.; Hattori, H.; Kanatani, Y.; Takase, B.; Kishimoto, S.; Amano, Y.; Aoki, H.; Kiyosawa, T.; et al. Effect of controlled release of fibroblast growth factor-2 from chitosan/fucoidan micro complex-hydrogel on in vitro and in vivo vascularization. *J. Biomed. Mater. Res. Part A* **2008**, *85*, 619–627. [CrossRef] [PubMed]
42. Zemani, F.; Benisvy, D.; Galy-Fauroux, I.; Lokajczyk, A.; Colliec-Jouault, S.; Uzan, G.; Fischer, A.M.; Boisson-Vidal, C. Low-molecular-weight fucoidan enhances the proangiogenic phenotype of endothelial progenitor cells. *Biochem. Pharmacol.* **2005**, *70*, 1167–1175. [CrossRef] [PubMed]
43. Marinval, N.; Morenc, M.; Labour, M.-N.; Samotus, A.; Mzyk, A.; Ollivier, V.; Maire, M.; Jesse, K.; Bassand, K.; Niemiec-Cyganek, A.; et al. Fucoidan/VEGF-based surface modification of decellularized pulmonary heart valve improves the antithrombotic and re-endothelialization potential of bioprostheses. *Biomateials* **2018**, *172*, 14–29. [CrossRef]
44. Wang, W.; Wang, S.-X.; Guan, H.-S. The Antiviral Activities and Mechanisms of Marine Polysaccharides: An Overview. *Mar. Drugs* **2012**, *10*, 2795–2816. [CrossRef] [PubMed]
45. Lee, J.-B.; Hayashi, K.; Hashimoto, M.; Nakano, T.; Hayashi, T. Novel Antiviral Fucoidan from Sporophyll of Undaria pinnatifida (Mekabu). *Chem. Pharm. Bull.* **2004**, *52*, 1091–1094. [CrossRef] [PubMed]
46. Jiang, C.; Knappe, S.; Reutterer, S.; Szabo, C.M.; Dockal, M.; Zhang, Z.; Till, S.; Scheiflinger, F. Structure-activity relationship of the pro- and anticoagulant effects of Fucus vesiculosus fucoidan. *Thromb. Haemost.* **2014**, *111*, 429–437. [CrossRef] [PubMed]
47. Bouvard, C.; Galy-Fauroux, I.; Grelac, F.; Carpentier, W.; Lokajczyk, A.; Gandrille, S.; Colliec-Jouault, S.; Fischer, A.-M.; Helley, D. Low-Molecular-Weight Fucoidan Induces Endothelial Cell Migration via the PI3K/AKT Pathway and Modulates the Transcription of Genes Involved in Angiogenesis. *Mar. Drugs* **2015**, *13*, 7446–7462. [CrossRef]
48. Fitton, J.H.; Stringer, D.N.; Karpiniec, S.S. Therapies from Fucoidan: An Update. *Mar. Drugs* **2015**, *13*, 5920–5946. [CrossRef] [PubMed]
49. Cumashi, A.; Ushakova, N.A.; Preobrazhenskaya, M.E.; D'Incecco, A.; Piccoli, A.; Totani, L.; Tinari, N.; Morozevich, G.E.; Berman, A.E.; Bilan, M.I.; et al. A comparative study of the anti-inflammatory, anticoagulant, antiangiogenic, and antiadhesive activities of nine different fucoidans from brown seaweeds. *Glycobiology* **2007**, *17*, 541–552. [CrossRef]
50. Ale, M.T.; Mikkelsen, J.D.; Meyer, A.S. Important Determinants for Fucoidan Bioactivity: A Critical Review of Structure-Function Relations and Extraction Methods for Fucose-Containing Sulfated Polysaccharides from Brown Seaweeds. *Mar. Drugs* **2011**, *9*, 2106–2130. [CrossRef]
51. Fitton, J.H. Therapies from Fucoidan; Multifunctional Marine Polymers. *Mar. Drugs* **2011**, *9*, 1731–1760. [CrossRef] [PubMed]
52. Masuoka, K.; Ishihara, M.; Asazuma, T.; Hattori, H.; Matsui, T.; Takase, B.; Kanatani, Y.; Fujita, M.; Saito, Y.; Yura, H.; et al. The interaction of chitosan with fibroblast growth factor-2 and its protection from inactivation. *Biomaterial* **2005**, *26*, 3277–3284. [CrossRef] [PubMed]
53. Mizuno, K.; Yamamura, K.; Yano, K.; Osada, T.; Saeki, S.; Takimoto, N.; Sakurai, T.; Nimura, Y. Effect of chitosan film containing basic fibroblast growth factor on wound healing in genetically diabetic mice. *J. Biomed. Mater. Res.* **2002**, *64*, 177–181. [CrossRef] [PubMed]
54. Benbow, N.L.; Sebben, D.A.; Karpiniec, S.; Stringer, D.; Krasowska, M.; Beattie, D.A. Lysozyme uptake into pharmaceutical grade fucoidan/chitosan polyelectrolyte multilayers under physiological conditions. *J. Colloid Interface Sci.* **2020**, *565*, 555–566. [CrossRef]
55. Ho, T.T.M.; Bremmell, K.E.; Krasowska, M.; Stringer, D.N.; Thierry, B.; Beattie, D.A. Tuning polyelectrolyte multilayer structure by exploiting natural variation in fucoidan chemistry. *Soft Matter* **2015**, *11*, 2110–2124. [CrossRef]

56. Benbow, N.L.; Webber, J.L.; Karpiniec, S.; Krasowska, M.; Ferri, J.K.; Beattie, D.A. The influence of polyanion molecular weight on polyelectrolyte multilayers at surfaces: Protein adsorption and protein–polysaccharide complexation/stripping on natural polysaccharide films on solid supports. *Phys. Chem. Chem. Phys.* **2017**, *19*, 23790–23801. [CrossRef]
57. Benbow, N.L.; Webber, J.L.; Pawliszak, P.; Sebben, D.A.; Karpiniec, S.; Stringer, D.; Tobin, M.J.; Vongsvivut, J.; Krasowska, M.; Beattie, D.A. Odd-even effects on hydration of natural polyelectrolyte multilayers: An in situ synchrotron FTIR microspectroscopy study. *J. Colloid Interface Sci.* **2019**, *553*, 720–733. [CrossRef]
58. Fadeeva, I.V.; Barinov, S.M.; Fedotov, A.Y.; Komlev, V.S. Interactions of calcium phosphates with chitosan. *Dokl. Chem.* **2011**, *441*, 387–390. [CrossRef]
59. Li, H.H. Refractive index of silicon and germanium and its wavelength and temperature derivatives. *J. Phys. Chem. Ref. Data* **1980**, *9*, 561–658. [CrossRef]
60. Kwan, C.-P.; Kaundinya, G.V.; Shriver, Z.; Raman, R.; Liu, D.; Qi, Y.; Varticovski, L.; Sasisekharan, R. Probing Fibroblast Growth Factor Dimerization and Role of Heparin-like Glycosaminoglycans in Modulating Dimerization and Signaling. *J. Biol. Chem.* **2001**, *276*, 23421–23429. [CrossRef]
61. Raman, R.; Venkataraman, G.; Ernst, S.; Sasisekharan, V.; Sasisekharan, R. Structural specificity of heparin binding in the fibroblast growth factor family of proteins. *Proc. Natl. Acad. Sci. USA* **2003**, *100*, 2357–2362. [CrossRef] [PubMed]
62. Ori, A.; Free, P.; Courty, J.; Wilkinson, M.C.; Fernig, D.G. Identification of Heparin-binding Sites in Proteins by Selective Labeling. *Mol. Cell. Proteom.* **2009**, *8*, 2256–2265. [CrossRef] [PubMed]
63. Musselman, C.A.; Kutateladze, T.G. Preparation, Biochemical Analysis, and Structure Determination of Methyllysine Readers. In *Methods Enzymology*; Marmorstein, R., Ed.; Academic Press: Cambridge, MA, USA, 2016; Volume 573, pp. 345–362.
64. Xu, R.; Ori, A.; Rudd, T.R.; Uniewicz, K.A.; Ahmed, Y.A.; Guimond, S.E.; Skidmore, M.A.; Siligardi, G.; Yates, E.A.; Fernig, D.G. Diversification of the Structural Determinants of Fibroblast Growth Factor-Heparin Interactions. *J. Biol. Chem.* **2012**, *287*, 40061–40073. [CrossRef]
65. Van De Weert, M.; Andersen, M.B.; Frokjaer, S. Complex Coacervation of Lysozyme and Heparin: Complex Characterization and Protein Stability. *Pharm. Res.* **2004**, *21*, 2354–2359. [CrossRef]
66. Kim, I.-Y.; Seo, S.-J.; Moon, H.-S.; Yoo, M.-K.; Park, I.-Y.; Kim, B.-C.; Cho, C.-S. Chitosan and its derivatives for tissue engineering applications. *Biotechnol. Adv.* **2008**, *26*, 1–21. [CrossRef] [PubMed]
67. Pillai, C.; Paul, W.; Sharma, C.P. Chitin and chitosan polymers: Chemistry, solubility and fiber formation. *Prog. Polym. Sci.* **2009**, *34*, 641–678. [CrossRef]
68. Kumorek, M.; Kubies, D.; Riedel, T. Protein Interactions With Quaternized Chitosan/Heparin Multilayers. *Physiol. Res.* **2016**, *65*, S253–S261. [CrossRef] [PubMed]
69. Hsu, B.B.; Jamieson, K.S.; Hagerman, S.R.; Holler, E.; Ljubimova, J.Y.; Hammond, P.T. Ordered and Kinetically Discrete Sequential Protein Release from Biodegradable Thin Films. *Angew. Chem. Intern. Ed.* **2014**, *53*, 8093–8098. [CrossRef]
70. Macdonald, M.; Rodriguez, N.M.; Smith, R.; Hammond, P.T. Release of a model protein from biodegradable self assembled films for surface delivery applications. *J. Control Release* **2008**, *131*, 228–234. [CrossRef]
71. Macdonald, M.L.; Samuel, R.E.; Shah, N.J.; Padera, R.F.; Beben, Y.M.; Hammond, P.T. Tissue integration of growth factor-eluting layer-by-layer polyelectrolyte multilayer coated implants. *Biomaterials* **2011**, *32*, 1446–1453. [CrossRef]
72. Laucirica, G.; Marmisollé, W.A.; Azzaroni, O. Dangerous liaisons: Anion-induced protonation in phosphate–polyamine interactions and their implications for the charge states of biologically relevant surfaces. *Phys. Chem. Chem. Phys.* **2017**, *19*, 8612–8620. [CrossRef] [PubMed]
73. Peng, C.; Liu, J.; Xie, Y.; Zhou, J. Molecular simulations of cytochrome c adsorption on positively charged surfaces: The influence of anion type and concentration. *Phys. Chem. Chem. Phys.* **2016**, *18*, 9979–9989. [CrossRef] [PubMed]
74. Kubota, T.; Namiki, A.; Fukazawa, M.; Ishikawa, M.; Moroi, M.; Ebine, K.; Yamaguchi, T. Concentrations of Hepatocyte Growth Factor, Basic Fibroblast Growth Factor, and Vascular Endothelial Growth Factor in Pericardial Fluid and Plasma. *Jpn. Heart J.* **2004**, *45*, 989–998. [CrossRef]
75. She, Z.; Wang, C.; Li, J.; Sukhorukov, G.B.; Antipina, M.N. Encapsulation of Basic Fibroblast Growth Factor by Polyelectrolyte Multilayer Microcapsules and Its Controlled Release for Enhancing Cell Proliferation. *Biomacromolecules* **2012**, *13*, 2174–2180. [CrossRef] [PubMed]

76. Shah, N.J.; Hyder, M.N.; Quadir, M.A.; Courchesne, N.-M.D.; Seeherman, H.J.; Nevins, M.; Spector, M.; Hammond, P.T. Adaptive growth factor delivery from a polyelectrolyte coating promotes synergistic bone tissue repair and reconstruction. *Proc. Natl. Acad. Sci. USA* **2014**, *111*, 2847–2852. [CrossRef]
77. Vrana, N.E.; Erdemli, O.; Francius, G.; Fahs, A.; Rabineau, M.; Debry, C.; Tezcaner, A.; Keskin, D.; Lavalle, P. Double entrapment of growth factors by nanoparticles loaded into polyelectrolyte multilayer films. *J. Mater. Chem. B* **2014**, *2*, 999–1008. [CrossRef]

Publisher's Note: MDPI stays neutral with regard to jurisdictional claims in published maps and institutional affiliations.

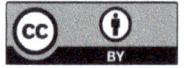

© 2020 by the authors. Licensee MDPI, Basel, Switzerland. This article is an open access article distributed under the terms and conditions of the Creative Commons Attribution (CC BY) license (http://creativecommons.org/licenses/by/4.0/).

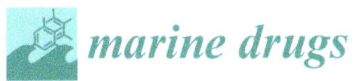

Article

Fucoidans of Moroccan Brown Seaweed as Elicitors of Natural Defenses in Date Palm Roots

Soukaina Bouissil [1,2], Zainab El Alaoui-Talibi [1], Guillaume Pierre [2], Halima Rchid [3], Philippe Michaud [2], Cédric Delattre [2,4,*] and Cherkaoui El Modafar [1]

1. Laboratoire d'Agrobiotechnologie et Bioingénierie, Faculté des Sciences et Techniques Marrakech, Université Cadi Ayyad, Marrakesh 40000, Morocco; soukaina.BOUISSIL@etu.uca.fr (S.B.); Z.elalaouitalibi@uca.ma (Z.E.A.-T.); elmodafar@uca.ac.ma (C.E.M.)
2. Institut Pascal, Université Clermont Auvergne, CNRS, SIGMA Clermont, F-63000 Clermont-Ferrand, France; guillaume.pierre@uca.fr (G.P.); philippe.michaud@uca.fr (P.M.)
3. Laboratoire de Biotechnologies et Valorisation des Ressources Végétales, Faculté des Sciences, Université Chouaib Doukkali, El Jadida 24000, Morocco; rchid.h@ucd.ac.ma
4. Institut Universitaire de France (IUF), 1 Rue Descartes, 75005 Paris, France
* Correspondence: cedric.delattre@uca.fr

Received: 9 November 2020; Accepted: 25 November 2020; Published: 26 November 2020

Abstract: Fucoidans from Moroccan brown seaweed *Bifurcaria bifurcata* and *Fucus spiralis* were tested for their elicitor activity after their purification and complete characterization. The fucoidans of *B. bifurcata* (BBF) and of *F. spiralis* (FSF) were extracted and purified then characterized by infrared spectroscopy, proton nuclear magnetic resonance spectroscopy and size exclusion chromatography. The results show that BBF and FSF are mainly sulfated with 45.49 and 49.53% (w/w) sulfate, respectively. Analysis of neutral sugars determined by gas chromatography–mass spectrometry showed that FSF and BBF were mainly composed of 64% and 91% fucose and 20% and 6% galactose, respectively, with a few other sugars such as glucose (8% in FSF), rhamnose (1% in BBF) and mannose (8% in FSF and, 2% in BBF). The eliciting activity of these sulfated polysaccharides in stimulating the natural defenses of the date palm was evaluated through the activity of phenylalanine ammonia-lyase (PAL), and the increase in phenols and lignin content in the roots. The results obtained clearly show that the two fucoidans early and intensely stimulate the natural defenses of the date palm after 24 h of treatments. This remarkable elicitor effect seems to be linked to the sulfated groups compared to non-sulfate alginates extracted from the same algae. These results open promising perspectives for a biological control approach against date palm diseases.

Keywords: sulfated polysaccharides; natural defenses; phenolic metabolism; phenylalanine ammonia-lyase

1. Introduction

Sulfated polysaccharides are increasingly recognized for their broad spectrum of biological activities. They usually found in large quantities in brown seaweeds. In addition, the polysaccharides structures depend on the algae species. Thus, various biological activities could be discovered with each new sulfated polysaccharide extraction [1].

Amongst these polysaccharides, the most studied was carrageenan [2], ulvan [3] and fucoidans. Fucoidans at the molecular level constitute a polymer of L-fucose linked by (1,3) and (1,4) with residues mainly sulfated on C-4 [4,5]. The characteristic structure of fucoidans rich in L-fucose and sulfated ester groups has generated widespread interest due to their therapeutic effects. Several works reported the biological proprieties of fucoidans [6], namely antioxidant [7,8], antitumor [9–12] and anticoagulant [13]. In addition to these biological applications, fucoidans and their oligosaccharides have also been the subject of other studies on biostimulants of defence mechanisms in plants [14,15]. They were also suggested as biological approaches to control plants disease [16], by benefiting from their stimulating effect of early and late defensive responses. It is reported that biological and biostimulant properties of fucoidans depend in particular on the degree of sulfation [8] and on their various physico–chemical properties [5].

The aim of this work is to study the potential activity of fucoidans to elicit the natural defence mechanisms in date palm (*Phoenix dactylifera* L.) roots as a monocotyledon plant. Through an innovative elicitation model allowing the treatment of the roots which are the site of infection of the date palm by *Fusarium oxysporum* f. sp. *albedinis* (Foa), a telluric pathogen causing the fatal disease (Bayoud) of date palm [17]. In response to Bayoud disease, date palm develops numerous defence mechanisms in roots such as the induction of phytoalexins [18], the accumulation of caffeoyl shikimic acids [19,20] and the reinforcement of the cell walls by lignin and phenolic compounds [21]. These defence mechanisms all depend on, phenylalanine ammonia-lyase (PAL) activity, triggering the phenlypropanoid pathway [17]. The activity of this enzyme governs the defence mechanisms induced in sensitive and resistant varieties during a date palm and Foa interactions [22]. In this context crude fucoidans, extracted from two brown algae *Bifurcaria bifurcata* and *Fucus spiralis* from the Atlantic coast of Morocco were structurally characterized and tested for their possible eliciting effect on the defence mechanisms of the date palm roots.

2. Results and Discussion

2.1. Chemical Composition of Crude Fucoidans

The abundance of the two brown algae *B. bifurcata* and *F. spiralis* on the Moroccan Atlantic coast was the reason for the choice of these two species. The yield as well as the chemical composition of the fucoidans extracted from these species are shown in Table 1. FSF and BBF yields were around 8 and 2%, respectively, based on algae dry weight.

Table 1. Chemical composition and yield of *F. spiralis* (FSF) and *B. bifurcata* (BBF) crude fucoidans.

Analytical Data (%, w/w)	FSF	BBF
Yield [a]	7.9	1.9
Neutral sugar [b]	51.16	45.23
Uronic acids [b]	14.68	21.79
Sulfates [b]	49.53	45.49
Protein [b]	Traces	Traces
M_w (g/mol) [c]	20×10^3	14×10^3

[a] Expressed on the weight of dry depigmented algae. [b] Expressed on the weight of dry fucoidans. [c] Molecular weight by High Performance Size Exclusion Chromatography (HPSEC) analysis.

Colorimetric assays show that FSF and BBF contained principally neutral sugar from 45.23 to 51.16 for *B. bifurcata* (BBF) and of *F. spiralis* (FSF), respectively, those extracted fucoidans were also highly sulfated (FSF, 49.53% and BBF, 45.49%).

The main neutral sugars which constitute FSF and BBF was determined by gas chromatography–mass spectrometry (GC-MS) analysis and the result reported in Table 2 shows that was the L-fucose with 63.98 and 90.68%, respectively, based on dry weight of sulfated polysaccharides (FSF and BBF).

The results obtained (Table 1) are different from those demonstrated for fucoidans of *B. bifurcata* from Britain with a higher extraction yield (17% w/w), 40–42% of carbohydrate with 22.2% of sulfates [23]. Compared to fucoidans extracted from other green algae, the BBF extraction yield remained much lower than that registered of fucoidans of *Cystoseira compressa* (5.2% w/w) [24] and *Cystoseira barbata* (5.45% w/w) [8], whereas, it is close to 2.8% of fucoidans purified from *C. crinite* and to 2.2% extracted from *Dictyota dichotoma* [25,26], while the FSF yield was more important than that reported for the algae mentioned above. On the other hand, the sulfates concentration of extracted polysaccharides (FSF and

BBF) was much higher than those reported for fucoidans extracted from *Cystoseira* and *Sargassum* species [8,24,27]. Elsewhere, fucoidans from *Alaria* sp. and *Saccharina japonica* at spore production was highly sulfated than fucoidans obtained at vegetative status of these brown algae species [28]. Thus, fucoidans' yield and their overall chemical composition could be influenced by the procreating status of seaweed [29]. L-fucose was the principal constitutive monosaccharide of FSF and BBF, with a Fuc_p/Gal_p ratio of 3.2 and 14.7, respectively (Table 2), indicating a predominate amount of L-fucose than galactose. This composition was similar to that found in fucoidans of *Saccharina cichorioides* (Fuc_p/Gal_p ratio of 13.84) related to 88.6% mol of L-fucose and 6.4% mol of galactose [27]. The ratio found in this work for BBF (14.7) appeared higher than that recorded for fucoidans of *S. japonica* with Fuc_p/Gal_p of 1.13 [27], and the ratio obtained from *Undaria pinnatifida* fucoidans which was equal to 1.39 [29]. More studies carried out on fucoidans reported the lower Fuc_p/Gal_p ratio for fucoidans of *C. compressa* (2.57) [24], *C. barbata* (1.3) [8], *Agarum cribrosum* (2.63) [30], *Lachemilla angustata* (3.93) [31] and *Fucus evanescens* (8.2) [27]. The monosaccharide composition obtained for FSF and BBF reported the presence of more than 50% of L-fucose; this can explain the higher sulfate concentration in FSF and BBF. It was reported that concentration of sulfated residues depend on the nature of fucoidans monosaccharide composition [27,31].

Table 2. Monosaccharide composition of *F. spiralis* (FSF) and *B. bifurcata* (BBF) crude fucoidans.

Monosaccharides [a] (% mol)	FSF	BBF
Fucose	63.98	90.68
Galactose	20.00	6.19
Glucose	8.00	nd
Mannose	7.99	1.65
Rhamnose	nd	1.46
Fuc_p/Gal_p ratio	3.2	14.7

[a] Monosaccharides composition by GC-MS analysis, expressed as molar % of the total identified peaks based on the weight of dry fucoidans.

2.2. Proton Nuclear Magnetic Resonance (^{1}H-NMR) and Infrared (ATR-FTIR) Spectroscopies

To better characterize the fucoidans, an ^{1}H NMR analysis was carried out. FSF and BBF spectra are presented in Figure 1. The two spectra exhibit five regions characteristic of fucoidans. The intense peaks at 1.34 and at 1.22 ppm are from the H6 methyl protons of L-fucopyranose [32]. Signal at 2.14 ppm refer to the methyl protons of the O-acetyl groups [32]. The spectrum between 4.1 and 3.7 ppm corresponds to the protons of the ring (H2-H5) [8]. The signal around 4.3 ppm, is related to the protons of the 4-O-sulfated monosaccharides [33,34]. It is more intense in the case of FSF than BBF, which corroborates the slight difference in sulfates proportions between the two samples (Table 1). Finally the signals region between 5.3 and 5.03 ppm, are attributed to the C-H proton of substituted O=C and to proton H1 of monosaccharides-α-L-fucopyranose [32]. The spectra obtained for FSF and BBF are very similar to those obtained for fucoidans of *Fucus vesiculosus* and *Ascophyllum nodosum* [33], *C. barbata* [8] and *C. compressa* [24].

In parallel, an infrared analysis was carried out. The Attenuated Total Reflectance ATR-FTIR spectra of BBF and FSF were represented in Figure 2. The two spectra showed characteristics bands at 3406–3403, 2941, 1635–1605, 1423–1420, 1222–1223, 1027–1013, 836–833, 577–574 and 479–748 cm^{-1} (Figure 2). The absorption peaks around 3406–3403 and 2941 cm^{-1} are attributed to the elongation of (O-H) and asymmetric vibrations of (C-H), respectively [35]. The signals around 1635 cm^{-1} were attributed to the elongation vibrations of (C=O) in uronic monosaccharides [36]. Asymmetric vibrations of elongation within O-S-O were revealed at 1222 and 1223 cm^{-1} indicating the presence of sulfate esters [37], whilst the elongation of sulfur dioxide (O=S=O) could be indicated by the signals at 1027 and at 1013 cm^{-1} for BBF (Figure 2A) and FSF (Figure 2B), respectively [37]. In addition, sulfate groups linked to C4 of fucosyl units seem to be revealed at 836 and 833 cm^{-1} characteristics bands of (C4-O-S) elongation [38]. However, the binding of sulfate groups with galactose residues was indicated by the absorption bands at 577 and 479 cm^{-1} [37].

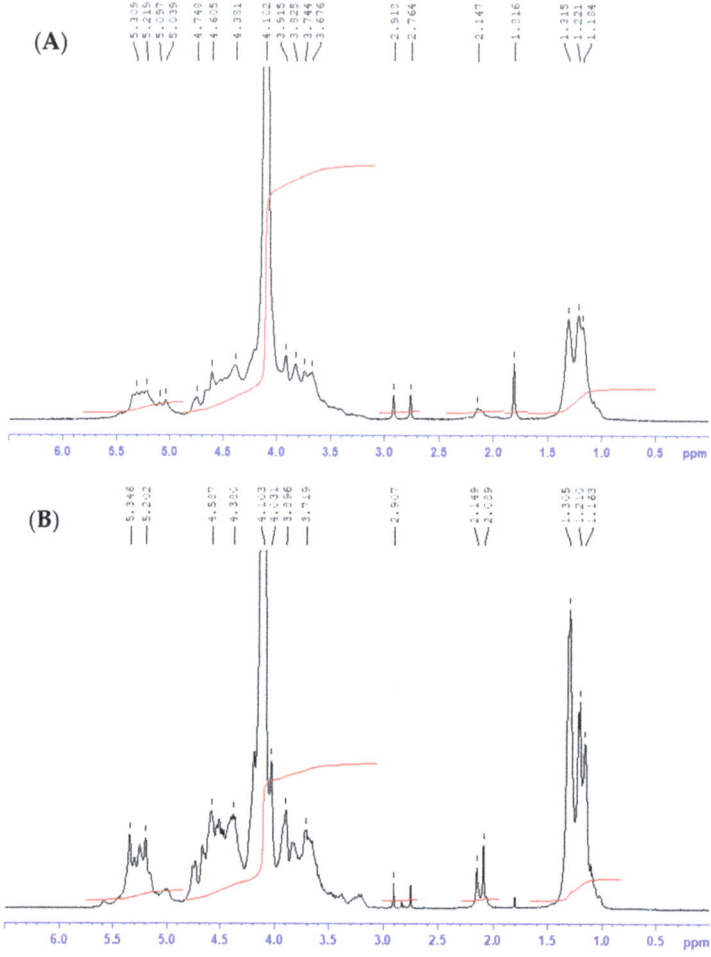

Figure 1. ^{1}H NMR spectra of sulfated polysaccharides from (**A**) *B. bifurcata* (BBF) and (**B**) *F. spiralis* (FSF) at 60 °C in D$_2$O solution.

2.3. Effect of Fucoidans (FSF and BBF) on the Natural Defence of Date Palm Roots

2.3.1. Phenylalanine Amonia-Lyase (PAL) Activity

Given the involvement of the phenolic metabolism in the natural defenses in date palm roots against Foa [17], the mobilization of the phenlypropanoids pathway was demonstrated by studying PAL activity, as the main enzyme of this metabolic pathway. As shown in Figure 3, PAL activity was induced by both *F. spiralis* (FSF) and *B. bifurcata* (BBF) fucoidans. A total of 12 h of FSF treatment were sufficient to significantly increase PAL activity compared to the control treatment ($p < 0.05$). This increase stayed significantly different from control plants over 24 h. A second narrower peak was obtained at 96 h, this could be explained by the elicitor solutions (fucoidans) remained in permanent contact with the roots for the duration of the experiment (4 days), leading to a second wave of induction of PAL activity. The BBF treatment intensely and significantly increased PAL activity after 24 h of treatment, 4.8 times higher than the response noted in control plants ($p < 0.05$).

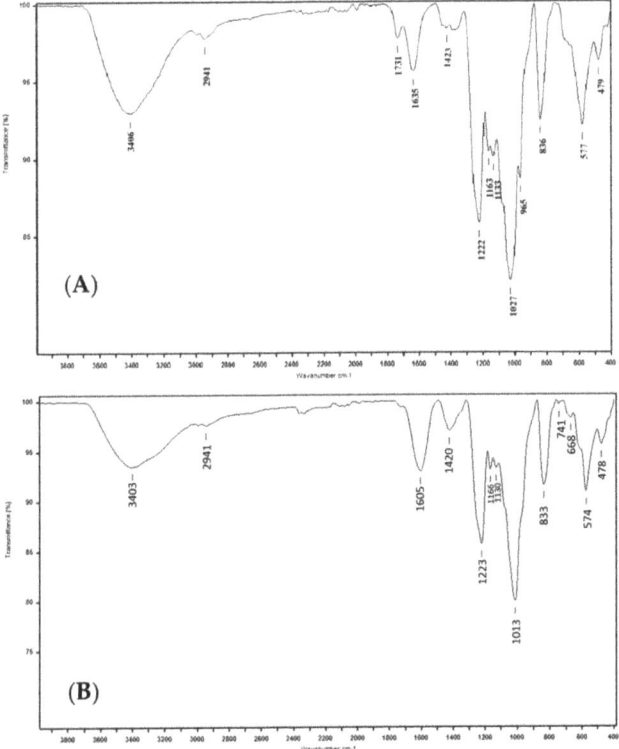

Figure 2. ATR-FTIR spectra of sulfated polysaccharides from (**A**) *B. bifurcata* (BBF) and (**B**) *F. spiralis* (FSF).

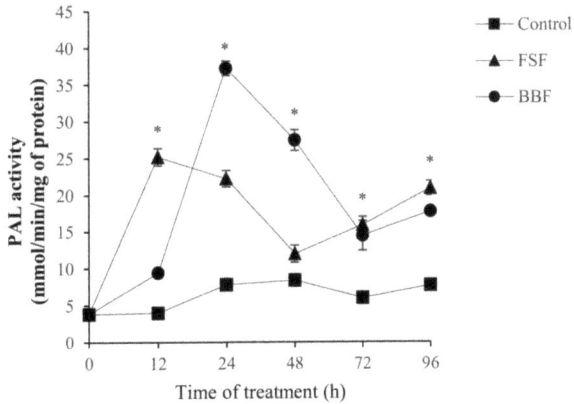

Figure 3. Induction of phenylalanine ammonia-lyase (PAL) activity in date palm roots treated with sulfated polysaccharides of *F. spiralis* (FSF) and *B. bifurcata* (BBF). Based on Tukey's test at 12 h, 24 h, 72 h and 96 h * Control vs. FSF: $p < 0.05$, at 24 h, 48 h, 72 h and 96 h * Control vs. BBF: $p < 0.05$.

2.3.2. Total Phenolic Compounds Content

The elicitor effect of the sulfated polysaccharides studied (FSF and BBF) on phenolic metabolism was also approached by the accumulation of total phenols in treated roots. The accumulation of phenolic compounds following FSF and BBF treatments was presented in Figure 4. Roots elicitation by FSF caused a significant ($p < 0.05$) and intense accumulation of phenolic compounds after 24 h compared to the control treatment (Figure 4). Second narrower accumulation of phenols was approved after 72 h of FSF treatment, this could be explained by the induction of PAL activity at the same time. However, a precocious and significant ($p < 0.05$) accumulation of these compounds was manifested just 12 h after following BBF treatment, this level of phenolic compounds remained higher than control plants during 24 h before decreasing at 48 h.

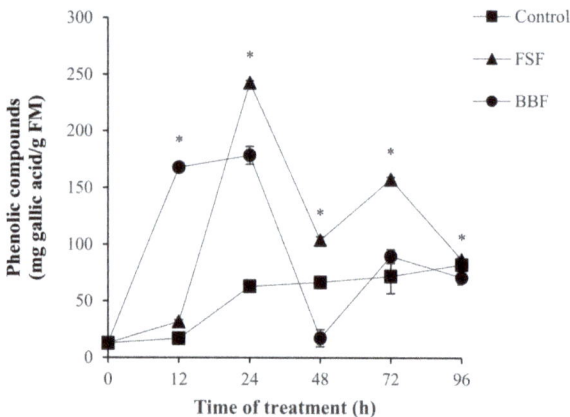

Figure 4. Effect of *F. spiralis* (FSF) and *B. bifurcata* (BBF) fucoidans on the accumulation of phenolic compounds in date palm roots. Means values ± SE. Based on Tukey's test at 12 h and 24 h * Control vs. BBF: $p < 0.05$, at 24 h, 48 h and 72 h * Control vs. FSF: $p < 0.05$.

2.3.3. Accumulation of Lignin Content

Different trend of the lignin deposition in treated roots was exhibited following elicitation by FSF and BBF (Figure 5). The level of this metabolite increased slightly after 12 h then greatly increased ($p < 0.05$) after 48 h of FSF treatment. This response was expected since lignin is a phenols polymer whose maximum accumulation was obtained after 24 h with FSF (Figure 4). On the other hand, with BBF treatment (Figure 5), the lignin contents undergo a weak increase after 24 h and 48 h of elicitation while after 96 h a higher increase was noted, this could be explained by the possibility of the polymerization of phenolic compounds increased after 72 h of BBF treatment. The highest content of lignin was obtained at 48 h in response to FSF and after 96 h of BBF treatment, it is three times higher than that obtained in control roots.

The crude fucoidans from *F. spiralis* (FSF) and *B. bifurcata* (BBF) were extracted and structurally characterized; the results obtained show a significant proportion of L-fucose in FSF and BBF with a higher degree of sulfation (45 and 49% w/w respectively). A biological test showed that the crude fucoidans (FSF and BBF) exhibit an eliciting effect of the defence mechanisms in date palm roots. These mechanisms were initiated by the induction of PAL activity. FSF and BBF expressed a slightly differential effect on PAL activity, which could be due to the difference in structure between the two fucoidans. Indeed, the structural characterization revealed differences in sulfate proportions within FSF and BBF, suggesting a difference in FSF and BBF affinity to membrane receptors. The perception and recognition of elicitors from pathogens, plants and algae called damage- or pathogen-associated molecular pattern molecules (DAMPs, PAMPs) by Pattern Recognition Receptors (PRRs) in plants induces a signalling cascade in the host cell through their cytosolic domains leading to the induction of defence mechanisms in the host plant [39]. This could be the cause of the early induction of PAL activity after treatment with FSF compared to BBF. In addition, following the induction of PAL activity, the phenolic metabolites were accumulated in the treated roots, as well as lignin deposition. Phenols and lignin are among the most involved defence elements during date palm–Foa interactions [15–20]. The results obtained are similar to the reaction observed in tobacco plants pretreated with fucoidans and sulfated oligofucoidans, in which PAL activity was also induced [14]. In addition, such tobaccos demonstrate an increase in the activity of lipoxygenase (LOX) and Pathogenesis-related protein (PR), as well as transient defence reactions such as acidification of the cytoplasm and accumulation of H_2O_2 [14]. Based on this, it is possible to assume similar effects in the case of date palm root response to FSF and BBF, including also the induction of glutathione-S-transferase (GST) activity, as shown for tobacco [15]. In addition, a fucoidans pre-treatment of carrot leaves protects them against *Alternaria radicina* and *Botrytis cinerea* attacks by stimulating the accumulation of phenolic compounds and by inducing peroxidase (POD) and polyphenol oxidase (PPO) activities [40]. Thus, fucoidans-treated date palm roots, besides phenolic compounds accumulation, may also activate the POD and PPO enzymes. Otherwise, we have shown in recent work, that alginates extracted from the same brown algae *F. spiralis* and *B. bifurcata* stimulate the natural defenses of date palm in the same way as fucoidans, but the latter seem to be more active at low concentrations (0.5 g/L) compared to 1 g/L of alginates [41]. This could be explained by the structural difference between alginates and fucoidans, in particular the presence of sulfated groups and the degree of sulfation. The structure–function relationship governing the induction of plant defence mechanisms in response to fucoidans stile less elucidated. However it was reported that sulfation of polysaccharides alters their affinity for receptors located in cell walls [42]. In addition, the desulfation of sulfated polysaccharides reduces or eliminates their eliciting effect on natural defenses in tomatoes [43], whereas oligo-carrageenans (λ) with a higher degree of sulfation reduce the impact of various viral, bacterial and fungal diseases [44]. Furthermore a sulfated ulvan and oligo-ulvans improve the induction of PAL activity and therefore the accumulation of the phenols in tomato leaves [43], apple fruit [3] and olive tree [45]. Numerous works on the other biological activities of fucoidans relate their effectiveness to their structural characteristics, notably sulfation and molecular weight. It has been widely documented that fucoidans owe their broad spectrum of biological activities to their sulfated nature and molecular weights [6,27,28,46,47]. Based on previous work, fucoidans with a molecular weight (Mw) between 10 and 300×10^3 g/mole showed significant anticoagulant activity than those with higher Mw > 850×10^3 g/mole [48–50]. Likewise, immune-regulation activities increased with low molecular weight fucoidans of *Laminaria japonica* [51]. It has been shown also that the immune-regulatory potential of fucoidan was influenced by the sulfate group as well as the acetyl one [52]. In short, the biological efficiency of fucoidans was modulated by several parameters, in particular the proportion of SO_4^{2-} groups and their position, the molecular weight, the acetylation degree and monosaccharides composition [6,53].

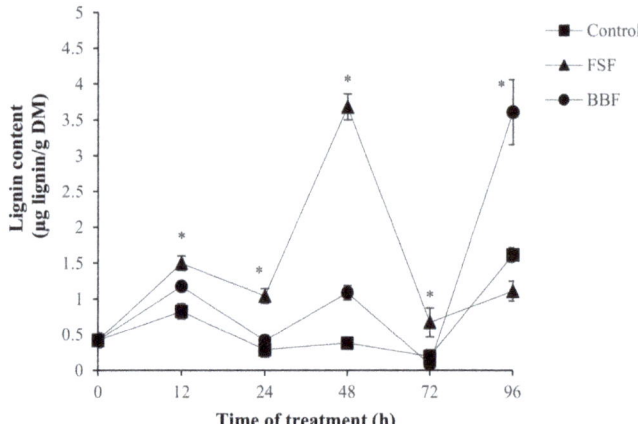

Figure 5. Effect of sulfated polysaccharides from *F. spiralis* (FSF) and *B. bifurcata* (BBF) on the accumulation of lignin in date palm roots. Means values ± SE. Based on Tukey's test at 12 h, 24 h, 48 h and 72 h * Control vs. FSF: $p < 0.05$, at 12 h, 48 h and 96 h * Control vs. BBF: $p < 0.05$.

3. Conclusions

The crude fucoidans from the brown algae, *F. spiralis* and *B. bifurcata* tested on the date palm roots, display potential elicitor activity on the phenolic metabolism due to the induction of PAL activity. Thus, leading to mobilisation of the phenlypropanoids pathway and to the accumulation of phenolic compounds and lignin. The elicitor effect of studied fucoidans was related to their highly sulfated structures with a small molecular weight (M_W). In addition, the simple and innovative elicitation model adopted in this paper highlighted the elicitor effect of fucoidans without stressing the roots, which could be applied in the field. These results open prospects for the formulation of a biological product, leading to a preventive control of date palm Bayoud disease.

4. Materials and Methods

4.1. Extraction, Purification and Chemical Analysis of Fucoidans (FSF and BBF)

Brown algae *B. bifurcata* and *F. spiralis* were harvested on the at El Jadida city (Morocco) in December 2017. The extraction and separation of sulfated polysaccharides were performed according to Ermakova et al. [54]. Samples of 25 g of each algae species were depigmented with formaldehyde 2% and then dried for 12 h at ambient temperature. Dried powders were then treated twice with HCl 0.1 M solution during 2 h (at 60 °C, 450 rpm). After centrifugation for 20 min at 5000 rpm, the recovered supernatants were neutralized to pH 7.5. Crude fucoidans were obtained with thrice ethanol 96% (3 v/v) precipitation and then freeze-dried to *B. bifurcata* and *F. spiralis* crude fucoidans powders (BBF and FSF, respectively). All chemical analysis of FSF and BBF was performed using colorimetric assays as described in previous paper [41].

4.2. GC-MS Analysis of FSF and BBF

Prior to GC-MS analysis, samples of 15 mg of BBF and FSF were hydrolyzed using Trifluoroacetic acid (TFA) under 120 °C for 90 min. Monosaccharides generated by this acid hydrolysis were then treated with N,O-Bis (trimethylsilyl) trifluoroacetamide (BSTFA) with 1% Trimethylchlorosilane (TMCS) according to Pierre et al.'s method [55,56]. After evaporation, monosaccharides constituting the fucoidans (FSF and BBF) as well as the standards were injected in GC-MS at 10 g/L of dichloromethne.

4.3. ATR-FTIR Spectroscopy

Infrared analysis of FSF and BBF was carried out using the Attenuated Total Reflectance (ATR) technique by a VERTEX 70 FTIR system. Spectra were obtained after 50 scans in a 500–400 cm^{-1} wave range.

4.4. ^{1}H NMR Spectroscopy Analysis

Twenty mg of crude fucoidans was prepared thrice in 0.5 mL of D$_2$O. With a 400 MHz Bruker AVANCE spectrometer, the ^{1}H NMR spectroscopy analysis was carried out at 60 °C.

4.5. Elicitation Test

Roots of three-month-old date palm plants (greenhouse model) were soaked in fucoidan solutions (FSF and BBF) at a concentration of 0.5 g/L and pH 6.5 over 4 days. Fucoidans-treated roots were compared to distilled water-treated roots as a control treatment. After 12 h and then every 24 h, biochemical assays of phenylalanine ammonialyase (PAL) activity, phenolic compounds and lignin content in treated roots were performed. Data were reported as the means values of 3 replicates, each replicate containing 3 plants.

4.6. Phenylalanine Ammonialyase (PAL) Activity

PAL activity was determined according to the method described by Liu et al. [57] with slight modifications. Enzyme extract was prepared at 4 °C, with 250 mg of crushed date palm roots in 3 mL of borate buffer (100 mM, pH 8.8, 4 °C) with EDTA (1 mM) and 5% (w/v) of insoluble polyvinyl polypyrrolidone (PVPP). The enzyme extract was recovered after centrifugation for 30 min and at 10,000× g. The reaction mixture of PAL activity assay composed of enzymatic extract (600 µL), L-phenylalanine at 20 mM (250 µL) and borate buffer (1 mL). An amount of 100 µL HCl was added after incubation (1 h, 30 °C). The results were obtained at 920 nm. The Bradford method [58] was then used to quantify the total protein in the enzyme extract.

4.7. Phenolic Compounds

The hydromethanolic phenolic extracts obtained according to Hagen et al.'s [59] method were then purified using the protocol described in previous paper [41]. Total phenolic determination was performed following the Folin–Ciocalteu method [60].

4.8. Extraction and Spectrophotometric Assay of Lignin Content

The lignin was extracted using the Bruce and West [61] protocol, with some modifications, in 0.5 mL of ethanol 90% (v/v), were grounded 500 mg of treated roots. Pellet obtained after centrifugation at 10,000× g for 20 min and at 4 °C was dried for 12 h at 35 °C. Samples of 25 mg of the dried residue were treated with 0.5 mL of thioglycolic acid and 1.25 mL of HCl solution at 2 M. The mixture was heated during 8 h at 100 °C. After cooling and centrifugation, 2.5 mL of NaOH was added to the pellet. The supernatant recovered after stirring for 18 h at 25 °C, was centrifuged (10,000× g, 20 min, 4 °C) treated with 0.5 mL of pure HCl, to precipitate lignin thioglycolic acid after incubation over 4 h at 4 °C. The absorbance at 280 nm was measured in 500 µL of NaOH. The lignin content was expressed in µg of lignin thioglycolic acid/g Dry Matter (DM).

4.9. Statistical Analysis

PAL activity, polyphenols and lignin contents results were tested by ANOVA analysis in SPSS software Version 20.0 using Tukey's test. The difference between treatments is significant at $p < 0.05$.

Author Contributions: Conceptualization, S.B., C.D., Z.E.A.-T. and C.E.M.; methodology, S.B., G.P., and. Z.E.A.-T.; supervision, C.D., C.E.M., and Z.E.A.-T.; Software, S.B.; Validation, S.B., C.D., Z.E.A.-T. and C.E.M.; writing—Original draft, S.B., C.D., Z.E.A.-T., and C.E.M., writing—Review and editing, S.B., C.D., Z.E.A.-T.; C.E.M, G.P., H.R., and P.M. All authors have read and agreed to the published version of the manuscript.

Funding: This research was funded by Hubert Curien Program (PHC TOUBKAL 18/63), and financially supported by Ministry of Europe and Foreign Affairs, and CNRST of Morocco within the French–Morocco bilateral program. Grant Number: 38964TM.

Conflicts of Interest: The authors declare no conflict of interest.

References

1. Wijesinghe, W.; Jeon, Y.-J. Biological activities and potential industrial applications of fucose rich sulfated polysaccharides and fucoidans isolated from brown seaweeds: A review. *Carbohydr. Polym.* **2012**, *88*, 13–20. [CrossRef]
2. Prajapati, V.D.; Maheriya, P.M.; Jani, G.K.; Solanki, H.K. Carrageenan: A natural seaweed polysaccharide and its applications. *Carbohydr. Polym.* **2014**, *105*, 97–112. [CrossRef]
3. Abouraïcha, E.; Alaoui-Talibi, Z.E.; Boutachfaiti, R.E.; Petit, E.; Courtois, B.; EL Modafar, C. Induction of natural defense and protection against Penicillium expansum and Botrytis cinerea in apple fruit in response to bioelicitors isolated from green algae. *Sci. Hortic.* **2015**, *181*, 121–128. [CrossRef]
4. Berteau, O. Sulfated fucans, fresh perspectives: structures, functions, and biological properties of sulfated fucans and an overview of enzymes active toward this class of polysaccharide. *Glycobiology* **2003**, *13*, 29R–40R. [CrossRef]
5. Bouissil, S.; Pierre, G.; El Alaoui-Talibi, Z.; Michaud, P.; El Modafar, C.; Delattre, C. Applications of Algal Polysaccharides and Derivatives in Therapeutic and Agricultural Fields. *Curr. Pharm. Des.* **2019**, *25*, 1187–1199. [CrossRef]
6. Wang, Y.; Xing, M.; Cao, Q.; Ji, A.; Liang, H.; Song, S. Biological Activities of Fucoidan and the Factors Mediating Its Therapeutic Effects: A Review of Recent Studies. *Mar. Drugs* **2019**, *17*, 183. [CrossRef]
7. Yuan, Y.; MacQuarrie, D.J. Microwave assisted extraction of sulfated polysaccharides (fucoidan) from Ascophyllum nodosum and its antioxidant activity. *Carbohydr. Polym.* **2015**, *129*, 101–107. [CrossRef] [PubMed]
8. Sellimi, S.; Kadri, N.; Barragan-Montero, V.; Laouer, H.; Mohamed, H.; Nasri, M. Fucans from a Tunisian brown seaweed Cystoseira barbata: Structural characteristics and antioxidant activity. *Int. J. Biol. Macromol.* **2014**, *66*, 281–288. [CrossRef]
9. Li, S.; Gao, A.; Dong, S.; Chen, Y.; Sun, S.; Lei, Z.; Zhang, Z. Purification, antitumor and immunomodulatory activity of polysaccharides from soybean residue fermented with Morchella esculenta. *Int. J. Biol. Macromol.* **2017**, *96*, 26–34. [CrossRef]
10. Mori, N.; Takeda, K.; Tomimori, K.; Kimura, R.; Ishikawa, C.; Nowling, T.K. Anti-tumor activity of fucoidan is mediated by nitric oxide released from macrophages. *Int. J. Oncol.* **2011**, *40*, 251–260. [CrossRef]
11. Park, H.S.; Kim, G.-Y.; Nam, T.-J.; Kim, N.D.; Choi, Y.H. Antiproliferative Activity of Fucoidan Was Associated with the Induction of Apoptosis and Autophagy in AGS Human Gastric Cancer Cells. *J. Food Sci.* **2011**, *76*, T77–T83. [CrossRef]
12. Park, H.Y.; Park, S.-H.; Jeong, J.-W.; Yoon, D.; Han, M.H.; Lee, D.-S.; Choi, G.; Yim, M.-J.; Lee, J.M.; Kim, D.-H.; et al. Induction of p53-Independent Apoptosis and G1 Cell Cycle Arrest by Fucoidan in HCT116 Human Colorectal Carcinoma Cells. *Mar. Drugs* **2017**, *15*, 154. [CrossRef] [PubMed]
13. Athukorala, Y.; Jung, W.-K.; Vasanthan, T.; Jeon, Y.-J. An anticoagulative polysaccharide from an enzymatic hydrolysate of Ecklonia cava. *Carbohydr. Polym.* **2006**, *66*, 184–191. [CrossRef]
14. Klarzynski, O.; Descamps, V.; Plesse, B.; Yvin, J.-C.; Kloareg, B.; Fritig, B. Sulfated Fucan Oligosaccharides Elicit Defense Responses in Tobacco and Local and Systemic Resistance against Tobacco Mosaic Virus. *Mol. Plant Microbe Interact.* **2003**, *16*, 115–122. [CrossRef] [PubMed]
15. Chandía, N.; Matsuhiro, B. Characterization of a fucoidan from Lessonia vadosa (Phaeophyta) and its anticoagulant and elicitor properties. *Int. J. Biol. Macromol.* **2008**, *42*, 235–240. [CrossRef]
16. Klarzynski, O.; Plesse, B.; Joubert, J.-M.; Yvin, J.-C.; Kopp, M.; Kloareg, B.; Fritig, B. Linear β-1,3 Glucans Are Elicitors of Defense Responses in Tobacco. *Plant Physiol.* **2000**, *124*, 1027–1038. [CrossRef]

17. EL Modafar, C. Mechanisms of date palm resistance to Bayoud disease: Current state of knowledge and research prospects. *Physiol. Mol. Plant Pathol.* **2010**, *74*, 287–294. [CrossRef]
18. EL Modafar, C.; Tantaoui, A.; Boustani, E.E. Cinetique d'accumulation et Fongitoxicite des Phytoalexines du Palmier Dattier vis-a-vis de Fusarium oxysporum f. sp. albedinis. *J. Phytopathol.* **1999**, *147*, 477–484. [CrossRef]
19. Ziouti, A.; EL Modafar, C.; Fleuriet, A.; Boustani, S.E.; Macheix, J. Les polyphénols, marqueurs potentiels de la résistance du palmier dattier (Phoenix dactylifera L.) au Fusarium oxysporum f. sp. albedinis. Compte rendu du Groupe Polyphénols. *J. Nat. Prod.* **1992**, *16*, 346–349.
20. Kidder, G.W.; Awayda, M.S.; Iii, G.W.K. Effects of azide on gastric mucose. *Biochim. Biophys. Acta Bioenerg.* **1989**, *973*, 59–66. [CrossRef]
21. EL Modafar, C.; Boustani, E.E. Cell Wall-Bound Phenolic Acid and Lignin Contents in Date Palm as Related to its Resistance to Fusarium Oxysporum. *Biol. Plant.* **2001**, *44*, 125–130. [CrossRef]
22. EL Modafar, C.; Tantaoui, A.; Boustani, E.-S.E. Differential induction of phenylalanine ammonia-lyase activity in date palm roots in response to inoculation with Fusarium oxysporum f. sp. albedinis and to elicitation with fungal wall elicitor. *J. Plant Physiol.* **2001**, *158*, 715–722. [CrossRef]
23. Mian, A.; Percival, E. Carbohydrates of the brown seaweeds himanthalia lorea, bifurcaria bifurcata, and Padina pavonia. *Carbohydr. Res.* **1973**, *26*, 133–146. [CrossRef]
24. Hentati, F.; Delattre, C.; Ursu, A.V.; Desbrières, J.; Le Cerf, D.; Gardarin, C.; Abdelkafi, S.; Michaud, P.; Pierre, G. Structural characterization and antioxidant activity of water-soluble polysaccharides from the Tunisian brown seaweed Cystoseira compressa. *Carbohydr. Polym.* **2018**, *198*, 589–600. [CrossRef]
25. Ammar, H.H.; Hafsa, J.; Cerf, D.L.; Bouraoui, A.; Majdoub, H. Antioxidant and gastroprotective activities of polysaccharides from the Tunisian brown algae (Cystoseira sedoides). *J. Tunis. Chem. Soc.* **2016**, *18*, 80–88.
26. Rabanal, M.; Ponce, N.M.; Navarro, D.A.; Gómez, R.M.; Stortz, C.A. The system of fucoidans from the brown seaweed Dictyota dichotoma: Chemical analysis and antiviral activity. *Carbohydr. Polym.* **2014**, *101*, 804–811. [CrossRef]
27. Prokofjeva, M.M.; Imbs, T.; Shevchenko, N.M.; Spirin, P.V.; Horn, S.; Fehse, B.; Zvyagintseva, T.; Prassolov, V.S. Fucoidans as Potential Inhibitors of HIV-1. *Mar. Drugs* **2013**, *11*, 3000–3014. [CrossRef]
28. Vishchuk, O.S.; Tarbeeva, D.V.; Ermakova, S.P.; Zvyagintseva, T.N. Structural Characteristics and Biological Activity of Fucoidans from the Brown Algae Alaria sp. and Saccharina japonica of Different Reproductive Status. *Chem. Biodivers.* **2012**, *9*, 817–828. [CrossRef]
29. Malyarenko, O.S.; Ermakova, S.; Zvyagintseva, T.N. Sulfated polysaccharides from brown seaweeds Saccharina japonica and Undaria pinnatifida: isolation, structural characteristics, and antitumor activity. *Carbohydr. Res.* **2011**, *346*, 2769–2776. [CrossRef]
30. Cho, M.; Lee, D.-J.; Kim, J.-K.; You, S. Molecular characterization and immunomodulatory activity of sulfated fucans from Agarum cribrosum. *Carbohydr. Polym.* **2014**, *113*, 507–514. [CrossRef]
31. Saha, S.; Navid, M.H.; Bandyopadhyay, S.S.; Schnitzler, P.; Ray, B. Sulfated polysaccharides from Laminaria angustata: Structural features and in vitro antiviral activities. *Carbohydr. Polym.* **2012**, *87*, 123–130. [CrossRef]
32. Synytsya, A.; Kim, W.-J.; Kim, S.-M.; Pohl, R.; Synytsya, A.; Kvasnička, F.; Čopíková, J.; Park, Y.I. Structure and antitumour activity of fucoidan isolated from sporophyll of Korean brown seaweed Undaria pinnatifida. *Carbohydr. Polym.* **2010**, *81*, 41–48. [CrossRef]
33. Pereira, M.S.; Mulloy, B.; Mourão, P.A.S. Structure and Anticoagulant Activity of Sulfated Fucans. *J. Biol. Chem.* **1999**, *274*, 7656–7667. [CrossRef]
34. Kariya, Y.; Mulloy, B.; Imai, K.; Tominaga, A.; Kaneko, T.; Asari, A.; Suzuki, K.; Masuda, H.; Kyogashima, M.; Ishii, T. Isolation and partial characterization of fucan sulfates from the body wall of sea cucumber Stichopus japonicus and their ability to inhibit osteoclastogenesis. *Carbohydr. Res.* **2004**, *339*, 1339–1346. [CrossRef] [PubMed]
35. Benaoun, F.; Delattre, C.; Boual, Z.; Ursu, A.V.; Vial, C.; Gardarin, C.; Wadouachi, A.; Le Cerf, D.; Varacavoudin, T.; El-Hadj, M.D.O.; et al. Structural characterization and rheological behavior of a heteroxylan extracted from Plantago notata Lagasca (Plantaginaceae) seeds. *Carbohydr. Polym.* **2017**, *175*, 96–104. [CrossRef]
36. Dammak, M.; Hadrich, B.; Miladi, R.; Barkallah, M.; Hentati, F.; Hachicha, R.; Laroche, C.; Michaud, P.; Fendri, I.; Abdelkafi, S. Effects of nutritional conditions on growth and biochemical composition of Tetraselmis sp. *Lipids Health Dis.* **2017**, *16*, 41. [CrossRef]

37. Sekkal, M.; Legrand, P. A spectroscopic investigation of the carrageenans and agar in the 1500–100 cm^{-1} spectral range. *Spectrochim. Acta Part A Mol. Spectrosc.* **1993**, *49*, 209–221. [CrossRef]
38. Dore, C.M.P.G.; Alves, M.G.D.C.F.; Will, L.S.E.P.; Costa, T.G.; Sabry, D.A.; Rêgo, L.A.R.D.S.; Accardo, C.M.; Rocha, H.A.O.; Filgueira, L.G.A.; Leite, E.L. A sulfated polysaccharide, fucans, isolated from brown algae Sargassum vulgare with anticoagulant, antithrombotic, antioxidant and anti-inflammatory effects. *Carbohydr. Polym.* **2013**, *91*, 467–475. [CrossRef]
39. Lotze, M.T.; Zeh, H.J.; Rubartelli, A.; Sparvero, L.J.; Amoscato, A.A.; Washburn, N.R.; Devera, M.E.; Liang, X.; Tör, M.; Billiar, T. The grateful dead: damage-associated molecular pattern molecules and reduction/oxidation regulate immunity. *Immunol. Rev.* **2007**, *220*, 60–81. [CrossRef]
40. Jayaraj, J.; Wan, A.; Rahman, M.; Punja, Z.K. Seaweed extract reduces foliar fungal diseases on carrot. *Crop. Prot.* **2008**, *27*, 1360–1366. [CrossRef]
41. Bouissil, S.; El Alaoui-Talibi, Z.; Pierre, G.; Michaud, P.; El Modafar, C.; Delattre, C. Use of Alginate Extracted from Moroccan Brown Algae to Stimulate Natural Defense in Date Palm Roots. *Molecules* **2020**, *25*, 720. [CrossRef] [PubMed]
42. Ménard, R.; De Ruffray, P.; Fritig, B.; Yvin, J.-C.; Kauffmann, S. Defense and Resistance-inducing Activities in Tobacco of the Sulfated β-1,3 glucan PS3 and its Synergistic Activities with the Unsulfated Molecule. *Plant Cell Physiol.* **2005**, *46*, 1964–1972. [CrossRef]
43. Modafar, C.E.; Elgadda, M.; Boutachfaiti, R.E.; Abouraicha, E.; Zehhar, N.; Petit, E.; Alaoui-Talibi, Z.E.; Courtois, B.; Courtois, J. Induction of natural defence accompanied by salicylic acid-dependant systemic acquired resistance in tomato seedlings in response to bioelicitors isolated from green algae. *Sci. Hortic.* **2012**, *138*, 55–63. [CrossRef]
44. Vera, J.; Castro, J.; Contreras, R.A.; González, A.; Moenne, A. Oligo-carrageenans induce a long-term and broad-range protection against pathogens in tobacco plants (var. Xanthi). *Physiol. Mol. Plant Pathol.* **2012**, *79*, 31–39. [CrossRef]
45. Ben Salah, I.; Aghrouss, S.; Douira, A.; Aissam, S.; El Alaoui-Talibi, Z.; Filali-Maltouf, A.; El Modafar, C. Seaweed polysaccharides as bio-elicitors of natural defenses in olive trees against verticillium wilt of olive. *J. Plant Interact.* **2018**, *13*, 248–255. [CrossRef]
46. Ale, M.T.; Mikkelsen, J.D.; Meyer, A.S. Important Determinants for Fucoidan Bioactivity: A Critical Review of Structure-Function Relations and Extraction Methods for Fucose-Containing Sulfated Polysaccharides from Brown Seaweeds. *Mar. Drugs* **2011**, *9*, 2106–2130. [CrossRef] [PubMed]
47. Wells, M.L.; Potin, P.; Craigie, J.S.; Raven, J.A.; Merchant, S.S.; Helliwell, K.E.; Smith, A.G.; Camire, M.E.; Brawley, S.H. Algae as nutritional and functional food sources: revisiting our understanding. *Environ. Biol. Fishes* **2016**, *29*, 949–982. [CrossRef]
48. Shanmugam, M.; Mody, K. Heparinoid-active sulphated polysaccharides from marine algae as potential blood anticoagulant agents. *Curr. Sci. India* **2000**, *79*, 1672–1683.
49. Zayed, A.; Hahn, T.; Rupp, S.; Kramer, R.; Ulber, R. Fucoidan as a natural anticoagulant, antiviral and anti-cancer drug. *Naunyn Schmiedebergs Arch. Pharmacol.* **2018**, *391*, S7–S8.
50. Yang, C.; Chung, D.; Shin, I.-S.; Lee, H.; Kim, J.; Lee, Y.; You, S. Effects of molecular weight and hydrolysis conditions on anticancer activity of fucoidans from sporophyll of Undaria pinnatifida. *Int. J. Biol. Macromol.* **2008**, *43*, 433–437. [CrossRef]
51. Sun, T.; Zhang, X.; Miao, Y.; Zhou, Y.; Shi, J.; Yan, M.; Chen, A. Studies on Antiviral and Immuno-Regulation Activity of Low Molecular Weight Fucoidan from Laminaria japonica. *J. Ocean Univ. China* **2018**, *17*, 705–711. [CrossRef]
52. Choi, E.-M.; Kim, A.-J.; Kim, Y.-O.; Hwang, J.-K. Immunomodulating Activity of Arabinogalactan and Fucoidan In Vitro. *J. Med. Food* **2005**, *8*, 446–453. [CrossRef] [PubMed]
53. Li, B.; Lu, F.; Wei, X.; Zhao, R. Fucoidan: Structure and Bioactivity. *Molecules* **2008**, *13*, 1671–1695. [CrossRef] [PubMed]
54. Ermakova, S.; Men'Shova, R.; Vishchuk, O.; Kim, S.-M.; Um, B.-H.; Isakov, V.; Zvyagintseva, T. Water-soluble polysaccharides from the brown alga Eisenia bicyclis: Structural characteristics and antitumor activity. *Algal Res.* **2013**, *2*, 51–58. [CrossRef]
55. Pierre, G.; Graber, M.; Rafiliposon, B.A.; Dupuy, C.; Orvain, F.; Crignis, M.D.; Maugard, T. Biochemical Composition and Changes of Extracellular Polysaccharides (ECPS) Produced during Microphytobenthic Biofilm Development (Marennes-Oléron, France). *Microb. Ecol.* **2011**, *63*, 157–169. [CrossRef]

56. Pierre, G.; Zhao, J.-M.; Orvain, F.; Dupuy, C.; Klein, G.; Graber, M.; Maugard, T. Seasonal dynamics of extracellular polymeric substances (EPS) in surface sediments of a diatom-dominated intertidal mudflat (Marennes–Oléron, France). *J. Sea Res.* **2014**, *92*, 26–35. [CrossRef]
57. Liu, H.; Jiang, W.; Bi, Y.; Luo, Y. Postharvest BTH treatment induces resistance of peach (*Prunus persica* L. cv. Jiubao) fruit to infection by Penicillium expansum and enhances activity of fruit defense mechanisms. *Postharvest Biol. Technol.* **2005**, *35*, 263–269. [CrossRef]
58. Bradford, M.M. A rapid and sensitive method for the quantitation of microgram quantities of protein utilizing the principle of protein-Dye binding. *Anal. Biochem.* **1976**, *72*, 248–254. [CrossRef]
59. Hagen, S.F.; Borge, G.I.A.; Bengtsson, G.B.; Bilger, W.; Berge, A.; Haffner, K.; Solhaug, K.A. Phenolic contents and other health and sensory related properties of apple fruit (Malus domestica Borkh., cv. Aroma): Effect of postharvest UV-B irradiation. *Postharvest Biol. Technol.* **2007**, *45*, 1–10. [CrossRef]
60. Budini, R.; Tonelli, D.; Girotti, S. Analysis of total phenols using the Prussian Blue method. *J. Agric. Food Chem.* **1980**, *28*, 1236–1238. [CrossRef]
61. Bruce, R.J.; West, C.A. Elicitation of Lignin Biosynthesis and Isoperoxidase Activity by Pectic Fragments in Suspension Cultures of Castor Bean. *Plant Physiol.* **1989**, *91*, 889–897. [CrossRef] [PubMed]

Publisher's Note: MDPI stays neutral with regard to jurisdictional claims in published maps and institutional affiliations.

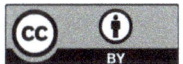

© 2020 by the authors. Licensee MDPI, Basel, Switzerland. This article is an open access article distributed under the terms and conditions of the Creative Commons Attribution (CC BY) license (http://creativecommons.org/licenses/by/4.0/).

MDPI
St. Alban-Anlage 66
4052 Basel
Switzerland
Tel. +41 61 683 77 34
Fax +41 61 302 89 18
www.mdpi.com

Marine Drugs Editorial Office
E-mail: marinedrugs@mdpi.com
www.mdpi.com/journal/marinedrugs

www.ingramcontent.com/pod-product-compliance
Lightning Source LLC
LaVergne TN
LVHW070444100526
838202LV00014B/1660